BASIC ENDOCRINOLOGY

An Interactive Approach

J. Matthew Neal, MD, FACP

Director of Endocrinology

Internal Medicine Residency

Ball Memorial Hospital;

Clinical Associate Professor of Medicine

Indiana University School of Medicine

Muncie Center for Medical Education

Muncie, Indiana

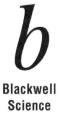

**Blackwell
Science**

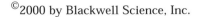
©2000 by Blackwell Science, Inc.

BLACKWELL SCIENCE, INC.

Editorial Offices:

Commerce Place, 350 Main Street
Malden, Massachusetts 02148, USA

Osney Mead, Oxford OX2 0EL, England

25 John Street, London WC1N 2BL, England

23 Ainslie Place, Edinburgh EH3 6AJ, Scotland

54 University Street, Carlton, Victoria 3053, Australia

Other Editorial Offices:

Blackwell Wissenschafts-Verlag GmbH
Kurfürstendamm 57, 10707 Berlin, Germany

Blackwell Science KK, MG Kodenmacho Building
7-10 Kodenmacho Nihombashi, Chuo-ku
Tokyo 104, Japan

Distributors:
USA   Blackwell Science, Inc.
            Commerce Place
            350 Main Street
            Malden, Massachusetts 02148
            (Telephone orders: 800-215-1000
            or 781-388-8250; fax orders: 781-388-8270)

Canada   Login Brothers Book Company
            324 Saulteaux Crescent
            Winnipeg, Manitoba, R3J 3T2
            (Telephone orders: 204-224-4068)

Australia   Blackwell Science Pty, Ltd.
            54 University Street
            Carlton, Victoria 3053
            (Telephone orders: 03-9347-0300;
            fax orders: 03-9349-3016)

Outside North America and Australia
            Blackwell Science, Ltd.
            c/o Marston Book Services, Ltd.
            P.O. Box 269, Abingdon
            Oxon OX14 4YN, England
            (Telephone orders: 44-01235-465500;
            fax orders: 44-01235-465555)

Acquisitions: Chris Davis
Production: Irene Herlihy
Manufacturing: Lisa Flanagan
Cover and interior design by: Leslie Haimes
Interior Images: composed by designer using
            Photodisc, Volume 4
Typeset by: Northeastern Graphic Services, Inc.
Printed and bound by: Sheridan Books

Printed in the United States of America
00 01 02 03 5 4 3 2 1

Library of Congress Cataloging-in-Publication Data
Neal, J. Matthew.
    Basic endocrinology : an interactive approach /
by J. Matthew Neal.
        p.   cm.
    Includes index.
    ISBN 0-632-04429-2
    1. Endocrine glands—Diseases Miscellanea.
2. Endocrine glands—Diseases Examinations,
questions, etc.   I. Title.
    [DNLM: 1. Endocrine Diseases Examination
Questions.   2. Endocrine Diseases.
WK 18.2 N341b 2000]
RC648.N38   2000
616.4'0076—dc21
DNLM/DLC
for Library of Congress   99-30331
                                           CIP

Notice: The indications and dosages of all drugs in this book have been recommended in the medical literature and conform to the practices of the general community. The medications described do not necessarily have specific approval by the Food and Drug Administration for use in the diseases and dosages for which they are recommended. The package insert for each drug should be consulted for use and dosage as approved by the FDA. Because standards for usage change, it is advisable to keep abreast of revised recommendations, particularly those concerning new drugs.

CONTENTS

PREFACE

This introductory textbook is intended as a problem-based teaching tool and self-assessment guide for medical students, residents, and others wishing a review of endocrinology. It is an outgrowth of my teaching sessions with medical students and residents. I have designed it as an interactive text, one that asks "why?", rather than just re-iterating material from lectures.

The purpose of this text is to provide a solid foundation of clinical endocrinology; thus, it is meant to supplement existing texts, not replace them. It is not meant to be a "cookbook of endocrinology," but rather is a guide to basic clinical principles and physiology. I have tried to not overload the reader with details, but at the same time not to be simplistic. For the most part, drug dosages and trade names have been omitted—these things can be retrieved from a standard textbook. I focus on pathophysiology rather than on the details of clinical medicine.

Each chapter is set up in a "frequently asked questions" (FAQ) format, to answer those questions that I have found to be most common. The questions are accompanied by pertinent diagrams and relevant clinical photographs. I have attempted to group endocrine disorders by organ system. There is some overlap, and I have tried to avoid duplication of material. My hope is that this will provide a solid foundation that will last throughout your career.

At the conclusion of each chapter is a series of review questions designed to facilitate learning. It has been demonstrated that students learn best when application of the reading material is required. The questions are an integral part of the book and should be studied for maximum learning. There are two types of questions. The first are relatively simple "fill in the blank" questions designed to help the reader review the text. The second are a mixture of multiple-choice, true-false, and matching questions, which help the reader integrate his or her knowledge into a practical situation. The clinical questions are actual case studies that I have seen in my practice.

Like computer software, this book went through several "beta versions" before release of the finished product. I would like to thank the many Indiana University medical students and Ball Memorial Hospital residents who "beta-tested" the material during its evolution and offered helpful comments. I would also like to thank my patients, who are the best teachers of all. Without them, this book would not exist. I would most of all like to thank my wife, Alexis, for her tremendous patience, support, and helpful ideas during this project.

J.M.N.

CHAPTER 1

INTRODUCTION TO ENDOCRINOLOGY

Q: What are hormones?

A: The word *hormone* is derived from the Greek word meaning "arouse to activity." As organisms become more complex, intercellular communication mechanisms are necessary for homeostasis. Hormones may act on the cell in which they were made (autocrine) or on adjacent cells (paracrine).

Q: What types of molecules make up hormones?

A: Most hormones are **protein** or **peptide** hormones made of multiple amino acids linked together. Most of these hormones are quite large and very complex. Large peptide hormones include insulin, glucagon, adrenocorticotrophic hormone (ACTH), and growth hormone. Some peptide hormones are quite small; however, thyroid-releasing hormone (TRH), a hypothalamic hormone, is a tripeptide.

Glycoproteins are large peptide hormones associated with a carbohydrate moiety. These include luteinizing hormone (LH), follicle-stimulating hormone (FSH), thyroid-stimulating hormone or thyrotropin (TSH), and human chorionic gonadotropin (β-hCG).

Amino acids may be modified to form hormones. The amino acid tyrosine is modified to form the **catecholamines,** such as epinephrine and norepinephrine. Two thyronine molecules are modified and joined to form the **iodothyronines,** such as thyroxine (T_4) and triiodothyronine (T_3).

Cholesterol is the precursor of steroid hormones, such as cortisol, estradiol, testosterone, and aldosterone. It is also the precursor of sterol hormones such as calcitriol.

Eicosanoids are hormones derived from fatty acids. The most important, the **prostaglandins,** are derived from arachidonic acid. Other eicosanoids include thromboxanes, leukotrienes, and prostacyclins. These molecules help regulate hormone release and action. They are important in smooth muscle contraction, hemostasis, inflammatory and immunologic responses, and circulatory, respiratory, and gastrointestinal systems.

Many hormones share biochemical homology although they have quite different actions. The glycoprotein hormones LH, FSH, TSH, and hCG are composed of alpha and beta subunits. They share a common alpha subunit (α-SU), but the beta subunits are quite different, giving a unique biologic effect to each hormone. Growth hormone and prolactin are very similar in structure, although they have vastly different actions.

Q: What are the types of hormones?

A: Some hormones bind directly to receptors *in* the cell (cytoplasm or nucleus) and mediate their effect in this fashion (Fig. 1-1). Others have no direct effect but instead bind to cell surface receptors, which initiates production of one or more **second messengers** that carry out the action (Fig. 1-2). The most common second messenger is cyclic adenosine monophosphate (cAMP).

Q: What hormones have intracellular receptors?

A: The hormones with intracellular receptors include steroid hormones, iodothyronines (thyroid hormones), and sterol hormones (e.g., calcitriol), and their receptors are part of the steroid receptor "superfamily." Because of their nonpolar nature and poor solubility in plasma, these hormones travel in

blood, attached to one or more types of **carrier proteins.** The protein binding typically allows these hormones to have a longer half-life than those that travel freely. They also tend to be fat-soluble, which contributes to their longer half-lives. The portion of the hormone bound to the carrier protein is **inactive**; only the free portion is biologically **active.**

Examples of hormones and their specific carrier proteins include

thyroxine—thyroid-binding globulin (TBG)

testosterone—sex hormone-binding globulin (SHBG)

cortisol—corticosteroid-binding globulin (CBG, transcortin)

Some carrier proteins (e.g., albumin, prealbumin) are nonspecific and may carry multiple hormones. Knowing which hormones are attached to carrier proteins is essential, as various disease states can alter protein binding and result in abnormalities of the **total** level of the hormone (bound + free) without affecting the **free** (active) portion. Many laboratory tests only measure the total rather than the free level.

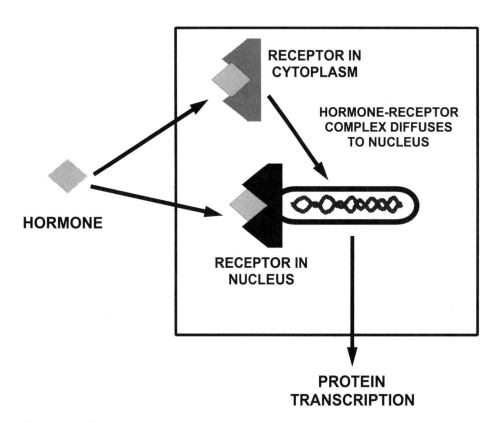

Figure 1-1. Hormones interacting with nuclear receptor.

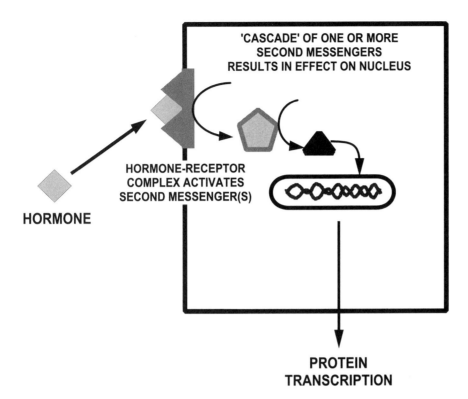

Figure 1-2. Hormones interacting with surface receptors.

Q: How does the steroid family of hormones work?

A: Hormones of the steroid family diffuse into the cell and bind to a receptor in the nucleus itself or to a cytoplasmic receptor (see Fig. 1-1). In the latter case, the hormone-receptor complex diffuses to the nucleus. After binding to a specific region, production of a specific protein (such as an enzyme) results.

Q: What is the surface receptor group of hormones?

A: Surface receptor hormones do not bind directly to the receptor but rather act via second messengers (see Fig. 1-2). These hormones also travel freely in plasma unbound to carrier proteins, and tend to be water soluble because of their polar (highly charged) properties. The surface receptor hormones include

    proteins (e.g., insulin, ACTH, somatostatin)

    glycoproteins (e.g., TSH, LH, FSH)

    catecholamines (e.g., epinephrine)

    eicosanoids (e.g., prostaglandins)

Of the vast number of hormones, most belong to the surface receptor group. They typically cannot travel into the cell, but rather bind to a surface receptor, which then activates one or more second messengers (via a "cascade"), which in turn exert an effect on the nuclear receptor.

The four major classes of surface receptor hormones are 1) seven-transmembrane domain receptors, 2) single-transmembrane domain growth-factor receptors, 3) cytokine receptors, and 4) guanylyl cyclase–linked receptors. The majority of receptors are of the seven-transmembrane domain type. The second messenger response from these receptors is modulated by **G-proteins,** a family of regulatory proteins.

Not all hormones **stimulate** production of second messengers; some hormones act to **inhibit** second messenger production. For example, the adenylyl cyclase-cAMP system is stimulated by hormones such as LH, FSH, ACTH, and glucagon, but is inhibited by somatostatin, dopamine, and angiotensin II.

Most peptide hormones degrade rapidly and have a short half-life. However, the second messenger controls the end effect, so the effect may be prolonged if the second messenger persists.

Q: What are the common second messenger systems?

A: The most common second messenger system is the adenylyl cyclase-cAMP system. Others include phospholipase C, protein kinase, tyrosine kinase, calcium, and guanylyl cyclase-cGMP.

Q: How is hormonal secretion regulated?

A: For each endocrine cell, there is typically a **trophic** (stimulatory) hormone and an **inhibitory** hormone (Fig. 1-3). Target organ hormones often do not have a specific inhibitory hormone. An increase in hormone concentration (e.g., T_4) is mediated by a decrease in the trophic hormone level (e.g., TSH) by a process known as **feedback inhibition.**

The inhibitory hormone for the trophic hormone may be its product. When the hormone level becomes high enough, it tells the trophic hormone to "shut off." Other hormones lack a well-defined trophic hormone and have only an inhibitory hormone (e.g., prolactin has only dopamine).

Paradoxically, the trophic hormone may actually inhibit hormone secretion by the target organ. In normal health, gonadotropin-releasing hormone (GnRH) is secreted in pulsatile fashion (every 90 minutes), which results in increased LH and FSH secretion by the pituitary. If GnRH is given continuously, however, suppression of LH and FSH secretion occurs. In certain cases, the inhibitory hormone may also augment trophic hormone secretion. An example of this is the normal female reproductive cycle. Normally, estrogen inhibits pituitary LH secretion; right before ovulation, estrogen actually causes positive feedback and stimulation of LH secretion.

Q: How and when should hormones be measured?

A: Hormones that have a relatively long half-life (e.g., T_4) may reliably be measured randomly. However, many hormones are secreted in a **circadian rhythm**—their levels vary throughout the day, so random measurements of their levels are less useful. Cortisol levels, for example, are typically highest in the morning and lowest in the evening. In fact, loss of the normal diurnal rhythm is seen in many endocrine disorders. For these hormones, it is necessary to do a **provocative** or **perturbation study** in which a substance is given to produce the desired result (Table 1-1).

In cases where hormonal *deficiency* is of concern, a **stimulatory test** is done in which a **secretagogue** is given that provokes a response. The hormone of interest is usually measured beforehand and at one or more intervals. For example, the rapid

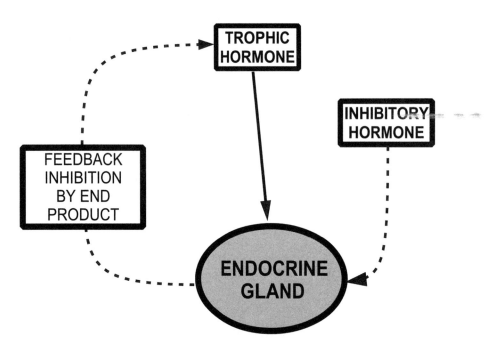

Figure 1-3. Normal hormonal regulation.

TABLE I-I.   Examples of Hormones and Their Regulation

HORMONE	SECRETAGOGUE	INHIBITOR	DEFICIENCY SYNDROME	EXCESS SYNDROME
Cortisol	ACTH	—	Addison's disease; congenital enzyme defects	Cushing's syndrome
Growth hormone	GHRH, hypoglycemia, arginine, L-dopa, clonidine, exercise	Hyperglycemia, somatostatin	GH deficiency	Acromegaly; gigantism
Aldosterone	Diuresis, erect posture, hypovolemia, hypotension	Volume infusion	Addison's disease; congenital enzyme defects	Hyperaldosteronism
ACTH	CRH	Cortisol	Secondary adrenal insufficiency	Cushing's disease; ectopic ACTH secretion
Thyroxine, triiodothyronine	TSH	Iodide (acute)	Primary hypothyroidism	Primary hyperthyroidism (e.g., Graves' disease)
TSH	TRH	Somatostatin, dopamine, T_4, T_3	Secondary hypothyroidism	Inappropriate TSH secretion (TSH-secreting pituitary tumor; pituitary resistance to thyroid hormone)
Sex steroids	LH	—	Hypergonadotropic hypogonadism	Precocious puberty; hirsutism; virilization, feminization syndromes
Insulin	Hyperglycemia	Hypoglycemia, somatostatin	Type I diabetes	Insulinoma, nesidioblastosis

ACTH test is used to exclude primary adrenal insufficiency. A basal cortisol level is measured, and a known amount of synthetic ACTH is given; repeat cortisol is measured in 30 and 60 minutes.

If hormone *excess* is expected, then a **suppression** or **inhibitory test** is done by giving a substance known to *suppress* hormone levels. For example, random growth hormone (GH) levels are often not useful in evaluating acromegaly because of the episodic secretion of pituitary hormones. Hyperglycemia is a known inhibitor of GH secretion, so a glucose suppression test can be done in which GH levels are measured before and after a 100-gram glucose load. In normal health, growth hormone GH is suppressed; in acromegaly, secretion is autonomous and it is not suppressed.

An alternative to a provocative test that eliminates some of the problems associated with random hormone measurements may be urine collection over a long period of time (e.g., 24 hours). For example, pheochromocytomas often secrete catecholamines intermittently, which can make random measurements less useful; a 24-hour urine collection for catecholamines and metabolites will usually be elevated in such persons. In patients suspected of having Cushing's syndrome, a good screening test is a 24-hour urine free cortisol (as an alternative to the overnight dexamethasone suppression test).

Some conditions may be differentiated by the extent that hormone levels increase or suppress in response to stimulus or suppression. For example, Cushing's syndrome may be caused by ACTH-secreting pituitary tumors or by ACTH-secreting ectopic tumors. After dexamethasone administration, the pituitary tumor typically suppresses to a greater degree than does the ectopic tumor, thus aiding the clinician in diagnosis.

For hormone excess, it may be desirable to precipitate hormone release via stimulatory tests. Patients suspected of insulinoma often undergo a prolonged fast in which an increase in insulin levels is observed. Infusion of pentagastrin is done to provoke calcitonin secretion in patients with medullary thyroid carcinoma.

Q: How are hormones measured?

A: Large hormones are typically measured using one of three basic methods: radioimmunoassay, immunoradiometric assay, and radioreceptor assay. Other methods include bioassay and chromatography.

The **radioimmunoassay** (RIA) is a type of competitive binding assay commonly used for small hormones, such as steroids and iodothyronines (Fig. 1-4). An antigen (the hormone) interacts with a specific antibody directed against the antigen, forming an antigen-antibody complex. The reaction is reversible and is dependent on the concentrations of the antigen and antibody:

$$[Ag] + [Ab] \leftrightarrow [Ag\text{-}Ab \text{ complex}]$$

A known amount of radiolabeled hormone—such as radioiodine-labeled thyroxine—is added to serum with antibody directed against the hormone (e.g., anti-T_4). A known amount of unlabeled standard T_4 is then added to several tubes in increasing amounts. The antibody-antigen complex is then separated, and the number of radioactive counts is measured, which is proportional to the amount of tracer present. This is a competitive-binding study, so both the radiolabeled and unlabeled T_4 will compete for the binding sites on the antibody. As the concentration of the unlabeled T_4

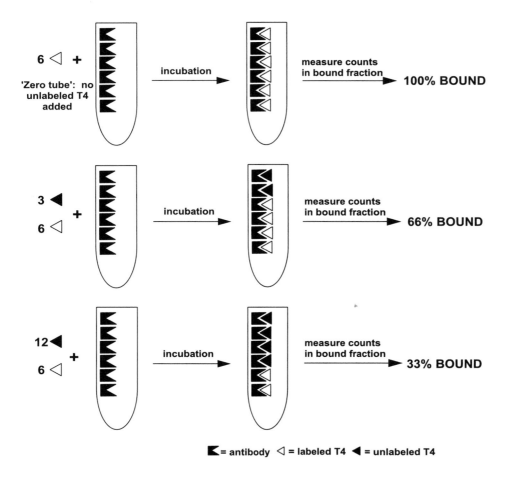

6 ◁ +

'Zero tube': no unlabeled T4 added

incubation → measure counts in bound fraction → **100% BOUND**

3 ◀
+
6 ◁

incubation → measure counts in bound fraction → **66% BOUND**

12 ◀
+
6 ◁

incubation → measure counts in bound fraction → **33% BOUND**

◀ = antibody   ◁ = labeled T4   ◀ = unlabeled T4

Figure 1-4. Radioimmunoassay (RIA).

increases, the proportion of radiolabeled antigen decreases. This is a logarithmic, not a linear, process: a standard curve can be plotted so that an unknown value can be predicted.

Immunoradiometric assays (IRMA) use two antibodies instead of one (Fig. 1-5). These two antibodies are directed against two different stearic parts of the molecule; thus, IRMA assays are more specific than RIA (in which the antibody only binds to one portion). Because the molecule must be very large to accommodate two different antibody binding sites, IRMA is used chiefly for large peptide hormones (e.g., growth hormone). The useful measurement range is several times that of RIA.

The first or "capture" antibody (which is not radiolabeled) is bound to a solid-phase matrix that is easily separable from the mixture. The unla-beled hormone (unknown or standard) is then added, and it interacts with the capture antibody. To this mixture, the second or "signal" antibody is added in excess (it is radiolabeled, usually with iodine 125); the excess ensures that there is enough antibody to bind to the mixture. A "sandwich" forms, in which the hormone is wedged between the solid-bound capture antibody and the radiolabeled antibody. Once the excess antibody is removed, the radioactive counts are measured in the mixture. IRMA is not a competitive binding assay like RIA, as only one hormone (unlabeled) is competing for the antibody, which is added in excess. Radioactive counts increase with increasing hormone concentration.

Immunochemiluminometric assays (ICMA) are similar to IRMA except that the signal antibody is

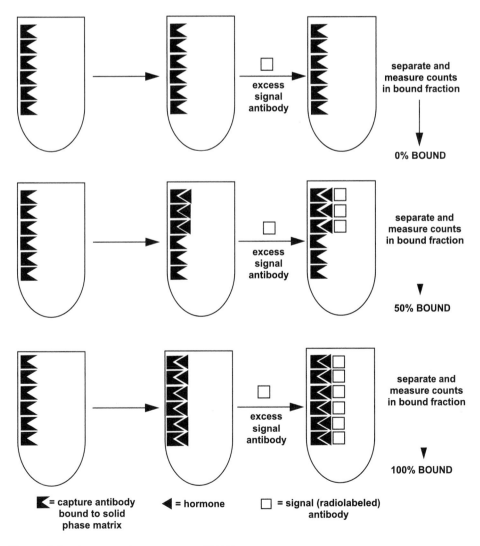

Figure 1-5. Immunoradiometric assay (IRMA).

labeled with a compound that emits light, rather than with a radioactive tracer. These tests often are quicker than IRMA and do not involve the hazards of using radioactive isotopes in the laboratory. Advanced techniques include the enzyme-linked immunosorbent assay (ELISA) and polymerase chain reaction (PCR) methods.

Radioreceptor assays (RRA) use a radiolabeled hormone receptor rather than an antibody. These are incubated with both radiolabeled and unlabeled hormone. Thus, RRA is a competitive-binding assay, similar to RIA. Due to the high specificity of receptors for hormones, however, RRA can be more specific than RIA. Examples of RRA include measurement of antibodies to hormone receptors (e.g., thyroid receptor antibodies seen in Graves' disease). RRA is not as widely used at this time as the other techniques.

Bioassays are functional tests in which the hormone is injected into an animal or in vitro cells and the effect is observed. These tests were common in the past before the advent of modern laboratory methods, but are rarely done today.

Chromatography uses the small difference in the charges of molecules to separate them. The unknown substance is placed in a chromatographic column; the media used in the columns include resins (ion exchange, affinity, and molecular sieve chromatography), liquids (high-performance liquid chromatography or HPLC), and gases (gas-liquid chromatography). Chromatography is used to separate such compounds as catecholamines, glycated hemoglobin, steroids, and vitamin D metabolites. After purification, the compounds are assayed by other means.

Q: How are hormones secreted?

A: Some hormones are stored in membrane vesicles, and released via exocytosis. Other hormones travel directly across the plasma membrane, either by diffusion or by means of a transporter. Hormones that are released by the vesicle mechanism include peptide hormones and catecholamines. Iodothyronines such as thyroxine are also released in this fashion. Hormones that typically travel directly across the cell membrane include steroids, vitamin D, and the eicosanoids (e.g., prostaglandins).

Q: How are endocrine disorders named?

A: A normal endocrine state is denoted by the prefix **eu** (e.g., euglycemia, euthyroid, eucalcemic). Hypofunctional states contain the prefix **hypo** (e.g., hypoparathyroidism, hypopituitarism). And the prefix **hyper** indicates a hyperfunctional state, as in hyperthyroidism, hyperparathyroidism, and hyperinsulinism.

These disorders may be classified more specifically. For example, there are many causes of hyperthyroidism, including Graves' disease, toxic nodular goiter, and subacute thyroiditis. Patients with elevated glucose levels are usually said to have diabetes mellitus rather than hyperglycemia.

Q: What is the basis of endocrine deficiency disorders?

A: Endocrine deficiency may occur in primary, secondary, or tertiary forms (Table 1-2). Endocrine deficiency occurs if insufficient hormone is present; this is a **primary deficiency disorder**. Examples include hypothyroidism due to Hashimoto's thyroiditis, Addison's disease (primary adrenal insufficiency), and type 1 diabetes mellitus. In primary disorders, the organ's trophic hormone level is elevated; for example, those with primary hypothyroidism have an elevated serum TSH level.

Secondary deficiency disorders occur when the trophic hormone for the target organ is deficient. This occurs in hypopituitarism, in which the target organs (e.g., thyroid, adrenal, gonads) are structurally intact, but are not stimulated properly. **Tertiary disorders** are similar to secondary syndromes except that the deficiency lies one step higher; the trophic hormone for the trophic gland is deficient. An example of this is hypothalamic dysfunction, in which the hypothalamic hormones are made in insufficient amounts to stimulate the pituitary, and in turn, the target organs.

The etiology of the deficiency is varied. It may of course occur if the organ producing the hormone is removed; a typical example is hypothyroidism caused by thyroidectomy for thyroid carcinoma.

TABLE 1-2.   Etiology of Endocrine Deficiency and Resistance Syndromes

CAUSE	EXAMPLE

Hormone deficiency	Autoimmune
	    Hypothyroidism (Hashimoto's disease)
	    Type 1 diabetes mellitus
	    Addison's disease
	Postsurgical
	    Hypothyroidism
	    Hypoparathyroidism
	Inflammation, infiltration, neoplasm
	    Hemochromatosis
	    Histoplasmosis
	    Nonfunctional pituitary tumors

Receptor defect/hormone resistance	Decreased receptors or sensitivity to hormone
	    Pseudohypoparathyroidism
	    Testicular feminization
	    Type 2 diabetes mellitus
	    Thyroid hormone resistance
	    Laron dwarfism

Abnormal hormone	Growth hormone deficiency

Autoimmune destruction is a common reason for hormone deficiency. Antibodies are produced against the target organ, causing destruction. Autoimmune processes appear to require two factors:

1. genetic predisposition

2. an environmental "trigger."

An example of genetic predisposition is the HLA type associated with the type II polyglandular autoimmune diseases (e.g., Hashimoto's thyroiditis, Graves' disease, Addison's disease, type 1 diabetes). The trigger has not been elucidated but appears to be some type of environmental insult, such as a viral infection or exposure to an antigen. This second event appears to be necessary to develop the autoimmune syndrome. For example, an identical twin of a patient with type 1 diabetes has only a 50% to 60% chance of developing the disease, suggesting a second, environmental factor in addition to genetic predisposition.

The autoantibodies that cause target organ abnormalities may also affect other parts of the body. In Graves' disease, hyperthyroidism results from autoantibody-induced stimulation of the thyroid. The antibodies also may attack the tissues behind the eye, resulting in protrusion of the eyes and extraocular muscle involvement (exophthalmos). Because the autoantibodies (not the thyroid hormone excess) cause the exophthalmos, treatment of thyroid disease does not result in improvement of the eye problem unless antibody levels decrease as well.

Inflammatory or infiltrative disease may also result in organ destruction and hormone deficiency. Patients with chronic pancreatitis may develop diabetes from insufficient insulin secretion. Those with hemochromatosis may develop adrenal insufficiency and diabetes from destruction of the adrenals and pancreas. Large tumors in or about the target organ may destroy enough cells to cause hormone deficiency. A common example is hypopituitarism, caused by large sellar or suprasellar tumors.

Another mechanism of hormone deficiency is production of a structurally abnormal hormone that does not have the desired effect. These disorders are extremely rare. An example is growth hormone deficiency resulting from an abnormal growth hormone molecule. Treatment with exogenous growth hormone corrects the problem.

Q: What is a hormone resistance syndrome?

A: Hormone resistance syndromes result in signs and symptoms of an endocrine deficiency disorder even though the hormone is made in sufficient amounts (see Table 1-2). This occurs if the patient's hormone receptors are insensitive to the hormone or are absent. The most common example is type 2 diabetes mellitus, in which patients are resistant to the effects of insulin; hyperglycemia results, even though insulin levels may be normal or even increased. Very large amounts of exogenous insulin may be required to overcome the insulin resistance.

Another less common example is testicular feminization, in which genetic males with absent testosterone receptors develop a female appearance due to deficient hormone action, despite normal or elevated testosterone levels. Laron dwarfism is an extremely rare disorder in which the liver lacks growth hormone (GH) receptors, leading to abnormally short stature despite normal GH levels.

Q: What is the treatment of hormone deficiency disorders?

A: The ideal therapy for hormone deficiency disorders is to replace the hormone so that normal physiologic levels are attained. This is relatively easy for orally absorbed hormones that have a long half-life (e.g., thyroxine). Patients with hypothyroidism may take a single thyroxine tablet by mouth daily. Other disorders that are easily treated with oral medication include adrenal insufficiency and estrogen deficiency.

Some hormones are not well absorbed orally, including most peptide hormones, which are degraded in the gastrointestinal tract. Many of these are given by injection, such as insulin and growth hormone. Nasal administration has proven successful for some hormones (e.g., desmopressin).

Other hormones may be absorbed orally but are degraded in the liver by the first-pass phenomenon. Testosterone, for example, must be given parenterally or transdermally. Synthetically modified derivatives such as methyltestosterone are resistant to degradation.

Even if we can administer the hormone, we may not be able to mimic the body's own secretion.

With insulin-dependent diabetes mellitus, it is impossible to mimic insulin secretion perfectly. The patient must learn to live with compromises, such as occasional hyperglycemia and hypoglycemia; the effects interfere with daily living, but the patient can minimize them by rigidly adhering to diet and exercise guidelines.

It is not always practical to administer the deficient hormone. For example, persons with hypopituitarism lack ACTH and TSH, resulting in deficient cortisol and thyroxine secretion. It is impractical to administer these hormones, as both are peptides and require parenteral administration. Replacing the end organ products, cortisol and thyroxine, which are inexpensive and easily absorbed orally, is much easier.

Finally, the native hormone may not be available to give as replacement. In hypoparathyroidism, for example, the parathyroid hormone (PTH) is deficient. PTH is not widely available at this time, and it would be impractical to administer as it is degraded within minutes. Instead, we administer one of the products of PTH stimulation, activated vitamin D metabolites (e.g., calcitriol).

Q: What is the basis of endocrine excess syndromes?

A: As with deficiency syndromes, endocrine excess may occur in primary, secondary, or tertiary forms (Table 1-3). A primary disorder occurs when the organ itself produces the excess hormone, without stimulation by a trophic gland. An example is primary hyperaldosteronism caused by an autonomous adrenal tumor. Examples of secondary and tertiary excess syndromes include overproduction of pituitary and hypothalamic hormones by tumors. Cushing's syndrome is a disorder of glucocorticoid excess caused by adrenocortical hypersecretion. It may be caused by a cortisol-secreting tumor of the adrenal gland (primary form), or by hypersecretion of the trophic hormone (ACTH) by the pituitary (secondary form, also called Cushing's disease).

Hormone excess syndromes are typically caused by tumors, benign or malignant. The tumors typically arise in the organ that normally produces the hormone. Hyperfunctioning tumors may also arise in an organ other than the one that normally pro-

TABLE 1-3.   Etiology of Endocrine Excess Syndromes

CAUSE	EXAMPLE
Hormone production by tumor	Pheochromocytoma
	Acromegaly
	Cushing's disease or syndrome
	Hyperthyroidism (toxic nodular goiter)
Autoimmune	Hyperthyroidism (Graves' disease)
	Autoimmune hypoglycemia
Exogenous hormone administration	Cushing's syndrome (iatrogenic)
	Hypoglycemia (diabetics on insulin; factitious insulin use)
	Hyperthyroidism (factitious)

duces the hormone; this is called a **paraneoplastic syndrome.**

Autoimmune syndromes usually result in hormone deficiency, not endocrine excess. An exception to this is Graves' disease, in which thyroid autoantibodies mimic the trophic hormone (TSH) and result in hyperthyroidism.

A third reason for hormone excess is exogenous administration of the hormone, either intentionally (**iatrogenic**) or by the patient without the physician's knowledge (**factitious**). For example, high doses of glucocorticoids are commonly used to treat transplant rejection; however, chronic administration results in iatrogenic Cushing's syndrome. Individuals who attempt to induce weight loss by taking unprescribed exogenous thyroid hormone are an example of factitious hormone use. Often, the latter are health care workers who have access to medication.

Q: How are hormones metabolized?

A: Most naturally occurring peptide hormones have a half-life of only a few minutes and are degraded rapidly (e.g., insulin, glucagon, ACTH). The enzymes inside the cell are the primary cause of degradation, although some degradation occurs in the bloodstream. Glycoproteins are degraded less rapidly, and may have a half-life of several hours (e.g., TSH, LH).

Thyroid hormones have relatively long half-lives due to their strong affinity for binding proteins. The half-lives of thyroxine (T_4) and triiodothyronine (T_3) are 7 days and 1 day, respectively. The

hormones are degraded in the microsomal systems by deiodinases. Most circulating T_3 is formed from the peripheral deiodination of T_4. Other inactive deiodination products occur.

Catecholamines have a half-life of only a few minutes and are primarily degraded inside the cell.

Q: What imaging modalities are useful in endocrinology?

A: Great strides in the advancement of endocrinology have been made with improved imaging techniques. Endocrinology makes heavy use of nuclear medicine, ultrasound, computed tomography, and magnetic resonance imaging.

Q: What is nuclear medicine?

A: A **nuclear medicine** study uses a radioactive substance that is administered to patients. It may be given orally (e.g., radioiodine), intravenously (technetium sulfur colloid), or inhaled (xenon). The element used is typically a radioactive counterpart of a nonradioactive element; for example, iodine 123 (^{123}I) and iodine 131 (^{131}I) are **isotopes** of the nonradioactive iodine 127 (^{127}I). Other elements do not occur in the natural compound but are similar in structure and chemical properties to the natural element. Technetium (^{99m}Tc), a synthetic element with radioactive properties, is very suitable for imaging and is probably the most widely used agent in nuclear medicine.

The radioactive element is either administered in its native form or is attached to a molecule that mimics the native substance (Table 1-4). Radioiodine is administered as the iodide ion (I⁻). Techne-

TABLE 1-4.   Commonly Used Radionuclides in Endocrinology

RADIONUCLIDE	FORM ADMINISTERED	ENDOCRINE ORGAN OF INTEREST
^{123}I	Sodium iodide (NaI)	Thyroid
^{111}In	Radiolabeled somatostatin analogue (octreotide)	Neuroendocrine tumors
^{99m}Tc	Sodium pertechnetate ($NaTcO_4$)	Thyroid
^{99m}Tc	^{99m}Tc-2-methoxy-isobutyl isonitrile (Sestamibi)	Parathyroid
^{131}I	^{131}I-metaiodobenzylguanidine (MIBG)	Pheochromocytoma

tium is often given as the pertechnetate (TcO_4^-) ion, whose ionic radius size is similar to iodide and is absorbed by the thyroid in a similar fashion.

Radionuclides may emit radiation in several ways. They may emit photons or **gamma rays** that are nonparticulate emissions. Gamma rays may be of very high energy or low energy, depending on the radionuclide. Low-energy gamma emitters are useful in imaging as they give very little radiation dose to the patient. Technetium, the ubiquitous element of nuclear medicine, is ideal for this purpose as it has very low gamma energy, a short half-life, and is easily incorporated into compounds. The monoenergetic ^{123}I is ideal for thyroid imaging because of its short half-life and low-energy gamma rays.

Radioactive decay is exponential in nature. If the half-life and amount (activity) at any time are known, the amount at another time can be calculated as follows:

$$A = A_0 e^{\frac{-0.693t}{t_{1/2}}}$$

where

A = the activity at time t

A_0 = activity at time zero

e = the base of the natural logarithm (2.71828 . . .)

$t_{1/2}$ = the half-life of the radionuclide.

Activity refers to an actual physical amount of a radionuclide and is proportional to the number of disintegrations per second. The traditional unit of radionuclide activity is the **curie,** which equals

3.7×10^{10} disintegrations per second (dps). The amounts used in nuclear medicine are in the millicurie (mCi) or microcurie (μCi) range. The SI unit (Système International d'Unités) of activity is the becquerel (Bq); 1 mCi = 37 MBq (megabecquerels), and 1 Ci = 37 GBq (gigabecquerels). The **delivered dose** depends on many factors, such as type of energy emitted, and energy of the gamma rays. For example, 30 mCi of ^{131}I delivers approximately 100 times as much radiation as 30 mCi of ^{123}I because of the increased energy and particulate emissions of the former.

The amount of radiation emitted can be detected by a radiation counter. This merely measures the amount of radiation coming from the patient and provides no spatial information. A **radionuclide uptake** may be calculated using these measurements to provide the fractional amount of nuclide accumulated at a given time. A much more complex device, a **gamma camera,** can be used to produce a two-dimensional image or **scan** of the organ radiating the energy. Gamma cameras are used to produce thyroid scan images, for example.

Other radionuclides emit **particulate radiation** in addition to gamma rays. The primary particle of interest is the beta (β) particle, which is an electron ejected from atomic orbit. These particles may cause significant tissue destruction, and thus these elements are less suitable for imaging. They are used when actual destruction of the target organ is desired. ^{131}I is a powerful beta emitter used to destroy thyroid tissue in patients with hyperthyroidism and thyroid cancer.

Q: What is ultrasound and how is it used in imaging?

A: **Ultrasound** uses very high frequency sound waves and takes advantage of their attenuation by various materials. Sound waves are generated by a transducer, which is placed in contact with the body after application of a conductive gel. As the sound waves propagate through the body, they are reflected back, refracted, or absorbed. The reflected or refracted echoes go back to the transducer. The distance between the transducer and the reflected echo can be calculated by measuring the time between the transmitted wave and the echo. Material that absorbs sound (such as air) transmits little or no sound back to the transducer.

Very sophisticated images can be obtained by using an array of multiple transducers, each transmitting ultrasound to the body part. High-speed computers collect and interpret the data in a two-dimensional form that can be seen on a display screen.

An advantage of ultrasound is that it uses no ionizing radiation. It also is a "real-time" modality that can be used to guide procedures (e.g., fine-needle aspiration biopsy or insertion of a catheter into a difficult area). The resolution of ultrasound, however, is less than that of magnetic resonance imaging or computed tomography. Ultrasound is also not useful for air-filled cavities such as the lungs.

Q: What are CT and MRI scans?

A: **Computed tomography** (CT) uses conventional x-ray beams to produce high-resolution cross-sections of a body part. The patient is placed between the x-ray tube and a series of x-ray detectors, which move in a circular fashion around the patient. After the detectors have completed a full circle around the patient, a computer analyzes the data and reconstructs an image, a virtual cross-section of the area of interest.

A recent development is **spiral computed tomography,** in which the x-ray tube and detectors move in a spiral fashion from one end of the area to the other, resulting in many more data points than are obtainable with conventional CT. **Single-photon emission computed tomography** (SPECT) uses an administered nuclear source rather than an x-ray beam for the radiation source. SPECT is therefore a hybrid technology, embracing both CT and nuclear medicine.

Because of its speed, CT is useful for imaging large body cavities (such as the chest, abdomen, or pelvis) that contain visceral organs. Iodine-containing contrast agents are often administered, although these are contraindicated in patients with renal insufficiency. Many patients are allergic to contrast agents and require pretreatment with corticosteroids and antihistamines. These agents also interfere with radioiodine imaging of the thyroid for at least 4 to 6 weeks.

Magnetic resonance imaging (MRI) takes advantage of the effect of hydrogen nuclei when exposed to a strong magnetic field. At rest, the nuclei are oriented at random. When exposed to a magnetic field, the nuclei "polarize" and oscillate at a certain frequency, unique to each atom. To obtain a nuclear magnetic resonance (NMR) signal, a radiofrequency (RF) pulse is applied at 90° to the magnetic field, resulting in a change of the magnetic moment. After the RF pulse stops, the nuclei return to their original orientation, resulting in another change in magnetic moment that can be detected by a coil. Water comprises most of the body, so hydrogen is by far the body's most common element. T_1 and T_2 "weighting" of MRI images refers to the time constants or relaxation times, which are beyond the scope of this book.

Sophisticated computer reconstruction of these faint MR signals results in detailed cross-sectional images of the body. A greater variety of imaging angles is available than with CT. Another advantage of MRI is the lack of ionizing radiation. The disadvantages of MRI include the relatively long scan times compared to CT, and the enclosure of the patient, which may be difficult for those with claustrophobia. Open MRI units now exist in which the patient is only partially enclosed, but these devices use weaker magnets and may be less suitable for precise imaging of very small structures (e.g., the pituitary).

MRI is extremely useful for imaging the nervous system. Gadolinium enhances pituitary imaging and is administered as a contrast agent. MRI is contraindicated in persons with ferromagnetic implants (e.g., orthopedic prostheses and metal skull plates) as the strong magnetic field can tear them apart.

Q: What is positron emission tomography?

A: **Positron emission tomography** (PET) uses short-lived positron-emitting radionuclides such as ^{18}F, ^{82}Rb, and ^{15}O. A positron is an electron with a positive charge; when a positron and electron strike each other, they are converted to energy by an **annihilation reaction,** which is detected by sensors. Positron emitters are easily incorporated into substances such as glucose (^{18}fluorodeoxyglucose) that can measure blood flow and other aspects of metabolism. PET has primarily been used to measure cerebral and myocardial blood flow, but it shows promise in certain endocrine applications. A disadvantage of PET is the extremely short half-lives of the radionuclides, mandating that they be made at the facility in a cyclotron. Because of the massive expense of a PET system, this imaging modality is limited primarily to large academic medical centers.

BIBLIOGRAPHY

Baxter JD. Introduction to endocrinology. In: Greenspan FS, Strewler GJ, eds., Basic and clinical endocrinology. 5th ed. Stamford, CT: Appleton & Lange, 1997:1–31.

Britton KE, Bomanji JB. Nuclear medicine imaging in endocrinology. In: Besser GM, Thorner MO, eds. Clinical endocrinology. 2nd ed. St. Louis, MO: Mosby-Wolfe, 1994:25.2–25.14.

Brook C, Marshall N. Appendix 1: Measurements of concentrations of hormones in blood. In: Brook C, Marshall N, eds. Essential endocrinology. 3rd ed. Cambridge, MA: Blackwell Science, 1996:155–161.

Marynick SP. Competitive-binding assays in clinical endocrinology. In: Moore WT, Eastman RC, eds. Clinical endocrinology. 2nd ed. St. Louis, MO: Mosby, 1996:15–32.

Norman AW, Litwack G. General considerations of hormones. In: Norman AW, Litwack G, eds. Hormones. 2nd ed. Orlando: Academic Press, 1997:1–44.

Patton JA, Pickens DR, Price R. Physics and instrumentation. In: Sandler MP, Patton JA, Gross MD, Shapiro B, Falke THM, eds. Endocrine imaging. Stamford, CT: Appleton & Lange, 1992:1–59.

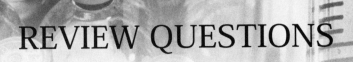

REVIEW QUESTIONS

I. SHORT ANSWER

1. Precursor molecules for hormones include
   _____, _____, and
   _____. _____ are peptide
   hormones attached to a sugar molecule.

2. The steroid "superfamily" hormones bind to
   receptors _____, resulting in
   _____. These hormones include
   _____, _____, and
   _____. These hormones typically are
   attached to _____ in serum.

3. The surface receptor hormone group includes
   the _____ and _____ hor-
   mones. Attachment of the hormone to the receptor results in formation of a _____
   and an effect on the nucleus. The most common substance formed is _____.
   These hormones are not attached to
   _____.

4. Hormones that increase an organ's hormone secretion are called _____ hormones or
   _____. Those that inhibit secretion
   are called _____ or _____
   hormones.

5. Many hormones are secreted in a _____
   rhythm and thus random measurements may
   be of little value. When hormone deficiency is
   suspected, a _____ test is usually performed; when a hormone excess is suspected, a
   _____ test is performed.

6. _____ is a competitive-binding assay
   in which radiolabeled and unlabeled hormones
   are mixed together. These hormones bind to an

unlabeled _____ after incubation. Radioactive counts _____ with increasing hormone concentration.

7. _____ assays are more sophisticated,
   requiring two different _____ directed at two distinct sites on the molecule.
   The first, or _____, binds the
   hormone to the matrix. The second, or
   _____ is radiolabeled. Radioactive
   counts _____ with increasing hormone concentration.

8. _____ use a radiolabeled receptor
   rather than an antibody. A test in which a biological effect of a hormone is observed after administration is called a _____.

9. A primary deficiency disorder occurs when the
   gland is _____ or _____.
   Causes include removal by _____
   and destruction by _____,
   _____, or _____ processes.

10. A secondary deficiency disorder occurs when
    the _____ hormone is deficient; the
    primary organ is structurally _____.

11. Normal or elevated hormone levels may pre-
    sent with a deficiency-like syndrome in the hor-
    mone _____ disorders. The most
    common example is _____, in which
    _____ utilization is impaired.

12. Endocrine excess syndromes are typically
    caused by hormone-secreting _____
    and only rarely by _____ stimula-
    tion. An example of the latter is _____.

13. Endocrine excess syndromes caused by ectopic tumors are called _____.

14. Hypothyroidism and adrenal insufficiency may be treated by _____ administration of hormones. Testosterone is degraded by the _____ and must be administered _____ or _____. Treatment of hypoparathyroidism requires _____, because _____ is not available at this time.

15. _____ uses radionuclides that are taken up by the organ of interest. Radionuclides may emit photons or _____ rays. Those with low energy are ideal for _____, while those with high energy are used for _____ purposes. The latter group also may emit particles such as _____.

16. _____ uses the properties of high-frequency sound waves to image the body. Solid tissues _____ sound, while air _____ sound. An advantage of this technique is that it does not expose the patient to _____.

17. _____ uses an array of x-ray beams to provide a cross-section of the area of interest. _____ uses an administered radionuclide rather than an x-ray beam as a source.

18. _____ takes advantage of the properties of _____ exposed to a strong magnetic field. It does not expose the patient to _____, but it is time-consuming. A contraindication to this study is the presence of _____ in the body.

II. MULTIPLE CHOICE

Select the one best answer.

19. The most common example of impaired hormone action due to a receptor defect is:
    a. Laron dwarfism
    b. type 1 diabetes mellitus
    c. type 2 diabetes mellitus
    d. hypothyroidism
    e. testicular feminization

20. In which one of the following disorders is the deficient hormone itself not used in treatment?
    a. primary hypothyroidism
    b. primary hypogonadism
    c. hypoparathyroidism
    d. type 1 diabetes mellitus
    e. primary adrenocortical insufficiency

21. Which of the following hormones interacts with a receptor in the nucleus rather than on the cell membrane?
    a. thyroid-stimulating hormone (TSH)
    b. estradiol
    c. parathyroid hormone
    d. prostaglandin E_1
    e. norepinephrine

22. In which one of the following disorders is the target organ hormone level elevated rather than decreased?
    a. hypoparathyroidism
    b. primary hypothyroidism due to Hashimoto's thyroiditis
    c. primary adrenal insufficiency (Addison's disease)
    d. pseudohypoparathyroidism
    e. hypogonadism due to orchiectomy

23. A sample of ^{123}I ($t_{1/2}$ = 13 hours) has an activity of 300 μCi. What will the activity be in 30 hours?
    a. 450 μCi
    b. 200 μCi
    c. 100 μCi
    d. 60 μCi
    e. 20 μCi

III. TRUE OR FALSE

24. Molecules that can serve as precursors for hormones include:
    ___ a.   amino acids
    ___ b.   fatty acids
    ___ c.   cholesterol
    ___ d.   sugars
    ___ e.   cyclic AMP

25. Hormone(s) that require a "second messenger" for action include:
    ___ a.   thyroxine
    ___ b.   insulin
    ___ c.   ACTH
    ___ d.   testosterone
    ___ e.   parathyroid hormone

26. Suppression or inhibitory tests are usually done to evaluate endocrine excess syndromes. Which of the following is (are) a stimulatory rather than inhibitory test(s)?
    ___ a.   dexamethasone suppression test (Cushing's syndrome)
    ___ b.   72-hour supervised fast (insulinoma)
    ___ c.   glucose tolerance test (acromegaly)
    ___ d.   saline infusion test (hyperaldosteronism)
    ___ e.   pentagastrin infusion test (medullary thyroid carcinoma)

27. Which of the following is (are) an example of a primary rather than a secondary or tertiary endocrine deficiency syndrome?
    ___ a.   hypogonadism due to pituitary gland destruction by tumor
    ___ b.   hypothyroidism due to thyroidectomy
    ___ c.   adrenal insufficiency due to hypothalamic destruction by craniopharyngioma
    ___ d.   adrenal insufficiency due to chronic suppression by exogenous glucocorticoids
    ___ e.   hypogonadism due to natural menopause

28. Advantages of immunoradiometric (IRMA) assays over radioimmunoassays (RIA) include:
    ___ a.   sensitive over a larger range
    ___ b.   can measure small hormones with more accuracy
    ___ c.   more specific for the hormone
    ___ d.   no use of hazardous radioisotopes
    ___ e.   not a competitive-binding assay

29. A 20-year-old woman takes oral contraceptives, which are known to increase serum-binding proteins. As a consequence, you would expect which hormone levels to be elevated?
    ___ a. T_4
    ___ b.   testosterone
    ___ c.   epinephrine
    ___ d.   cortisol
    ___ e.   thromboxane A_2
    ___ f.   LH

30. Regarding autoantibodies in endocrine disease, which of the following statements are true?
    ___ a.   They cause the type II polyglandular endocrine disorders.
    ___ b.   They cause the typical form of type 2 diabetes.
    ___ c.   Only endocrine organs can be affected.
    ___ d.   There may be a genetic predisposition.
    ___ e.   Genetic predisposition plus an environmental trigger is typically necessary for antibody response to occur.

31. Regarding feedback mechanisms, which of the following statements are true?
    ___ a.   Destruction of the target organ leads to low levels of trophic hormones.
    ___ b.   The inhibitory hormone for trophic hormones is often the product of the end organ.
    ___ c.   The trophic hormone can cause inhibition of the target organ under certain circumstances.

___ d. Suppressive tests are usually done to evaluate possible hormone deficiency.

___ e. All hormones have both a trophic and inhibitory hormone.

IV. MATCHING

Match each item with the appropriate answer. Each may be used only once.

32. ___ A. Bioassay

___ B. Radioimmunoassay (RIA)

___ C. Radioreceptor assay (RRA)

___ D. Immunoradiometric assay (IRMA)

a. Radiolabeled hormone competes with unknown hormone on antibody site; used for small hormones.

b. Effect of hormone is observed after injecting it into an animal or into cells in vitro.

c. Two different antibodies bind to unlabeled hormone forming a "sandwich"; very specific because antibodies bind to two different sites on the hormone.

d. A receptor preparation is used as the binding agent for the hormone to be measured.

33. ___ A. Magnetic resonance imaging (MRI)

___ B. Nuclear medicine

___ C. Ultrasound

___ D. Computed tomography (CT)

___ E. Positron emission tomography.

a. Useful for measurement of blood flow and metabolism; uses short-lived nuclides that are expensive to generate.

b. Uses an x-ray tube and a series of detectors to obtain cross-sections of the area of interest.

c. Measures reflected sound waves.

d. Radioactive substance is administered to the patient in a form assimilated into the body for diagnostic or therapeutic use.

e. Strong magnetic fields are used to orient hydrogen nuclei so that subtle changes in their magnetic fields can be measured.

ANSWERS

1. amino acids, fatty acids, cholesterol; glycoproteins

2. inside the cell, protein transcription and hormone effect; steroids, sterols, iodothyronines; carrier or binding proteins

3. peptide, catecholamine; second messenger; cyclic AMP (cAMP); carrier proteins

4. stimulatory, trophic; secretagogues; inhibitory

5. circadian; provocative, stimulatory, perturbation; suppressive, inhibitory

6. radioimmunoassay (RIA); antibody; decrease

7. immunoradiometric, antibodies; capture; signal; increase

8. radioreceptor assays; bioassay

9. defective, absent; surgery, autoimmune, inflammatory, infiltrative

10. trophic; intact

11. resistance; type 2 diabetes; insulin

12. tumors, autoimmune; Graves' disease

13. paraneoplastic syndromes

14. oral; first-pass phenomenon, parenterally, transdermally; vitamin D, parathyroid hormone (PTH)

15. nuclear medicine; gamma; imaging; therapeutic (destructive); β-particles (electrons)

16. ultrasound; reflect, absorbs; ionizing radiation

17. computed tomography (CT); single-photon emission computed tomography (SPECT)

18. magnetic resonance imaging (MRI), hydrogen nuclei (protons); ionizing radiation; ferromagnetic metallic objects

19. (c). Type 2 diabetes is predominantly a disorder of impaired hormone action due to insulin resistance. Levels of insulin are typically normal or elevated. Obesity contributes to insulin resistance in many patients. Laron dwarfism (a) and testicular feminization (e) are also receptor defects but are much less common. Type 1 diabetes (b) and hypothyroidism (d) result from hormone deficiency, not impaired action.

20. (c). Parathyroid hormone is not widely available to treat patients with hypoparathyroidism; vitamin D is given instead. In each of the other disorders, the deficient hormone itself is given.

21. (b). Steroid hormones interact with a nuclear receptor. Peptide hormones (a, c), prostaglandins (d), and catecholamines (e) interact with a surface receptor with formation of a second messenger.

22. (d). Pseudohypoparathyroidism is a hormone resistance syndrome, and parathyroid hormone levels are elevated. The same is true of type 2 diabetes (insulin), peripheral resistance to thyroid hormone (thyroxine), and testicular feminization (testosterone). The others are true endocrine deficiency syndromes.

23. (d). $A = A_0 e^{\frac{-0.693t}{t_{1/2}}} = 300 e^{\frac{-0.693t}{13}} = 300(0.2) = 60 \mu\text{Ci}$

24. True (a, b, c, d); False (e). Proteins, catecholamines, and iodothyronines are derived from amino acids (a); eicosanoids are derived from fatty acids; steroids and sterol hormones are made from cholesterol; sugars are necessary for formation of glycoproteins. Cyclic AMP (e) is a second messenger and not a hormone precursor.

25. True (b, c, e); False (a, d). Steroids, sterols, and thyroid hormones interact with a nuclear receptor; neurotransmitters, prostaglandins, and peptides attach to a surface receptor with second messenger formation.

26. True (b, e); False (a, c, d). The goal of the supervised fast (b) is to *stimulate* insulin secretion in insulinoma, because it may not be apparent under basal conditions. Calcitonin levels may be normal in medullary thyroid carcinoma, but increase dramatically after pentagastrin infusion (e).

27. True (b, e); False (a, c, d). A primary deficiency disorder is caused by the gland's inability to produce the hormone, despite normal levels of the trophic hormones. This may occur if the gland is removed (b) or nonfunctional (e). The disorders in (a) and (c) are caused by an absence of trophic hormones due to tumor destruction. Disorder (d) is caused by an absence of the trophic hormone due to chronic suppres-

sion, and is thus a secondary rather than primary disorder.

28. True (*a*, *c*, *e*); False (*b*, *d*). IRMA uses two antibodies that bind to two different stearic sites on the hormone. This increases specificity and increases the useful range of the assay. RIA is a competitive-binding assay in which two hormones (labeled and unlabeled) compete for antibody sites; thus, the reaction is subject to the laws of mass action. IRMA adds the antibody in excess, and thus all hormone is "captured." This also improves the quality of the assay. IRMA cannot be used to measure small hormones such as thyroxine (*b*), as the molecule must be large enough to accommodate two binding sites. IRMA and RIA both use radioisotopes (usually ^{125}I). Immunochemiluminometric assays (ICMA) use fluorescent compounds rather than radionuclides, avoiding the hazards of ionizing radiation.

29. True (*a*, *b*, *d*); False (*c*, *e*, *f*). Levels of hormones that travel attached to binding proteins (iodothyronines, steroids, sterols) would be elevated as the binding protein levels increase. This only refers to the *total* fraction; levels of *free* or unbound hormone would stay the same. Levels of hormones that travel freely in plasma (catecholamines, peptides, glycoproteins, eicosanoids) would not change.

30. True (*a*, *d*, *e*); False (*b*, *c*). Type 2 diabetes is usually a disorder of insulin resistance, not autoimmunity. Very rarely, autoantibodies may cause insulin resistance (type B insulin resistance with acanthosis nigricans). Autoantibodies may affect other organs (*c*). Patients with Graves' disease may have exophthalmos, due to autoantibody stimulation.

31. True (*b*, *c*); False (*a*, *d*, *e*). Target organ destruction (*a*) results in high trophic hormone levels. For example, patients with primary hypothyroidism have high thyrotropin (TSH) levels. High levels of the target organ hormone usually lead to suppression of the trophic hormone (*b*). Occasionally, the trophic hormone may cause suppression; GnRH given continuously leads to low FSH and LH levels. Suppressive tests (*d*) are typically done to evaluate hormone *excess*. Not all hormones have specific trophic and stimulatory hormones (*e*); many have either one or the other.

32. A (*b*); B (*a*); C (*d*); D (*c*).

33. A (*e*); B (*d*); C (*c*); D (*b*); E (*a*).

CHAPTER 2

PITUITARY GLAND

Q: What is the function of the hypothalamus and pituitary gland?

A: The hypothalamus and pituitary gland are "master glands" that exert control over many endocrine glands (such as the thyroid gland, adrenal gland, ovaries, and testes). The hypothalamic-pituitary axis (HPA) serves to integrate the central nervous system and the endocrine system.

Q: Where is the pituitary gland?

A: The pituitary gland lies in a part of the skull called the sella turcica at the base of the skull. The optic chiasm lies about 5 to 10 mm above a membrane called the diaphragma sellae, the "roof" of the pituitary, which is composed of dura mater. It is extremely vascular, supplied by the hypophyseal arteries and drained from the petrosal sinuses. It is divided into the anterior lobe or adenohypophysis, and the posterior lobe or neurohypophysis.

Q: What cells exist in the anterior pituitary gland?

A: Somatotrophs account for 50% of anterior pituitary cells and are acidophilic in appearance. They are usually located in the lateral portions, and they secrete somatotropin (growth hormone). Despite their large number, because of their location they are usually the first to become deficient in hypopituitarism.

Lactotrophs secrete prolactin and account for 10% to 25% of anterior pituitary cells. The hormone prolactin is necessary for normal lactation in the female. Like somatotrophs, lactotrophs are acidophilic in appearance.

Gonadotrophs comprise 10% to 15% of cells and are basophilic. They secrete the gonadotropins luteinizing hormone (LH) and follicle-stimulating hormone (FSH).

Corticotrophs represent 15% to 20% of cells and are basophilic in appearance. They secrete adrenocorticotrophic hormone (ACTH or corticotropin).

Thyrotrophs are the least common cell type (10%) and secrete thyroid-stimulating hormone (TSH or thyrotropin). They are basophilic in appearance.

Q: What tumors arise in the pituitary gland?

A: Most tumors of the pituitary gland are benign, and classified as either **microadenomas** or **macroadenomas.** Microadenomas are less than 1 cm in diameter, and do not generally cause compressive symptoms such as headaches or blindness. Macroadenomas are greater than 1 cm in diameter and are apt to produce compressive symptoms; the most feared complication is bitemporal hemianopsia (from compression of the optic chiasm), which can cause permanent blindness if untreated. Headaches are also common with large tumors.

Tumors may be functional and produce a hormone in excess, or may be nonfunctional. Large tumors (functional or nonfunctional) may result in cell destruction and hypopituitarism. Pituitary carcinomas are exceedingly rare and may be either functional or nonfunctional.

Q: What is the hypothalamus?

A: The hypothalamus is a group of neurons in the midbrain that secretes a variety of substances. The hormones can be divided into two types.

The **hypothalamic** or **hypophyseotropic hormones** are secreted by the arcuate neurons into the portal hypophyseal circulation. As their name implies, they exist to increase or inhibit secretion of anterior pituitary hormones.

The **posterior pituitary hormones** are secreted by the supraoptic and paraventricular nuclei of the hypothalamus; these hormones are secreted directly into the circulation.

Q: What are the hypothalamic hormones?

A: Hypothalamic hormones (Table 2-1) stimulate or inhibit the anterior pituitary gland.

Q: What are the anterior pituitary hormones?

A: The anterior pituitary hormones and their trophic and inhibitory hormones are described in Table 2-2. Their target organs are shown in Figure 2-1.

Q: What are the posterior pituitary hormones?

A: The posterior pituitary hormones are antidiuretic hormone (ADH, or arginine vasopressin) and oxytocin.

Q: What is growth hormone, and what is its function?

A: **Growth hormone** (GH) is a 191-amino acid peptide hormone synthesized by the somatotroph cells of the anterior pituitary. Its primary function is promotion of linear growth. GH has several direct effects on tissues. It causes an increase in protein synthesis, amino acid uptake, and free fatty acid release. A decrease in carbohydrate utilization due to its anti-insulin effects also occurs. Its effects on bone and cartilage are mediated through somatomedin C (insulin-like growth factor I or IGF-I).

Q: What are somatomedins?

A: **Somatomedins** are produced in the liver after stimulation by GH. Because their biologic activity is similar to insulin, they are also called insulin-like growth factors (IGFs). The somatomedin of interest is **somatomedin C** (IGF-I), which causes stimulation of epiphyseal cartilage and growth of

TABLE 2-1.   Hypothalamic Hormones

HORMONE	ACTION
Corticotropin-releasing hormone (CRH)	stimulates ACTH
Growth hormone-releasing hormone (GHRH)	stimulates growth hormone
Dopamine (prolactin-inhibiting hormone)	inhibits prolactin and TSH
Thyrotropin-releasing hormone (TRH)	stimulates TSH
Gonadotropin-releasing hormone (GnRH)	stimulates LH and FSH
Somatostatin	inhibits GH and TSH

TABLE 2-2.   Anterior Pituitary Hormones

HORMONE	TROPHIC HORMONE	INHIBITORY HORMONE	HORMONE PRODUCED BY TARGET ORGAN
ACTH	CRH	Cortisol	Cortisol
TSH	TRH	Somatostatin, dopamine, T_4, T_3	T_4, T_3
GH	GHRH	Somatostatin	IGF-I
Prolactin	? (TRH)	Dopamine	—
LH and FSH	GnRH (pulsatile secretion); activin (FSH)	GnRH (constant secretion), sex steroids, inhibin (FSH)	Sex steroids

long bones. Absence produces dwarfism, even if GH levels are normal (Laron type dwarfism). Pygmies, who lack IGF-I receptors, have short stature.

Q: How is growth hormone secreted?

A: Like many pituitary hormones, GH is secreted in circadian fashion, with peak levels occurring during sleep. Many factors increase or decrease secretion (Table 2-3).

Q: How is growth measured?

A: A **growth curve** is constructed by plotting linear height against age. Charts are available for boys (Fig. 2-2) and girls (Fig. 2-3), and for patients with congenital disorders known to be associated with growth problems, such as Turner's and Down syndromes. In the standard growth charts, the middle line represents the 50th percentile, and upper and lower lines represent the 95th and 5th percentiles, respectively.

Although the curves of the standard growth chart give information about growth over time, they do not directly give information about the rate of growth, which is important in assessing growth disorders. To visualize this, a **growth velocity curve** is made by computing the rate of growth between each growth point (expressed in cm/year) and plotting against age (Figs. 2-4, 2-5). For example, if a child grew from 140 to 145 cm in 6 months, the rate of growth would be (145 − 140) cm = 5 cm per 6 months or 12 cm/year. Many data points are necessary to create an accurate curve.

The growth rate is highest during infancy and falls off steadily, taking a "prepubertal dip" before in-

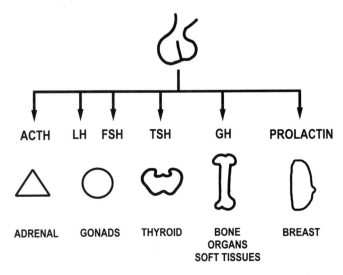

Figure 2-1. Anterior pituitary and target glands.

TABLE 2-3.   Factors Affecting Growth Hormone Secretion

STIMULATE GH SECRETION	INHIBIT GH SECRETION
Exercise	Hyperglycemia
Stress	Elevated free fatty acids
Hypoglycemia	Somatostatin
Dopamine agonists (L-dopa, bromocriptine)	Dopamine antagonists (phenothiazines)
L-Arginine	
Clonidine	

creasing again at puberty (the pubertal growth spurt). As final adult height is attained, the growth velocity falls to zero. The middle line represents the 50th percentile, and upper and lower lines represent the 95th and 5th percentiles, respectively.

Q: How can final adult height be estimated?

A: A convenient parameter for estimating final adult height is the **target height,** an average height based on the heights of both parents. This is merely an estimate and children may be shorter or taller than this:

$$\text{Male: TH} = \frac{[\text{FH} + (\text{MH} + 5)]}{2}$$

$$\text{Female: TH} = \frac{[\text{MH} + (\text{FH} - 5)]}{2}$$

where

TH = target height (inches)

FH = father's height (inches)

MH = mother's height (inches).

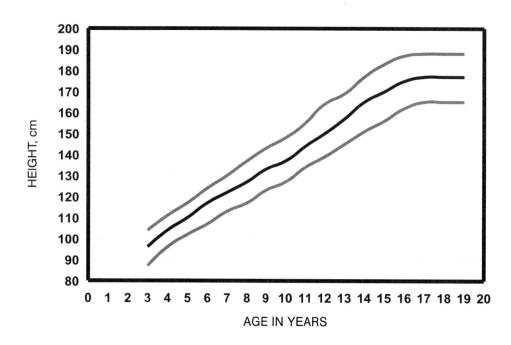

Figure 2-2. Growth chart for boys.

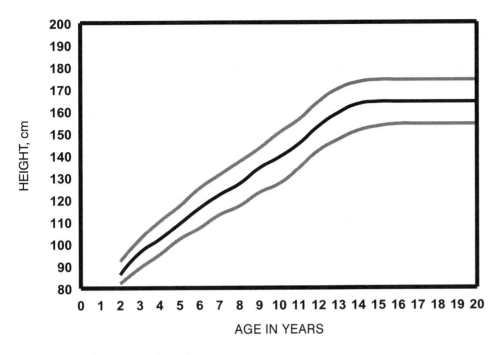

Figure 2-3. Growth chart for girls.

Q: What are some causes of short stature?

A: **Constitutional short stature** is just a variation from normal for the population. Height—like weight, intelligence, and many other parameters—is normally distributed; it stands to reason that a small percentage of patients will fall at the lower end, just as a few will be taller than normal. Genetic short stature is a type of constitutional short stature occurring in children of short parents.

Q: What do growth curves look like with constitutional short stature?

A: Most normal patients stay at and do not cross a percentile. In constitutional short stature, the

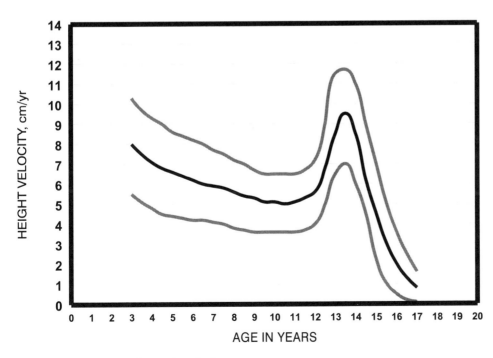

Figure 2-4. Growth velocity chart for boys.

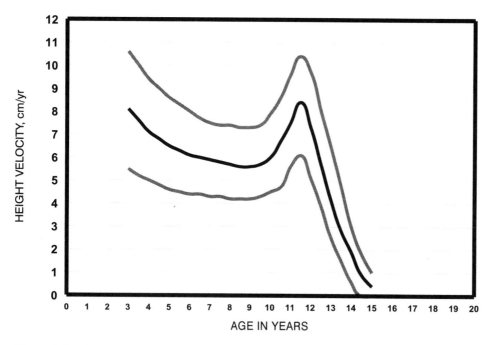

Figure 2-5. Growth velocity chart for girls.

growth curve is consistently at or below the 5th percentile (Fig. 2-6). Growth velocity is normal.

Q: What are some pathologic causes of short stature?

A: There are several pathologic causes of short stature:

- Growth hormone deficiency

- Intrauterine growth retardation

- Infections, such as rubella and cytomega-lovirus (CMV)

- Maternal drug usage

- Genetic syndromes, such as Turner's syndrome, Laurence-Moon-Biedl syndrome, Prader-Willi syndrome, and Noonan's syndrome

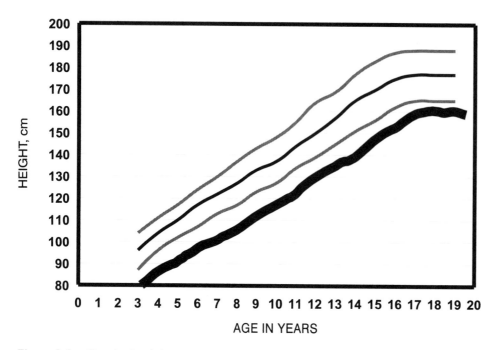

Figure 2-6. Constitutional short stature.

- Skeletal dysplasias, such as achondroplastic dwarfism

- Chronic systemic disease, such as renal insufficiency, gastrointestinal disease, cancer, and cystic fibrosis

- Psychosocial dwarfism—poor growth associated with emotional and nutritional deprivation. (Growth often improves after the patient is removed from the dysfunctional environment.)

Q: What is achondroplastic dwarfism?

A: **Achondroplastic dwarfism,** the most common form of skeletal dysplasia, is inherited in autosomal dominant fashion. These patients have short limbs but relatively normal-sized trunk and head. GH secretion is normal. GH therapy has been used with limited success, but it is not an indicated therapy. The disorder may also arise as a spontaneous mutation.

Q: What are the etiologies of growth hormone deficiency?

A: The incidence of **GH deficiency** is approximately 1 per 4000, so it should not be considered rare. Hypothalamic causes include decreased GHRH secretion and hypothalamic tumors. Pituitary etiolo-gies include pituitary tumors, trauma, pituitary removal by surgery, pituitary irradiation, and secretion of abnormal GH molecules.

Q: What is the growth curve appearance in GH deficiency?

A: Typically, the growth curve appears normal until GH deficiency occurs, and then growth velocity falls off (Fig. 2-7). Once the deficiency is treated, linear growth and velocity should again increase.

Q: How is GH deficiency diagnosed?

A: As with many pituitary hormone measurements, random GH levels are not useful because of diurnal variations. A provocative or perturbation study must be done by administering a secretagogue (see Table 2-3). In response to testing, normal children increase GH secretion to greater than 10 ng/mL. At least two different tests should be done before establishing the diagnosis.

Q: How is GH deficiency treated?

A: Human GH is available as a recombinant DNA preparation and is usually given once daily as a subcutaneous injection. Treatment must be started before the epiphyses close, or there will be no benefit. Treatment is very expensive, but it is usu-

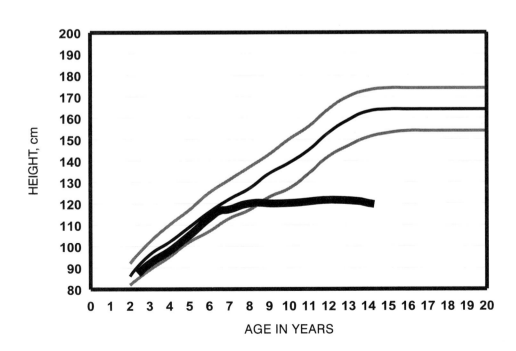

Figure 2-7. Growth hormone deficiency.

ally covered by insurance. Somatomedin C (IGF-I) is available for experimental use but is not available clinically.

Q: Are adults with GH deficiency treated?

A: In adults with hypopituitarism, treatment has traditionally been aimed at replacement of the hormones necessary for life (adrenal steroids and thyroid hormone) and sex steroids. GH is not necessary for life, but it does facilitate beneficial metabolic changes; adults with GH deficiency have decreased muscle mass and bone density as compared to normal persons. Human GH, now an approved therapy for GH deficiency in adults, should be considered for these patients.

Q: Are any other patients treated with growth hormone?

A: GH is used to treat children with short stature as a result of chronic renal insufficiency, even though their GH secretion is normal. Girls with Turner's syndrome also benefit, although their GH secretion is normal as well.

Q: Are there any defects of somatomedin C secretion?

A: **Laron dwarfism** is a condition in which patients lack GH receptors; although these individuals have normal GH secretion, inadequate IGF-I is produced, resulting in short stature. Pygmies cannot produce IGF-I and thus have short stature. IGF-I can be produced by recombinant DNA technology and would be of theoretical benefit, but it is yet to be widely used.

Q: What is the most common cause of tall stature?

A: As with short stature, **constitutional tall stature** is just a variation from normal for the population: someone without organic disease who falls statistically at one extreme (Fig. 2-8). Genetic tall stature is a form of constitutional tall stature in which the child's height is similar to his or her parents, who are tall.

Children with constitutional tall stature are taller than their peers and have accelerated growth velocity and moderately advanced bone age. The predicted height is in upper normal adult range. Growth hormone testing is normal. Obesity may lead to moderate advancement of bone age; obesity with short stature is uncommon.

Q: Are there any genetic syndromes associated with tall stature?

A: **Klinefelter's syndrome** is the most common cause of congenital hypogonadism in the male and typi-

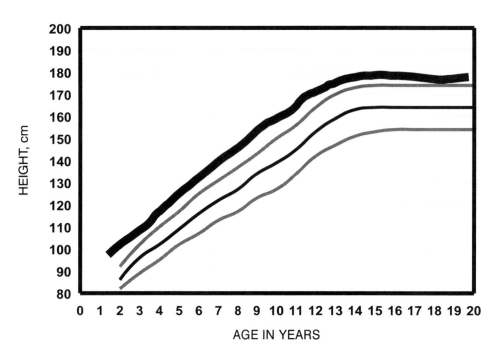

Figure 2-8. Constitutional tall stature.

cally results in "eunuchoidal" proportions (disproportionately long arms and legs). **Marfan's syndrome** is an inherited (autosomal dominant) disorder of connective tissue. These patients typically have tall stature with long, thin fingers, hyperextensibility of joints, and lens subluxation. They are at risk of fatal events such as aortic dissection. Other rare conditions include cerebral gigantism (Sotos syndrome) and homocystinuria; the latter patients have a marfanoid appearance.

Q: What are the endocrine causes of tall stature?

A: Pituitary gigantism, precocious puberty, and hyperthyroidism are endocrine causes of tall stature.

Pituitary gigantism is a rare disorder caused by growth hormone excess (usually a GH-secreting pituitary adenoma). GH excess prior to epiphyseal fusion results in rapid growth rate and excessive size for age. Until epiphyseal fusion occurs, the body is proportional; after that, the growth of soft tissues characteristic of acromegaly may be present. Growth curves show normal growth until GH excess occurs, at which time linear growth and growth velocity increase (Fig. 2-9). These patients may have symptoms of tumor (headache or visual field involvement). Treatment is resection of the pituitary tumor and/or GH antagonists (octreotide, bromocriptine). Radiotherapy may be necessary in refractory cases.

Precocious puberty causes early tall stature as a result of early sex steroid secretion and accelerated growth velocity, with marked advancement of bone age (Fig. 2-10). As early sex steroid secretion accelerates bone development, epiphyseal closure will occur earlier, resulting in adult short stature.

Hyperthyroidism (exogenous or endogenous) may cause increased growth and advanced bone age. If the condition is left untreated, the patient's final height will be reduced.

Q: What is acromegaly?

A: **Acromegaly** is a term derived from the Greek words *akros* meaning extremity, and *mega* meaning large. It is the end result of growth hormone excess, after the long bones of the skeleton have no further potential for growth. Some bones (the skull, mandible, and hands) can grow further, as can organs and soft tissues of the body. Some clinical features of acromegaly may include acral (hand and foot) enlargement (with a fleshy, doughy consistency) (Fig. 2-11), facial bone and cartilage enlargement (Fig. 2-12), weight gain, goiter, hypertension, cardiomegaly, renal calculi, hy-

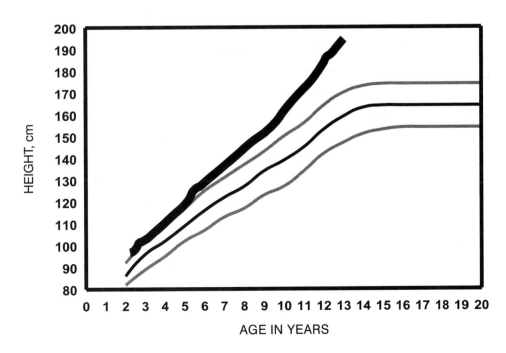

Figure 2-9. Gigantism.

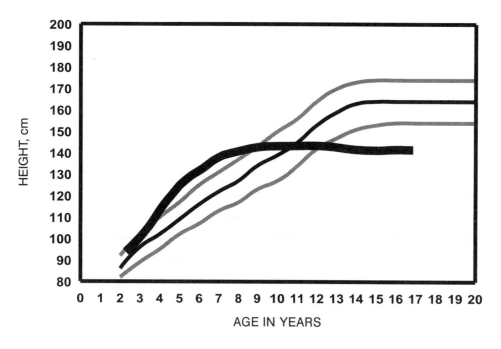

Figure 2-10. Precocious puberty.

perhidrosis, photophobia, hyperinsulinemia (due to anti-insulin effects of GH), glucose intolerance, amenorrhea (due to hypopituitarism), galactorrhea (due to hyperprolactinemia), gynecomastia, and hypoadrenalism (due to hypopituitarism).

Q: What are the causes of acromegaly?

A: The most common cause of acromegaly is a GH-secreting tumor of the pituitary gland. Rarely, hypothalamic or ectopic tumors can secrete excess growth hormone-releasing hormone (GHRH), re-

sulting in increased GH levels. Very rarely, ectopic GH secretion itself can occur.

Q: How is acromegaly diagnosed?

A: In many cases acromegaly is clinically obvious. In others, the changes are quite subtle, as they have

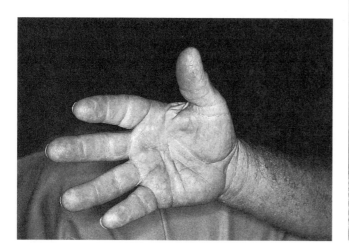

Figure 2-11. Hand of patient with acromegaly.

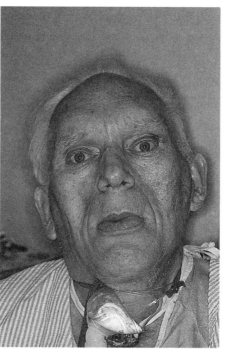

Figure 2-12. Facial features of acromegalic patient.

developed slowly over a number of years. It is common for the family not to notice acromegalic features, so it may be useful to review old photographs of the patient.

As with most pituitary disorders, random hormone measurements are typically of little value, as the hormones may be secreted sporadically. When endocrine excess is suspected, a suppression test is typically done. The most readily available physiologic suppressor of GH secretion is hyperglycemia, so typically the test is glucose suppression.

The glucose suppression test is done by giving a 100-gram dose of glucose orally, then measuring GH before and 1 hour afterward. In normal patients, GH suppresses to less than 2 ng/mL. In acromegaly, GH levels may show no suppression or may even paradoxically increase. IGF-I is usually elevated as well. Many GH-secreting tumors also secrete prolactin, so this should also be measured.

If clinical examination and laboratory studies confirm acromegaly, magnetic resonance imaging (MRI) of the pituitary is the next step, because acromegaly is almost always caused by a pituitary adenoma. Occasionally, the tumor may be too small to be seen on MRI.

Q: What is the treatment for acromegaly?

A: The primary treatment for acromegaly is surgical removal of the tumor. Small tumors can be removed by transsphenoidal resection, whereas larger tumors may require transfrontal craniotomy or may be unresectable. The prognosis for cure is poorer when the tumor is a macroadenoma (> 1 cm in diameter).

If the tumor is greater than 1 cm in diameter, it is beneficial to try and reduce the tumor size before surgery. The best medical treatment is the long-acting somatostatin analog octreotide. Typically octreotide is given as a subcutaneous injection or continuous infusion, and it effectively decreases GH levels, IGF-I levels, and tumor size. The tumor may shrink enough to allow surgical resection; other patients are not good candidates for surgery, and will require prolonged therapy. Octreotide must be given several times daily, although a long-acting depot preparation that can be given every 4 weeks is now available.

In persons with both GH and prolactin excess, the dopamine agonist bromocriptine may be effective. Bromocriptine is less effective with solitary GH-secreting tumors.

External beam radiotherapy may be used when medical or surgical treatment is unsuccessful. This therapy is helpful in over 50% of patients but does not work quickly—normalization of GH may take years. There is also a high incidence of panhypopituitarism.

Q: The dopamine agonist L-dopa increases GH secretion, so why is the GH agonist bromocriptine used to treat acromegaly?

A: In normal, healthy individuals, bromocriptine and other dopamine agonists do indeed increase GH secretion. In acromegalic individuals, these agents cause a paradoxical fall.

Q: What is the natural course of untreated acromegaly?

A: Patients with chronic, uncontrolled GH hypersecretion can be severely disfigured. Diabetes and hypertension commonly result. As the pituitary tumor enlarges, compression of the optic chiasm can lead to bitemporal visual defects and blindness. Death may occur from cardiovascular disease.

Q: What is prolactin?

A: **Prolactin,** a peptide hormone secreted by lactotrophs of the anterior pituitary, is important in mammalian lactation. It is biochemically related to growth hormone. Its deficiency results only in the lack of postpartum lactation. Its secretion is inhibited by dopamine. Thus far, a releasing factor for prolactin has not been elucidated, although thyroid-releasing hormone (TRH) may play a role.

Q: How is normal lactation regulated?

A: In normal lactation, breast size increases with ductal proliferation, and the increase in estrogen secretion causes stimulation of prolactin secretion. Milk secretion does not occur during pregnancy, however, as high estrogen levels also inhibit milk production.

After delivery, estrogen and progesterone levels abruptly decrease. In the postpartum period, milk production is stimulated by falling of estrogen and progesterone levels. The suckling reflex stimulates and helps maintain elevated prolactin during lactation (by inhibiting dopamine secretion); prolactin levels return to normal after several months of nursing. Lactation may continue after normalization of prolactin, due to the increased sensitivity of the breast to lower prolactin levels. Prolactin also helps maintain postpartum amenorrhea by inhibiting gonadotropin secretion.

Q: What conditions result from hyperprolactinemia (prolactin excess)?

A: **Hyperprolactinemia,** or prolactin excess, may result in galactorrhea (female) and hypogonadism (male or female).

Q: What is galactorrhea?

A: **Galactorrhea** is abnormal lactation, that is, lactation other than in the postpartum period. As this condition requires significant amounts of circulat-

ing estrogen and a developed breast, it is rare in males. About 50% of patients with galactorrhea have hyperprolactinemia. Idiopathic galactorrhea may also occur, in which prolactin levels are normal.

Q: Why do patients with hyperprolactinemia have hypogonadism?

A: Hyperprolactinemia inhibits gonadotropin secretion, causing hypogonadotropic hypogonadism. In women, it also interferes with the "positive" estrogen feedback on the pituitary just before ovulation, preventing the LH surge. Sex steroid levels are low. Patients with large, invasive tumors may have destruction of the gonadotroph cells themselves, resulting in permanent hypogonadotropic hypogonadism.

Q: What are the causes of hyperprolactinemia?

A: The causes of hyperprolactinemia are listed in Table 2-4.

TABLE 2-4.   Causes of Hyperprolactinemia

Pregnancy/postpartum period
Pituitary adenoma
Prolactin-secreting
Pituitary stalk compression (decreased dopaminergic inhibition)
Medications
Exogenous estrogens
Antidepressants (tricyclics, SSRIs)
Dopamine antagonists (phenothiazines, metoclopramide, methyldopa, reserpine)
Opioids
Monoamine oxidase inhibitors
Verapamil
Primary hypothyroidism (due to increased TRH secretion)
Chest wall lesions (from surgery, herpes zoster, etc.)—stimulates nerve endings (similar to infant suckling)
Renal or hepatic failure (decreased clearance)
Macroprolactinemia—abnormal prolactin molecule with very high molecular weight
Idiopathic

Q: What types of pituitary tumors cause hyperprolactinemia?

A: Prolactin-secreting tumors or **prolactinomas** may be micro- or macroadenomas, and are usually benign. Serum prolactin level roughly correlates with tumor size; prolactin levels in microadenomas are commonly in the 100 to 300 ng/mL range, whereas macroadenomas may produce levels of 1000 to 10,000 ng/mL or greater. Tumors larger than 3 to 4 mm are readily visible on MRI scan (Fig. 2-13). Small microadenomas (< 3 mm) are below the resolution of present-day equipment.

Q: How are prolactinomas treated?

A: Medical therapy is typically preferred, because of its ease and high efficacy. Dopamine agonists inhibit prolactin secretion, and the most widely used drug is bromocriptine. Other dopamine agonists used in treatment are pergolide and cabergoline. The latter has the advantage of twice-weekly dosing.

Patients with microadenomas may go into remission, and may not require long-term therapy. Those with large macroadenomas often need lifetime therapy. Surgery is typically reserved for patients that have large, invasive tumors that do not respond to medical therapy. Radiation therapy is used for those with recurrence after surgery. Both treatments carry a risk of hypopituitarism.

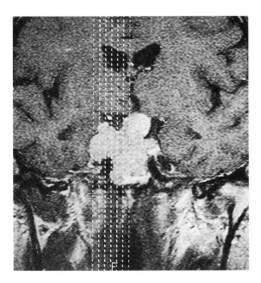

Figure 2-13. MRI of patient with large prolactinoma.

Q: What are the consequences of untreated hyperprolactinemia?

A: The major risk of prolactin excess is the effect of prolonged hypogonadism. In addition to the distressing symptoms of hypogonadism (such as amenorrhea and infertility), both men and women are at risk for osteoporosis. Galactorrhea, although distressing, is not life threatening. Large tumors can cause space-occupying problems, which may result in vision loss.

Q: Does an elevated prolactin level mean that the tumor is a prolactinoma?

A: An elevated prolactin level does not necessarily indicate a prolactinoma. Prolactin levels usually correlate with tumor size. Mild hyperprolactinemia (< 100 ng/mL) in a person with a macroadenoma is probably due to pituitary stalk compression. Prolactin is inhibited by dopamine, and has no well-defined trophic hormone; if the hypothalamic flow of dopamine is decreased by stalk compression, the prolactin level will elevate. This is in contrast to a prolactin-secreting macroadenoma, which usually presents with prolactin levels of 1000 to 10,000 ng/mL or more. GH-secreting tumors may also secrete prolactin.

Q: What are incidental pituitary tumors?

A: **Incidental** or **nonfunctional pituitary tumors** account for about 10% of pituitary tumors. They may be found on a computed tomography (CT) or MRI scan done for another reason. Large nonfunctional tumors may cause headache and/or visual field defects and are often investigated for that reason. Hypopituitarism may result from large, destructive tumors. Since these tumors are non-hormone-secreting, they do not respond to specific medical treatment. Small tumors may be followed with serial MRI studies; large tumors may need to be reduced surgically or with radiotherapy.

Q: What are gonadotropin-secreting tumors?

A: **Gonadotropin-secreting tumors** are generally large, bulky tumors that usually present with compressive symptoms (visual impairment, headaches). They most typically secrete excess FSH and alpha subunit (α-SU). There is no known consequence of FSH excess in men or postmenopausal women; it may cause menstrual irregularity in younger women. LH secretion usually is low, leading to symptoms of hypogonadism. LH rarely may be secreted in excess, but this usually has no clinical significance. Precocious puberty rarely has been reported.

Q: What is hypopituitarism?

A: **Hypopituitarism** is the deficiency of one or more pituitary hormones. **Panhypopituitarism** is the deficiency of all pituitary hormones.

Q: What are the causes of hypopituitarism?

A: The most common cause of hypopituitarism is destruction of the gland by a pituitary adenoma. Parapituitary tumors such as craniopharyngiomas may cause destruction, as can other benign tumors such as meningiomas. Metastatic tumors, such as those of the breast and lung, only rarely cause hypopituitarism.

Surgery and irradiation of the pituitary also commonly cause hypopituitarism. Severe head trauma can damage the pituitary stalk.

Isolated deficiencies of either hypothalamic or pituitary hormones may occur without structural damage. Typically, these are congenital defects. A well-known example is Kallmann's syndrome, in which GnRH (gonadotropin-releasing hormone) deficiency occurs with olfactory lobe hypoplasia and anosmia. Secretion of other hormones is normal.

Q: With structural damage to the pituitary, does deficiency of some hormones precede others, or do they all diminish at the same time?

A: After structural damage, the hormones tend to fail in a certain order, based on the relative density of each type of cell and their location in the pituitary. GH secretion is typically lost first, then gonadotropins (LH and FSH), then TSH, then ACTH. Prolactin is typically the last hormone to be lost; deficiency is rare except in Sheehan's syndrome (postpartum pituitary necrosis).

Fortunately, the two hormones necessary for life (TSH and ACTH) occur relatively late in hypopituitarism. Secretion of the posterior pituitary hormones (oxytocin and arginine vasopressin) are typically preserved in hypopituitarism caused by pituitary tumors. (Remember that these hormones are made in the hypothalamus; they are only stored in the pituitary.)

Isolated deficiencies of pituitary hormones are rare. Therefore, symptoms of one deficiency are usually accompanied by symptoms of other deficiencies. For example, ACTH deficiency in a man would likely be accompanied by hypogonadism and secondary hypothyroidism.

Q: What are the signs and symptoms of ACTH deficiency?

A: ACTH deficiency leads to secondary adrenal insufficiency, with inadequate cortisol production. Weakness, hypotension, hyponatremia, hypoglycemia, and death may occur when the condition is left untreated. Aldosterone secretion is normal with ACTH deficiency, and therefore hyperkalemia (seen in primary adrenal insufficiency) does not occur.

Q: How is ACTH deficiency diagnosed?

A: Random ACTH and cortisol levels are often of little value in diagnosing ACTH deficiency. The rapid ACTH test is done by measuring cortisol levels before, 30 minutes after, and 60 minutes after injection of 0.25 mg synthetic ACTH (cosyntropin). A normal response is increase in cortisol to greater than 18 μg/dL, or increase from baseline of more than 7 μg/dL. This test is more reliable in diagnosing primary rather than secondary adrenal insufficiency, as it does not directly measure ACTH reserve. Early in the course of ACTH deficiency, the adrenal may still respond adequately to exogenous ACTH, giving a normal reading. Eventually the adrenal will atrophy and not respond normally.

A better test is one that measures ACTH reserve. The traditional method is to provoke ACTH release by producing hypoglycemia. This is done by giving regular insulin, 0.1 unit/kg intravenously, which produces hypoglycemia. The serum cortisol should increase to over 20 μg/dL if hypoglycemia occurs. This can be a hazardous test and should only be done in a setting with adequate preparation (intravenous line, glucose, and hydrocortisone).

Another method is to inject corticotropin-releasing hormone (CRH) and measure cortisol levels. This is a very safe procedure, with none of the hazards of the insulin tolerance test. Synthetic ovine CRH is given intravenously as a bolus injection (1 μg/kg); ACTH and cortisol levels are measured at 0, 15, 30, and 60 minutes. Serum cortisol should rise to greater than 20 μg/dL.

Q: What is the treatment of secondary adrenal insufficiency?

A: The treatment for secondary adrenal insufficiency is glucocorticoid, preferably naturally occurring forms (hydrocortisone or cortisone). Mineralocorticoids such as fludrocortisone are unnecessary, as the renin-aldosterone system is intact.

Q: What are the signs and symptoms of secondary hypothyroidism?

A: The signs and symptoms of secondary hypothyroidism are similar to those of primary hypothyroidism: fatigue, cold intolerance, edema, sluggish speech and thinking, and dry skin and hair.

Q: What are the laboratory findings in secondary hypothyroidism?

A: In secondary hypothyroidism, peripheral hormones (T_4 and T_3) should be low, with a TSH that is inappropriately low (i.e., not elevated). The TSH may still be within the normal range; no elevation in the face of decreased hormone levels is evidence of pituitary insufficiency. TSH levels are elevated in primary hypothyroidism.

In equivocal cases, a **TRH stimulation test** may be done by measuring TSH before and after intravenous administration of TRH (500 μg IV) (Fig. 2-14). Patients with primary hypothyroidism show an exaggerated response of TSH to TRH, with values often exceeding 60 μU/mL. Normal patients show a moderate increase to between 10 and 20 μU/mL. Those with hypothalamic or pituitary disease show a minimal increase. Persons with primary hyperthyroidism have virtually no response at all, as TSH has been inhibited for long periods of time by high T_4 and T_3 levels.

Q: What disorders may be confused with secondary hypothyroidism?

A: The common **euthyroid sick syndrome,** in which abnormalities of thyroid hormone binding result

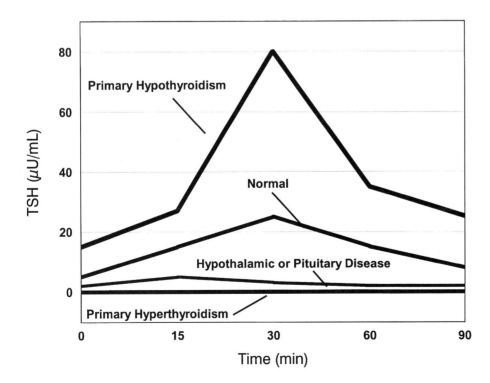

Figure 2-14.   TRH stimulation test.

in decreased total hormone levels but normal free levels, is often mistaken for secondary hypothyroidism. These patients by definition are euthyroid, and do not benefit from treatment. The euthyroid sick syndrome can be distinguished from hypopituitarism as free hormone levels are normal in the euthyroid sick syndrome. The alternative monodeiodination product of T_4, reverse T_3, is typically elevated in euthyroid sick syndrome, but is low in hypopituitarism.

Q: How do the treatments of primary and secondary hypothyroidism differ?

A: Both primary and secondary hypothyroidism are treated with synthetic thyroid hormone (L-thyroxine). In primary hypothyroidism, TSH is the most sensitive indicator to follow, and doses are titrated until TSH normalizes. In hypopituitarism, TSH is already deficient; because TSH is not a useful index to follow, peripheral hormone levels (free T_4) are monitored instead.

Patients with TSH deficiency should be tested for ACTH deficiency before beginning treatment, as the adrenal insufficiency must be treated first. Treating such a patient with thyroid hormone before glucocorticoids are administered may provoke an adrenal crisis.

Q: What is the empty sella syndrome?

A: The **empty sella syndrome** is a relatively common condition caused by a congenital defect in the diaphragma sella, resulting in enlargement of the sella and flattening of the anterior pituitary by cerebrospinal fluid (CSF). Patients are often middle-aged obese women with hypertension. Pituitary function is usually normal, and most patients are asymptomatic. A coexisting pituitary tumor may be present; biochemical testing should be done to exclude hypofunction and/or hyperfunction (e.g., hyperprolactinemia). Mild hyperprolactinemia from stalk compression is sometimes seen.

Q: What is Sheehan's syndrome?

A: **Sheehan's syndrome** (postpartum pituitary necrosis) occurs rarely in women following severe postpartum hemorrhage and results in ischemic damage to the pituitary. The pituitary is thought to

be more vulnerable to ischemic damage during pregnancy than it is normally. Women with this disorder have varying amounts of pituitary hormone deficiency. A typical presentation is lack of postpartum lactation or failure to resume menses.

Q: What is pituitary apoplexy?

A: **Pituitary apoplexy** is caused by a spontaneous hemorrhage into the pituitary, resulting in hypopituitarism; typically it is associated with a preexisting pituitary tumor. Patients usually present with severe headache, ophthalmoplegia, and decreased mentation. Without treatment, permanent visual damage, hypopituitarism, and death may occur. Emergency decompression of the pituitary may preserve visual and pituitary function. Immediate treatment with thyroxine and hydrocortisone is required, as these hormones are necessary for life. Diabetes insipidus is uncommon.

Q: What is the function of antidiuretic hormone?

A: **Antidiuretic hormone** (ADH, arginine vasopressin) is produced in the hypothalamus and secreted by the posterior pituitary gland (neurohypophysis). It acts through two receptors, V_1 and V_2.

- The effect on the V_1 receptor results in vascular smooth muscle contraction, prostaglandin synthesis, and liver glycogenolysis. This accounts for the pressor activity (hence the name *vasopressin*) and increased blood pressure.

- Effects on the V_2 receptor result in increased permeability of the renal collecting duct epithelium to water, enhancing free-water retention. In the absence of ADH, free-water absorption decreases, and polyuria results.

The stimuli for ADH secretion include hypotension, increased serum osmolality, and nausea. Decreased osmolality inhibits ADH secretion.

Q: What disorder occurs from deficiency of antidiuretic hormone (arginine vasopressin)?

A: Complete or partial ADH deficiency results in the polyuric state of **central** or **neurogenic diabetes insipidus** (CDI), in which the kidney is unable to concentrate urine, and large amounts of dilute urine are excreted. The patient complains of incessant thirst (polydipsia) and urination (polyuria), and may consume in excess of 10 liters of fluid per day. Lifestyle and sleep are constantly interrupted by frequent drinking and urination.

Q: What syndrome occurs from resistance to ADH?

A: **Nephrogenic diabetes insipidus** (NDI) is a condition in which ADH is made normally, but the kidney is resistant to it. In this case, ADH levels are elevated in the face of hypertonic plasma and dilute urine.

Q: What are the causes of central diabetes insipidus?

A: Hypothalamic tumors (such as craniopharyngiomas) or other tumors that press on the pituitary stalk may cause CDI. Pituitary tumors themselves only rarely result in CDI. Trauma, or surgery for pituitary or hypothalamic tumors may cause CDI by disruption of the pituitary stalk.

CDI following head trauma typically follows a "triphasic" response. Initially, there is a period of antidiuresis (excess ADH released from damaged neurons), followed by ADH deficiency and diabetes insipidus. The third phase is recovery, although CDI may persist in some patients.

CDI may also be autoimmune, caused by pituitary infections or infarctions, or it can be idiopathic (no cause can be found). A relative state of ADH deficiency may occur during pregnancy, due to consumption of vasopressin by placental vasopressinase. This condition is usually benign and abates after delivery.

Q: What are the causes of nephrogenic diabetes insipidus?

A: Nephrogenic diabetes insipidus may have several causes:

Drugs, such as lithium, demeclocycline, methoxyflurane, or colchicine

Chronic hypokalemia

Chronic renal disease

Sickle cell anemia

Hypercalcemia

Congenital defect (vasopressin resistance)

Familial

Q: How is diabetes insipidus diagnosed?

A: The diagnosis of diabetes insipidus requires assessment of ADH secretion. Measurement of ADH secretion is often difficult, as a random level is of little use. Any ADH measurement must take into account serum and urine osmolality. The two tests used are indirect and direct.

The **indirect test** is done by measuring the effect of dehydration on serum and urine osmolality. It is called "indirect," because it measures the effect of ADH, not the ADH level itself. The patient is dehydrated until the serum becomes hypertonic. If the patient has diabetes insipidus, the urine should remain dilute. When the plasma is hypertonic while urine is dilute, there is a defect in ADH secretion or action (indirect measurement of ADH secretion). ADH (arginine vasopressin) or the synthetic analog desmopressin is then given to the patient. If the patient has absence of ADH (CDI), the urine should concentrate and the plasma osmolality decrease. If there is ADH present but inadequate action (NDI), there is no effect.

The **direct test** is done by measuring ADH after dehydration. The patient is made hypertonic (either through dehydration or hypertonic saline infusion). ADH levels are then measured while the patient is hypertonic. In normal persons, serum ADH increases in a relatively linear fashion with serum osmolality. In diabetes insipidus, this linearity is lost. If ADH levels are decreased while the patient is hypertonic, the patient has CDI; if they are elevated, NDI is present.

Q: What is the treatment of diabetes insipidus?

A: Patients with diabetes insipidus who have an intact thirst mechanism do not require medication to live as long as they have free access to water. However, this can be very disruptive to their lifestyle, and in time can result in renal damage. CDI is most easily treated with the long-acting vasopressin analog desmopressin (DDAVP). The advantages of desmopressin include its long half-life and absence of vasopressor activity. It typically is given once or twice daily as a nasal spray or oral tablet. It also may be given subcutaneously or intravenously (usually in the hospital for patients who cannot eat). The dose is titrated to minimize thirst and polyuria. Routine laboratory studies are typically not needed in the patient with an intact thirst mechanism.

Patients who do not sense thirst pose a difficult management problem. They may become dehydrated and hypertonic if they do not drink enough. They also may become water intoxicated and develop hyponatremia and even seizures if they drink too much and use desmopressin. Such patients must meticulously measure their fluid intake to avoid these problems, and they require frequent laboratory monitoring.

Other agents exist that enhance the action of ADH, and are useful for partial CDI. These drugs are not useful for complete CDI because they require the presence of some ADH. The most commonly used agent is the sulfonylurea chlorpropamide. This is also used for the treatment of type 2 diabetes mellitus, but its tendency to potentiate ADH action has led to its decreased use for this purpose. Other agents include the lipid-lowering agent clofibrate, and the anticonvulsant carbamazepine.

Desmopressin is ineffective for NDI, as the problem is defective ADH action. If the offending drug (e.g., lithium) can be discontinued, this is of benefit. If not, medications exist that help free-water reabsorption, including diuretics such as hydrochlorothiazide and amiloride. Prostaglandin synthesis inhibitors (indomethacin) may also be useful.

Q: What other conditions are in the differential diagnosis of polyuria?

A: Common disorders such as diabetes mellitus should be excluded. A common cause of polyuria with dilute urine is water intoxication or **psychogenic polydipsia** (PP). This is common in psychiatric patients, who may feel a compulsion to drink water, often in excess of 10 liters per day. PP is distinguished from diabetes insipidus in that patients with PP are often hyponatremic (from water excess), rather than hypernatremic (due to dehydration in DI). After a period of fluid deprivation, the urine should concentrate in patients with PP, and serum does not become hypertonic as in DI.

Q: What problems result from ADH excess?

A: The **syndrome of inappropriate antidiuretic hormone** (SIADH) results in decreased free-water clearance and hyponatremia. By definition, although there is increased free water, the patient is euvolemic and not edematous. The term "inappropriate" means that the ADH excess occurs without the presence of an appropriate stimulus (e.g., hyperosmolality).

Q: What disorders can cause SIADH?

A: SIADH is a relatively common condition caused by many disorders:

Malignancy (lung carcinoma)

Chronic lung disease

Central nervous system trauma

Drugs (chlorpropamide, carbamazepine, clofibrate, vincristine)

Idiopathic

Q: How is the diagnosis of SIADH made?

A: SIADH is a diagnosis of exclusion, made after other causes of hyponatremia have been ruled out. Hyponatremia may be divided into hypovolemic, euvolemic, and hypervolemic forms (Table 2-5). Adrenal insufficiency and hypothyroidism as well as the other causes must be ruled out first. If no other cause can be found in a euvolemic patient, the patient is presumed to have SIADH.

Q: What is the treatment of SIADH?

A: Secondary causes (e.g., lung tumors) of SIADH should be treated, and any offending drugs removed. Often, as with acute head trauma, the condition is self-limiting and resolves eventually. If SIADH persists, a fluid restriction (1000–1500 mL per day) is usually effective in controlling the hyponatremia. If not, drugs that antagonize ADH action (such as demeclocycline) are useful. Without treatment, confusion, coma, and seizures may occur, although many patients tolerate chronic hyponatremia well.

TABLE 2-5. Causes of Hyponatremia

EUVOLEMIC	HYPOVOLEMIC	HYPERVOLEMIC
Hypothyroidism	Extrarenal losses	Congestive heart failure
Renal salt wasting	Vomiting	Renal failure
"Reset" hyponatremia	Diarrhea	Cirrhosis
Glucocorticoid deficiency	Renal losses	
SIADH	Diuretics	
	Mineralocorticoid deficiency	
	Hyperglycemia	

BIBLIOGRAPHY

Aron DC, Findling JW, Tyrrell JB. Hypothalamus and pituitary. In: Greenspan FS, Strewler GJ, eds. Basic and clinical endocrinology. 5th ed. Stamford, CT: Appleton & Lange, 1997:95–125.

Chrousos GP. Secondary adrenal insufficiency. In: Lamberts SWJ, ed. The diagnosis and treatment of pituitary insufficiency. Bristol, UK: BioScientifica, 1997:39–57.

Laws ER. Craniopharyngioma: transsphenoidal surgery. In: Bardin CW, ed. Current therapy in endocrinology and metabolism. 6th ed. St. Louis: Mosby, 1997:35–38.

Melmed S. Acromegaly. In: Melmed S, ed. The pituitary. Cambridge, MA: Blackwell Science, 1995:413–437.

Molitch ME. Prolactinoma. In: Melmed S, ed. The pituitary. Cambridge, MA: Blackwell Science, 1995:448–469.

Snyder PJ. Gonadotroph adenomas. In: Mazzaferri EL, Samaan NA, eds. Endocrine tumors. Cambridge, MA: Blackwell Scientific, 1993:152–164.

Thapar K, Kovacs K, Horvath E. Morphology of the pituitary in health and disease. In: Becker KL, ed. Principles and practice of endocrinology and metabolism. 2nd ed. Philadelphia: Lippincott-Raven, 1995:103–118.

Wass JAH, Sönksen PH. Hypopituitarism and growth hormone deficiency. In: Besser GM, Thorner MO, eds. Clinical endocrinology. 2nd ed. St. Louis: Mosby-Wolfe, 1994:2.2–2.15.

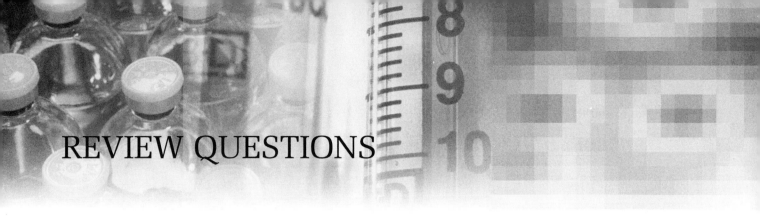

REVIEW QUESTIONS

I.   SHORT ANSWER

1. The hypothalamus and pituitary gland serve to integrate the central nervous system and the endocrine system via the _____. The pituitary gland lies in a part of the skull called the _____. Blood is supplied to the pituitary via the _____ and drained by the _____. The pituitary is divided into the _____ and _____ lobes.

2. Fill in the hormone(s) that each anterior pituitary cell type secretes:
    a. Lactotrophs: _____
    b. Somatotrophs: _____
    c. Corticotrophs: _____
    d. Thyrotrophs: _____
    e. Gonadotrophs: _____

3. The hypothalamus secretes two types of hormones: 1) the _____ hormones, which act to stimulate or inhibit anterior pituitary hormone secretion; and 2) the _____ hormones, _____ and _____.

4. Fill in the blanks for the following table:

HYPOTHALAMIC HORMONE	HORMONE STIMULATED OR INHIBITED
	stimulates ACTH
	stimulates growth hormone
	stimulates LH and FSH
	inhibits GH and TSH
	inhibits prolactin
	stimulates TSH

5. Fill in the blanks for the following table:

ANTERIOR PITUITARY HORMONE	END ORGAN
ACTH	
LH and FSH	
TSH	
GH	
Prolactin	

6. The anterior pituitary hormone required for linear growth is _____. It has several direct effects on tissues, including increased _____ and _____, increased _____, and decreased _____. It stimulates the liver to produce _____, which has the effect of stimulating cartilage and bone growth.

7. Hyperglycemia, elevated serum fatty acids, and somatostatin _____ GH secretion. Arginine, clonidine, exercise, and stress _____ GH secretion.

8. Linear growth is measured on a _____, where height is plotted against age. A _____ curve shows the rate of growth with respect to age. Growth rate is highest during _____, then falls off steadily until _____ when it increases dramatically.

9. The most common cause of short stature is _____, which typically occurs in individuals whose parents are _____. Short stature is seen in _____ deficiency; because the body habitus looks normal except for small size, the short stature is said to be _____. Achondroplastic dwarf-

ism is an example of _____ short stature, in which the limbs are abnormally short.

10. Short stature may be seen in chronic disease states such as _____, _____, or _____. It also may be seen in malnourished children or those in a dysfunctional environment, a condition known as _____.

11. GH deficiency is diagnosed with a perturbation study by administering a _____. Commonly used agents include _____, _____, _____, _____, and _____.

12. In addition to patients with GH deficiency, GH is also administered to patients with short stature caused by _____ and _____.

13. A condition resulting from lack of GH receptors is _____. This results in normal GH but low _____ levels.

14. The most common cause of tall stature is _____, which usually occurs in individuals whose parents are _____.

15. _____ is tall stature resulting from excess GH secretion before growth ends. If GH excess occurs in adulthood, the result is the syndrome _____. Treatment of these conditions includes _____, _____, and _____.

16. Excess sex steroid secretion during childhood results in early tall stature; this condition is known as _____. When left untreated, the excess sex steroids cause early _____ of the long bones and result in adult _____ stature.

17. List six signs and symptoms of acromegaly.

18. The most common cause of acromegaly is _____. Levels of _____ also may be elevated. Diagnosis is established by obtaining a GH level before and after _____, administered orally. A normal response is suppression of GH to less than _____ ng/mL at 1 hour.

19. A hormone necessary for lactation is _____. It is biochemically related to _____. Increase in _____ during pregnancy results in stimulation of this hormone. In the postpartum period, _____ occurs. Abnormal lactation (not postpartum) is called _____.

20. List five causes of hyperprolactinemia.

21. Tumors that produce excess prolactin are called _____. Pituitary tumors less than 1 cm in size are called _____; those greater than 1 cm are called _____. Large tumors may cause _____ and _____ due to compression of the optic chiasm.

22. The therapies for prolactinomas include _____, _____, and _____. The most widely used medical treatment is _____. Radiation therapy and surgery carry a risk of permanent _____, depending on the size of the tumor.

23. Hyperprolactinemia also causes _____ by inhibiting LH and FSH secretion. In women, lack of menses or _____ may occur; if it is long standing, prolonged deficiency of _____ may result in _____ and increased risk of fracture.

24. In addition to pregnancy and prolactinomas, a common cause of hyperprolactinemia is _____, especially _____. _____ may also result in hyperprolac-

tinemia, due to increased TRH secretion. Neurologic stimulation of prolactin secretion may also occur in persons with _____ from surgery or infections (e.g., herpes zoster).

25. The deficiency of one or more pituitary hormones is called _____. Deficiency of all hormones is called _____.

26. The most common cause of hypopituitarism is destruction of pituitary cells by a _____. A rare syndrome occurring in women with severe postpartum hemorrhage is _____.

27. An isolated deficiency of GnRH secretion associated with anosmia is _____, associated with low LH and FSH levels.

28. When structural damage to the pituitary occurs, the first hormone to be lost is typically _____. Deficiency of _____ is uncommon and is usually the last to occur.

29. Patients with deficiency of _____ develop secondary adrenal insufficiency. Unlike in primary adrenal insufficiency, _____ secretion is intact, so _____ does not occur.

30. ACTH reserve is traditionally tested by provoking secretion with _____. This produces hypoglycemia and normally increases ACTH and cortisol levels. This test may be hazardous. A safer test is to administer _____ and measure ACTH and cortisol levels afterward.

31. Secondary adrenal insufficiency is treated with _____. _____ are unnecessary because aldosterone secretion is normal.

32. Primary and secondary hypothyroidism can be distinguished in that TSH levels are _____ in the former, but _____ in the latter. TSH reserve can be tested by per-

forming a _____. An exaggerated response of TSH to TRH likely indicates _____, whereas a blunted response in a patient with low T_4 levels likely indicates _____.

33. A disorder commonly confused with secondary hypothyroidism is _____. Free hormone levels should be _____ in this disorder, whereas they are _____ in secondary hypothyroidism. Levels of _____ are typically elevated in this disorder.

34. Patients with secondary hypothyroidism are treated with _____. Unlike primary hypothyroidism, _____ is not a useful index to follow, and _____ should be monitored instead. Patients with panhypopituitarism must also be treated with _____ to avoid precipitation of _____.

35. _____ is an endocrinologic emergency resulting from hemorrhage into the pituitary. It is associated with severe headache and vision loss. Patients often have a preexisting _____. Without treatment, _____ may occur.

36. _____ is secreted by the posterior pituitary and results in _____ free-water balance. It also _____ vascular smooth muscle contraction, resulting in _____ blood pressure.

37. Deficiency of vasopressin results in the syndrome of _____. The symptoms include severe _____ and _____. Tumors that cause this syndrome are usually _____, not _____, in origin. After administration of vasopressin, serum osmolality should _____ and urine osmolality should _____.

38. Deficiency in the peripheral action of vasopressin results in _____, despite normal or elevated vasopressin levels. A common cause is the psychotropic drug _____. After administration of vasopressin, serum osmolality should _____ and urine osmolality should _____.

39. ADH replacement is usually given as the synthetic analog _____, in nasal spray or tablet form. It is long lasting and lacks the _____ activity of ADH. In those with partial ADH deficiency, drugs that potentiate ADH action such as _____, _____, or _____ can be given.

40. Nephrogenic diabetes insipidus can be treated with drugs such as _____, which increase free-water reabsorption. Prostaglandin synthesis inhibitors such as _____ may also be useful.

41. Complete the following table for patients with polyuric states (increased ↑, decreased ↓, or no change).

	CENTRAL DI	NEPHROGENIC DI	PRIMARY POLYDIPSIA
Serum osmolality			
Urine osmolality after water deprivation			
Urine osmolality after vasopressin			
Serum vasopressin			

42. ADH excess results in _____, with increased free body water and _____. By definition, even though free-water clearance is decreased, the patient is _____.

43. List three common causes of SIADH.

44. In addition to treatment of the underlying disorder, treatment of SIADH involves _____ and drugs such as _____.

II. MULTIPLE CHOICE

Select the one best answer.

45. Which of the following are necessary for normal growth?
    a. thyroxine
    b. growth hormone
    c. sex steroids
    d. adequate nutrition
    e. all of the above

46. The first hormone deficiency to develop in hypopituitarism is usually:
    a. TSH
    b. prolactin
    c. LH
    d. ACTH
    e. growth hormone

47. You are asked to evaluate a 16-year-old male for tall stature. He stands 6 feet 7 inches (201 cm) and weighs 240 lb (108 kg). His father is 5 feet 7 inches (170 cm), and his mother is 5 feet 4 inches (163 cm). The physical examination is unremarkable except for his large size. Puberty occurred at age 13, and he has normal secondary sexual development and potency. The arm span equals height. A growth hormone level drawn 60 minutes after a 100-gram glucose load is 32.1 ng/mL. You inform the patient that the most likely diagnosis is:
    a. Marfan's syndrome
    b. gigantism
    c. constitutional tall stature
    d. Ehlers-Danlos syndrome
    e. McCune-Albright syndrome

48. A 19-year-old male is evaluated because of a diagnosis of hypogonadism. Which of the follow-

ing findings would suggest hypothalamic or pituitary disease rather than primary testicular disease?

   a. eunuchoidal proportions

   b. increased serum LH

   c. low serum T_4 and TSH

   d. low serum testosterone

   e. loss of libido and potency

49. Complete transection of the pituitary stalk would result in deficiency of all the following hormones except which one?

   a. IGF-I

   b. triiodothyronine

   c. aldosterone

   d. estradiol (female)

   e. cortisol

50. You are asked to see a 12-year-old girl for short stature. She was at the 50th percentile until the last 3 years; now her height is at the 5th percentile. There is no sign of sexual development. She complains of excessive thirst and polyuria. On examination, she is well proportioned except for decreased sexual maturation. Her serum glucose is normal. Her serum growth hormone peaks to less than 3 ng/mL after L-dopa and arginine stimulation. The most likely diagnosis is:

   a. empty sella syndrome

   b. pituitary macroadenoma

   c. craniopharyngioma

   d. SIADH

   e. diabetes mellitus

51. Disproportionate short stature—extremities shorter than the trunk—should raise the suspicion of:

   a. psychosocial dwarfism

   b. growth hormone deficiency

   c. achondroplastic dwarfism

   d. constitutional short stature

   e. precocious puberty

52. A 12-year-old boy has grown exactly two inches in the last 15 months. His growth

velocity based on this information is approximately:

   a. 1.6 cm/year

   b. 2 cm/year

   c. 4 cm/year

   d. 6 cm/year

   e. 8 cm/year

53. A 13-year-old boy is seen for short stature. His mother is 5 feet 5 inches (165 cm) tall; his father is 6 feet 2 inches (188 cm) tall. His predicted target height is:

   a. 5 feet 8 inches

   b. 5 feet 10 inches

   c. 6 feet

   d. 6 feet 2 inches

   e. 6 feet 3 inches

54. After the administration of synthetic TRH (thyrotropin-releasing hormone), TSH levels would rise the highest in a person with which disorder?

   a. hyperthyroidism due to Graves' disease

   b. panhypopituitarism

   c. Kallmann's syndrome

   d. hypothyroidism due to Hashimoto's thyroiditis

   e. thyrotoxicosis factitia

III. TRUE OR FALSE

55. Drugs known to cause hyperprolactinemia include:

   ___ a.   oral contraceptives

   ___ b.   haloperidol (a phenothiazine)

   ___ c.   bromocriptine

   ___ d.   metoclopramide

   ___ e.   amoxicillin

56. A 63-year-old man complains of severe headache, fatigue, anorexia, and bitemporal vision loss. Serum cortisol and TSH levels are low. Sellar MRI demonstrates a 21-mm pituitary

mass with a blood-fluid level in it. *Immediate* treatment should include:

— a. testosterone

— b. thyroxine

— c. DDAVP

— d. hydrocortisone

— e. growth hormone

57. A 34-year-old woman takes lithium carbonate for bipolar disorder. She complains of persistent polyuria and polydipsia. Her serum glucose is normal. After overnight fluid deprivation, her serum osmolality is elevated at 305 mOsm/kg (normal: 270–290) with dilute urine (183 mOsm/kg). After administration of vasopressin, the urine does not concentrate, and serum osmolality remains elevated. Which of the following is/are true about this condition?

— a. Vasopressin levels are decreased.

— b. It may be effectively treated with thiazide diuretics.

— c. It may be effectively treated with desmopressin (DDAVP).

— d. It is likely caused by lithium.

— e. The patient has SIADH.

58. Treatment of SIADH might include:

— a. demeclocycline

— b. carbamazepine

— c. chemotherapy for a lung carcinoma

— d. fluid restriction

— e. amiloride

59. Clinical findings in secondary, but not primary, adrenal insufficiency include which of the following?

— a. fatigue

— b. hyperkalemia

— c. hypoglycemia

— d. hyperpigmentation

— e. anorexia

60. A 39-year-old woman presents with hand and foot enlargement, hyperhidrosis, and head-

aches. MRI of the pituitary gland demonstrates a 15-mm pituitary tumor. Which of the following would be typical findings in this patient?

— a. serum growth hormone of 43.7 ng/mL after 100-gram glucose load

— b. prolactin level of 75.9 ng/mL (normal: 3.3–21.0)

— c. glucose intolerance

— d. IGF-I level of 1069 ng/mL (normal: 90–360)

— e. serum T_4 of 20.2 μg/dL (normal: 4.5–12.0)

61. Acidophil pituitary adenomas may cause the following signs or symptoms:

— a. precocious puberty

— b. gigantism

— c. galactorrhea

— d. diabetes mellitus

— e. hyperthyroidism

62. Destruction of the hypothalamus by a tumor is expected to result in *decreased* levels of which pituitary hormones?

— a. ACTH

— b. prolactin

— c. TSH

— d. vasopressin

— e. growth hormone

63. Treatment of central (neurogenic) diabetes insipidus may include:

— a. desmopressin

— b. chlorpropamide

— c. fluid restriction

— d. clofibrate

— e. thiazide diuretics

IV. MATCHING

Match each item with the appropriate answer. Each may be used only once.

64. Match the following girls with their appropriate growth charts in Figure 2-15:

    ___ A. 1.5-cm pituitary tumor and growth hormone level of 45.2 ng/mL, 1 hour after a 100-gram glucose load

    ___ B. volleyball and basketball player highly recruited by colleges

    ___ C. large craniopharyngioma diagnosed at age 7; peak growth hormone of 2 ng/mL after challenge with L-dopa and clonidine

    ___ D. breast budding at age 4, menses at age 6; history of hydrocephalus.

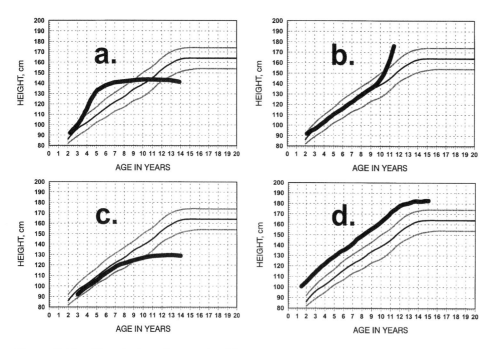

Figure 2-15.   Growth charts for question 64.

ANSWERS

1. hypothalamic-pituitary axis (HPA); sella turcica; hypophyseal arteries, petrosal sinuses; anterior, posterior

2. (*a*) prolactin; (*b*) growth hormone (GH); (*c*) corticotropin (ACTH); (*d*) thyrotropin (TSH); (*e*) luteinizing hormone (LH), follicle-stimulating hormone (FSH)

3. hypothalamic; posterior pituitary, arginine vasopressin (antidiuretic hormone, ADH), oxytocin

4.

HYPOTHALAMIC HORMONE	HORMONE STIMULATED OR INHIBITED
CRH (corticotropin-releasing hormone)	stimulates ACTH
GHRH (growth hormone-releasing hormone)	stimulates growth hormone
GnRH (gonadotropin-releasing hormone	stimulates LH and FSH
Somatostatin	inhibits GH and TSH
Dopamine	inhibits prolactin
TRH (thyrotropin-stimulating hormone)	stimulates TSH

5.

ANTERIOR PITUITARY HORMONE	END ORGAN
ACTH	adrenal cortex
LH & FSH	ovary or testis
TSH	thyroid
GH	liver (IGF-I), organs, soft tissue
Prolactin	breast

6. growth hormone; protein synthesis, amino acid uptake, free fatty acid release, carbohydrate utilization; insulin-like growth factor I (IGF-I, somatomedin C)

7. inhibit; increase

8. growth curve; growth velocity; infancy; puberty (adolescence)

9. constitutional; short; growth hormone; proportional; disproportionate

10. renal insufficiency, cystic fibrosis, malignancy; psychosocial dwarfism

11. secretagogue; insulin, arginine, clonidine, L-dopa, exercise

12. Turner's syndrome, chronic renal insufficiency

13. Laron dwarfism; IGF-I

14. constitutional, tall

15. gigantism; acromegaly; medication (octreotide or bromocriptine), surgery, radiotherapy

16. precocious puberty; epiphyseal fusion; short

17. List six: acral enlargement (hands and feet), weight gain, goiter, hypertension, cardiomegaly, renal calculi, hyperhidrosis, photophobia, hyperinsulinemia, glucose intolerance, irregular/absent menses, galactorrhea, gynecomastia, hypoadrenalism

18. GH-secreting pituitary tumor; prolactin; 100 gram glucose; 2

19. prolactin; growth hormone; estrogen; lactation; galactorrhea

20. List five: pregnancy, prolactinoma, medications, primary hypothyroidism, chest wall lesions, renal or hepatic failure, macroprolactinemia, idiopathic

21. prolactinomas; microadenomas; macroadenomas; bitemporal hemianopsia, blindness

22. medication, surgery, radiation therapy; bromocriptine; hypopituitarism

23. hypogonadotropic hypogonadism; amenorrhea; estrogen, osteoporosis

24. medication, psychotropic drugs (e.g., phenothiazines); primary hypothyroidism; chest wall lesions

25. hypopituitarism; panhypopituitarism

26. pituitary tumor; postpartum pituitary necrosis (Sheehan's syndrome)

27. Kallmann's syndrome

28. growth hormone (GH); prolactin

29. ACTH; mineralocorticoid (aldosterone), hyperkalemia

30. insulin; CRH

31. glucocorticoids; mineralocorticoids

32. elevated, low; TRH stimulation test; primary hypothyroidism, hypothalamic or pituitary disease

33. euthyroid sick syndrome; normal, low; reverse T_3

34. thyroxine; TSH, peripheral hormones (T_4); glucocorticoids, adrenal insufficiency

35. pituitary apoplexy; pituitary adenoma; death

36. antidiuretic hormone (vasopressin); increases; increases; increased

37. central (neurogenic) diabetes insipidus (CDI); polyuria, polydipsia; suprasellar, pituitary; decrease, increase

38. nephrogenic diabetes insipidus (NDI); lithium; not change, not change

39. DDAVP (desmopressin); pressor; clofibrate, chlorpropamide, carbamazepine

40. diuretics; indomethacin

41.

	CENTRAL DI	NEPHROGENIC DI	PRIMARY POLYDIPSIA
Serum osmolality	↑	↑	↓
Urine osmolality after water deprivation	no change	no change	↑
Urine osmolality after vasopressin	↑↑	no change	↑
Serum vasopressin	↓	↑	↓

42. syndrome of inappropriate antidiuretic hormone (SIADH), hyponatremia; euvolemic

43. List three: malignancy (lung carcinoma), chronic lung disease, central nervous system trauma, drugs (chlorpropamide, carbamazepine, clofibrate, vincristine), idiopathic, autoimmune

44. fluid restriction, demeclocycline

45. (e).

46. (e). GH deficiency typically occurs first, followed by gonadotropins, TSH, ACTH, and finally, prolactin.

47. (b). GH should suppress to less than 2 ng/mL after a glucose load. The level of 32.1 ng/mL suggests gigantism. Marfan's syndrome (a) may result in disproportionate tall stature.

48. (c). Hypogonadotropic hypogonadism (due to deficient GnRH and/or gonadotropin secretion) usually is associated with other pituitary hormone deficiencies, such as TSH deficiency. However, isolated deficiencies of hypothalamic or pituitary hormone secretion do occur (e.g., Kallmann's syndrome). Eunuchoidal proportions (a), low testosterone (d), and lack of libido (e) would be seen in either type of hypogonadism. Increased LH (b) is seen only with primary gonadal disease.

49. (c). Aldosterone secretion occurs normally in the absence of pituitary stimulation; it is dependent on the renin-angiotensin system (RAS). IGF-I (a) requires growth hormone for normal secretion. T_3 (b) requires TSH. Sex steroids (d) require LH, and cortisol (e) requires ACTH.

50. (c). She likely has growth hormone deficiency and central diabetes insipidus, common with large suprasellar tumors (craniopharyngiomas). Empty sella syndrome (a) commonly causes hyperprolactinemia but not GH deficiency. Pituitary tumors (b) may cause GH deficiency but only rarely cause diabetes insipidus. SIADH (d) results from too much, not too little, ADH. Diabetes mellitus (e) is excluded by normoglycemia.

51. (c). All the other conditions result in *proportional* short stature.

52. (c). 2 in = 5.08 cm growth in 15 months. Growth in 12 months = (5.08)(12)/15 = 4.06 cm/year.

53. $(c). \mathrm{TH} = \frac{[(65+5)+74]}{2} = \frac{70+74}{2} = \frac{144}{2} = 72$ inches

54. (d). Thyrotroph cells are most sensitive to TRH when hypothyroidism (d) is present, due to the low circulating hormone levels. The TSH response to TRH is most blunted in hyperthyroid-

ism (*a, e*). It is also blunted in hypopituitarism (*b*). The response is normal in Kallmann's syndrome (*c*), an isolated defect in GnRH secretion.

55. True (*a, b, d*); False (*c, e*).

56. True (*b, d*); false (*a, c, e*). This man has pituitary apoplexy and must receive hormones necessary for life (glucocorticoids and thyroxine). Testosterone (*a*) and GH (*e*), although beneficial, are not necessary for life, and thus are not immediately necessary. Central diabetes insipidus rarely occurs in this disorder; if it does, it is not life-threatening as long as the patient is alert and can drink fluids.

57. True (*b, d*); False (*a, c, e*). Nephrogenic diabetes insipidus is commonly a result of long-term lithium therapy and may be treated with thiazides or indomethacin. ADH is ineffective, and ADH levels are elevated.

58. True (*a, c, d*); False (*b, e*). Carbamazepine (*b*) potentiates ADH action and may be used for partial central diabetes insipidus. Amiloride (*e*) is used for nephrogenic diabetes insipidus.

59. True (*a, c, e*); False (*b, d*). Hyperkalemia (*b*) is only seen with mineralocorticoid deficiency (primary only). Hyperpigmentation is due to ACTH excess (primary only).

60. True (*a, b, c, d*); False (*e*). This woman has acromegaly. Many tumors produce excess prolactin in addition to growth hormone. Prolactin levels may also be elevated because of pituitary stalk compression. Although goiter may occur in acromegaly, patients are euthyroid and hyperthyroidism is not a feature.

61. True (*b, c, d*); false (*a, e*). Acidophils produce growth hormone and prolactin, excess of which can cause gigantism and galactorrhea, respectively. GH excess (acromegaly or gigantism) can also result in glucose intolerance and diabetes mellitus (*d*). Diabetes also could result from a basophilic ACTH-secreting adenoma (Cushing's disease). Gonadotroph and thyrotroph adenomas can cause precocious puberty (*a*) and hyperthyroidism (*e*), respectively, but are basophil adenomas.

62. True (*a, c, d, e*); False (*b*). Prolactin lacks a well-defined stimulatory hormone, and has only an inhibitory hormone (dopamine). Removal of the inhibitory hormone by hypothalamic destruction may result in increased levels. Vasopressin itself is made in the hypothalamus, and levels are decreased with its destruction. The other hormones require stimulatory hormones for proper release from the pituitary.

63. True (*a, b, d*); False (*c, e*). Desmopressin (*a*) is the treatment of choice for central diabetes insipidus. Chlorpropamide (*b*) and clofibrate (*d*) potentiate ADH action and may be used in partial neurogenic DI. Fluid restriction (*c*) is used for SIADH, not diabetes insipidus. Thiazides (*e*) are used for nephrogenic diabetes insipidus.

64. A (*b*); B (*d*); C (*c*); D (*a*). Girl A has gigantism, and her growth chart exhibits a dramatic sudden acceleration in growth. In contrast, Girl B has constitutional tall stature; she has been tall for her age throughout her lifetime, and does not deviate from the curve. Girl C, with the craniopharyngioma, has growth hormone deficiency. Girl D exhibits precocious puberty, which leads to initial accelerated growth and tall stature, followed by premature epiphyseal closure and short stature.

CHAPTER 3

THYROID GLAND

Q: What is the thyroid gland? Where is it located?

A: The thyroid is the largest endocrine organ in the body, and secretes thyroid hormones, which are required for normal growth and metabolism. It is located in the neck, anterior to the trachea and below the thyroid cartilage. It has two lobes with an isthmus, plus an embryonic remnant, the pyramidal lobe, in the midline. Each lobe is pear-shaped and measures about 3 to 4 cm in length, 1.5 to 2.0 cm in width, and 1.0 to 1.5 cm thick. The average weight of the thyroid in humans is about 20 grams. It may enlarge to many times this size in states of disease.

Q: What are the thyroid hormones?

A: The thyroid primarily secretes 3,5,3′,5′-L-tetraiodothyronine (T_4, L-thyroxine) (Fig. 3-1), plus a lesser amount of 3,5,3′-L-triiodothyronine (T_3) (Fig. 3-2). The D-isomers are inactive. T_4 is the primary secretory product of thyroid; 99.96% is protein bound, and 0.04% is free. As with all protein-bound hormones, only the free or unbound portion is biologically active. T_4 has an extremely long biologic half-life of 1 week.

T_3 (triiodothyronine) is secreted in small amounts by the thyroid but is mainly produced by peripheral **monodeiodination** of T_4 after it has left the thyroid. Like T_4, it is also highly protein bound. It is *much* more potent than T_4 on a molar basis and is the principal active thyroid hormone. It has a much shorter half-life than T_4 (1 day). A major function of T_4 is to be a long-lasting reservoir for production of T_3.

Q: How is thyroid function regulated?

A: Trophic hormones include hypothalamic thyrotropin-releasing hormone (TRH) and pituitary thyroid-releasing hormone (TSH, thyrotropin). High levels of T_4 and T_3 inhibit secretion of TSH and TRH by feedback inhibition (Fig. 3-3). Low T_4 and T_3 levels result in increased TRH and TSH.

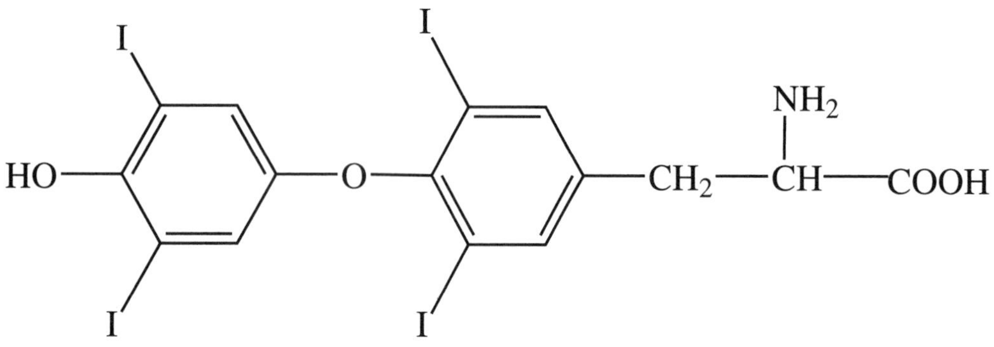

Figure 3-1. Thyroxine.

Q: How does thyroid hormone synthesis occur?

A: Iodothyronines are synthesized in the **follicle,** the functional unit of the thyroid. Follicles contain a proteinaceous gel called **colloid,** upon which thyroid hormones are synthesized.

The first step is called **trapping,** in which inorganic iodine is brought into the follicular cell (Fig. 3-4). It then undergoes **organification,** where it is incorporated into tyrosine residues, the eventual precursor of T_4. T_4 is formed on a protein (thyroglobulin) by coupling of the iodinated tyrosine residues. These hormones attached to thyroglobulin are stored in the colloid. TSH stimulates all these processes, including the release of T_4 into the bloodstream via proteolysis.

T_4 is the primary secretory product of the thyroid, although T_3 is secreted in small amounts. Most T_3 in the body is formed from peripheral monodeiodination of T_4.

Q: What proteins carry the highly bound thyroid hormones in the blood?

A: The major proteins that carry highly bound thyroid hormones in the blood are

thyroid-binding globulin (TBG): 70%

albumin: 20%

transthyretin (thyroid-binding prealbumin): 10%

Thus, the total portion of T_4 and T_3 measured in the blood is affected by conditions altering protein concentrations. Most common T_4 and T_3 assays will report the total hormone.

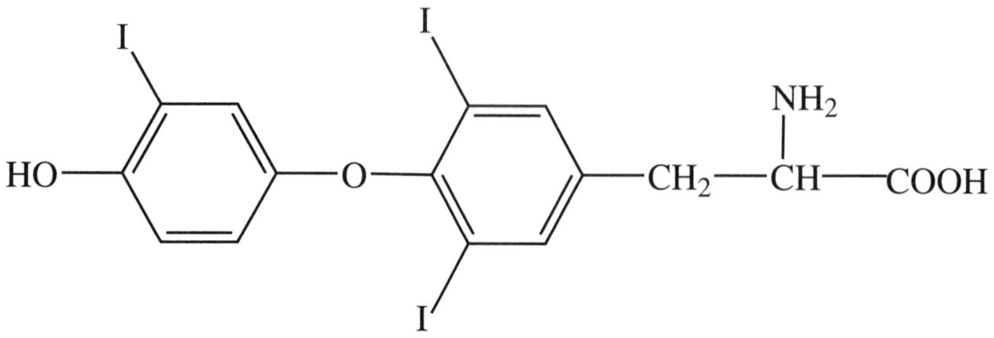

Figure 3-2. Triiodothyronine.

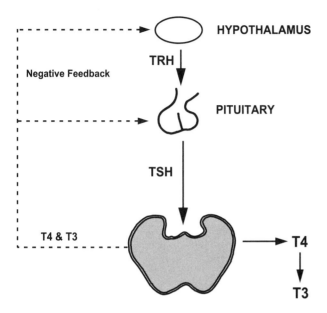

Figure 3-3. Normal thyroid function.

Q: What are the biological effects of thyroid hormone?

A: T_3 is the active hormone and binds to a receptor complex in nucleus, where protein transcription occurs. T_4 is a "prohormone" and its biologic activity is due to deiodination to T_3. Table 3-1 lists the biologic effects of iodothyronines.

Q: What autoantibodies are found in thyroid disease?

A: The common thyroid autoantibodies and their associated disorders are found in Table 3-2.

Q: What conditions cause increased binding protein concentrations, leading to increased total T_4 and T_3 levels?

A: The conditions that can increase binding protein concentrations are estrogen therapy, pregnancy, congenital protein abnormalities, acute liver disease, and hypothyroidism. A common presentation is a woman taking oral contraceptives who presents with a high total T_4 but normal free T_4 level.

Q: What clinical consequences result from altered protein concentrations?

A: The altered protein concentrations have no clinical consequences. Only the *free* portion is biologically active; the hypothalamus and pituitary are regulated by this free portion and will keep it at the correct level. The body does not care about the protein-bound, inactive fraction; we only need to be aware of the latter because such conditions can result in abnormal values when there is no problem.

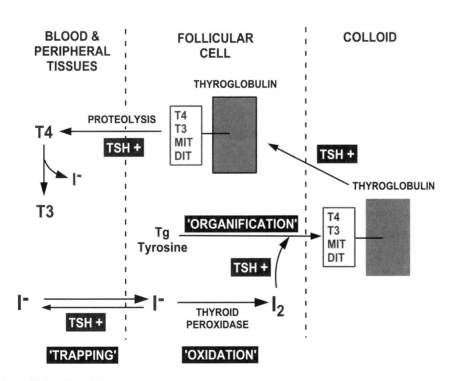

Figure 3-4. Thyroid hormone synthesis.

TABLE 3-1.   Biological Effects of Iodothyronines

Increased O_2 consumption and heat production
Increased cardiac muscle contractility
Increased sensitivity to catecholamines
Maintenance of hypoxic and hypercapnic drive in respiratory center
Increased gut motility
Increased erythropoiesis
Increased bone turnover
Increased protein turnover and loss of muscle tissue
Increased cholesterol degradation
Increased metabolic turnover of many hormones and drugs

Q: **What inherited protein disorders can cause elevated thyroid hormone levels?**

A: The most common is **familial dysalbuminemic hyperthyroxinemia** (FDH), in which an abnormal albumin-like protein has an extremely high affinity for T_4. Because a greater portion of T_4 is bound than normal, the total levels are increased (to maintain a normal free T_4 level). The patients are euthyroid, as the free T_4 and TSH are normal. Interestingly, the abnormal protein has a normal affinity for T_3, so the T_3 resin uptake may be normal. This is a benign disorder, but it must be recognized so that mistaken treatment for hyperthyroidism can be avoided.

Q: **Are there any conditions that can cause decreased protein levels?**

A: Conditions that can decrease protein levels include congenital protein abnormalities, androgen

therapy, glucocorticoids, protein malnutrition, nephrotic syndrome, and hyperthyroidism.

Q: **How can we correct for these protein abnormalities?**

A: The best way is to measure the *free* instead of the *total* hormone level, as the former is unaffected by protein concentrations. Free T_4 and T_3 are still not available in many laboratories.

Another, older way is to obtain a **free thyroxine index** or **FT_4I**, which is sometimes also (misleadingly) called a "T7." This is a derived product of the total T_4 and the T_3 resin uptake (T_3RU):

$$FT_4I = \text{Total } T_4 \times T_3 \text{ resin uptake}$$

Q: **What is a T_3 resin uptake?**

A: The **T_3 resin uptake (T_3RU)** is an older test used to indirectly quantitate the amount of thyroid binding protein. It is not to be confused with a triiodothyronine (T_3) level.

A known amount of radiolabeled T_3 (T_3*) is added to serum. A proportion of T_3* will attach to the protein binding sites for T_3. The amount left over (not protein bound) is taken up by a resin and measured. If the protein concentration is higher than normal, a greater proportion of T_3* will bind to the proteins, and less will be left over to bind to the resin (the amount of T_3* measured) (Fig. 3-5). Therefore, with increased proteins, T_3RU will be decreased. If proteins are decreased, the opposite occurs: less binds to the proteins, and more is left over, leading to an increased T_3RU. So, *the T_3RU is inversely proportional to the number of protein binding sites*. The free thyroxine index (FT_4I) is the product of T_4 and T_3RU, and is an approximation of the free T_4 level (Fig. 3-6).

TABLE 3-2.   Autoantibodies and Thyroid Disease

AUTOANTIBODY	ASSOCIATED THYROID DISEASE
Antithyroid peroxidase (anti-TPO; anti-microsomal)	Hashimoto's thyroiditis
Antithyroglobulin	Hashimoto's thyroiditis
Anti-TSH receptor antibody (TRAb)	Graves' disease
Thyroid-stimulating immunoglobulin (TSIg)	Graves' disease

Box = amount of thyroid binding proteins; larger box = larger amount of proteins

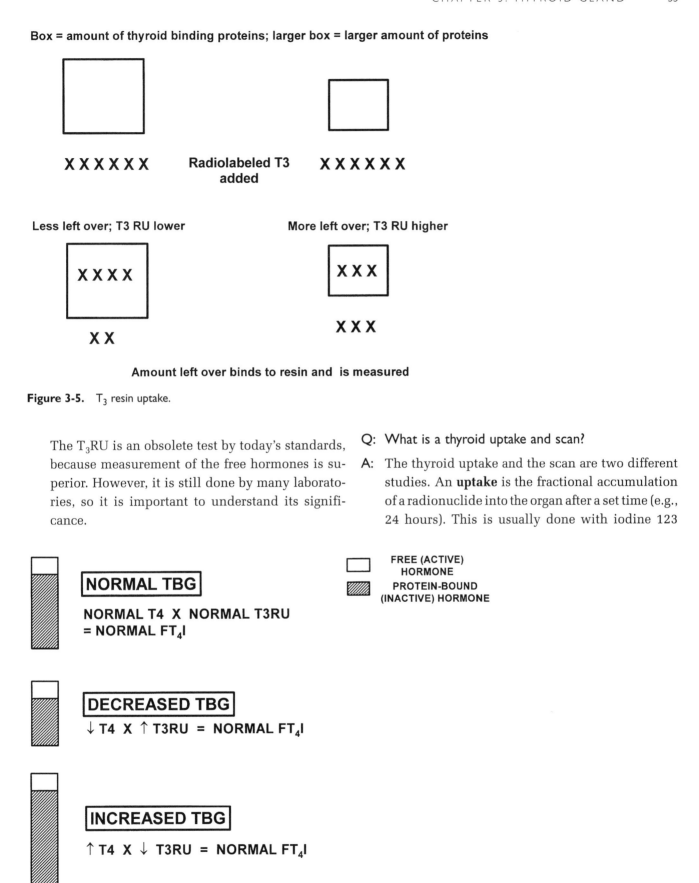

Figure 3-5. T₃ resin uptake.

The T$_3$RU is an obsolete test by today's standards, because measurement of the free hormones is superior. However, it is still done by many laboratories, so it is important to understand its significance.

Q: What is a thyroid uptake and scan?

A: The thyroid uptake and the scan are two different studies. An **uptake** is the fractional accumulation of a radionuclide into the organ after a set time (e.g., 24 hours). This is usually done with iodine 123

Figure 3-6. Thyroid hormone levels in different protein states.

(^{123}I). First, a certain amount is given orally to the patient. Then at 24 hours, the amount remaining is assessed with a gamma counter, and compared to a control capsule (which corrects for the amount lost due to natural disintegration). This gives an index of how active the thyroid is at the trapping of iodine, and thus it is often useful in assessing thyroid activity. Normal iodine uptake varies by geographic region, as a consequence of different amounts of iodine in the diet. In the United States, a typical normal value is 20% to 35% at 24 hours. Values are typically higher in countries where less iodine is consumed in the diet.

A **scan** is an actual two-dimensional image taken with a device called a **gamma camera.** A permanent record of the scan can be placed onto film for later viewing. Because scans provide some functional as well as anatomic information, they are useful in certain thyroid disorders. Scans may also be done with other substances, such as ^{131}I and technetium (^{99m}Tc). These usually yield less satisfactory images. Technetium can be given intravenously to patients who cannot eat.

Q: Do any agents interfere with a radioiodine uptake and scan?

A: Many commonly used substances interfere with the study. Administration of large amounts of iodine will suppress uptake and render the study invalid. Therefore, patients who have received intravenous contrast for an x-ray study should not have a scan for at least 4 to 6 weeks. Patients are encouraged not to take iodide-containing multivitamins for 2 weeks prior to the study. Those undergoing imaging for thyroid cancer are asked to follow a low-iodine diet.

Thyroid hormone suppresses iodide trapping and thus patients on thyroxine therapy cannot have a scan. Lithium also inhibits iodide uptake and the test cannot be reliably done on persons taking this medication. Amiodarone contains iodine and also inhibits iodide uptake.

Q: Is the thyroid uptake a reliable indicator of thyroid hormone output?

A: Thyroid uptake is not always a reliable indicator of hormone output. The uptake only measures iodine trapped by the thyroid, and not necessarily iodine converted to thyroid hormone. Trapping could occur without organification, so it is possible to have a normal or even a high uptake in hypothyroidism when **organification defects** are present. Thus the concept of "hypothyroid," "euthyroid," or "hyperthyroid" uptake is incorrect, as uptake information must always be correlated with thyroid hormone status.

Q: What is the difference between the types of radioiodine?

A: ^{123}I and ^{131}I are commonly used in nuclear medicine. ^{123}I is superior for imaging because of its monoenergetic low-energy gamma rays. There are no particulate emissions (β-particles). Because of the low-energy gamma rays and lack of particulate emissions, the patient receives a very low radiation dose. ^{123}I has a very short half-life (13 hours), so it is difficult to keep on hand in large quantities.

^{131}I is primarily used for therapeutic purposes where actual thyroid tissue destruction is desired, as in treatment of hyperthyroidism and thyroid cancer. Unlike ^{123}I, ^{131}I emits multi-spectrum high-energy gamma rays plus β-particles, making the delivered radiation dose much higher. ^{131}I has a much longer half-life (8 days) than ^{123}I. It can be used for imaging, but poorer quality is obtained because of the multiple gamma energies. It is sometimes preferred for thyroid cancer imaging, where long imaging times are needed.

Q: What is hypothyroidism?

A: **Hypothyroidism** is the condition in which thyroid hormone levels are abnormally low.

Q: What are the types of hypothyroidism?

A: There are three types of hypothyroidism: **primary,** the result of the absence or dysfunction of the thyroid; and **secondary** and **tertiary,** both the result of pituitary or hypothalamic dysfunction.

Q: What are the causes of primary hypothyroidism?

A: The autoimmune disorder **Hashimoto's thyroiditis** is the most common cause of primary hypothyroidism in the United States. Hashimoto's thyroiditis is a result of autoimmune destruction, leading to lymphocytic infiltration, often with enlargement of the thyroid (goiter). A less common autoimmune cause is **autoimmune atrophic thyroiditis,** which is more typical in older patients. The autoantibodies cause atrophy rather than enlargement.

Patients who have undergone thyroidectomy obviously have hypothyroidism. Those who have received ^{131}I treatment for hyperthyroidism frequently develop hypothyroidism. Persons receiving external beam radiation for other malignancies also occasionally develop hypothyroidism.

Congenital enzyme defects (very rare) or thyroid agenesis (1 in 4000 births) may result in neonatal hypothyroidism. Endemic hypothyroidism due to iodine deficiency is seen in underdeveloped countries, but it is rare in the United States.

Various drugs may also cause hypothyroidism, including iodine, inorganic or organic (iodide, iodinated contrast agents, amiodarone); lithium; and thionamides (propylthiouracil and methimazole).

Q: How is the diagnosis of primary hypothyroidism established?

A: Because the end organ (the thyroid) has failed, the trophic hormones (TRH and TSH) increase. The most sensitive indicator of primary hypothyroidism is an elevated TSH level. (TRH would be elevated also, but it is not typically measured.)

T_4 and T_3 levels typically are decreased. As the range of "normal" T_4 is quite large (5.0–12.0 μg/dL), it is possible to be mildly hypothyroid with a low normal T_4 (or T_3). In this case, the TSH would still be elevated. *The TSH, therefore, is the most sensitive indicator of thyroid function.*

Q: What are the thyroid uptake and scan results in hypothyroidism?

A: In hypothyroidism, the uptake may be low, normal, or elevated. In cases where the thyroid mass is decreased or absent, uptake would be decreased. In Hashimoto's thyroiditis (the most common cause of acquired hypothyroidism), organification defects occur, leading to inefficient thyroid hormone synthesis despite adequate trapping of iodine. Because the TSH is high, trapping increases despite low T_4 output; thus, patients with Hashimoto's may have an increased uptake despite being hypothyroid. In Hashimoto's disease, a "salt and pepper" appearance may also be noted, due to the irregular functioning of thyroid tissue.

The scan may show an absence of thyroid tissue (as a result of surgery, agenesis, etc.). The thyroid uptake and scan thus add little to the diagnosis and treatment of hypothyroidism and should not be done in most cases.

Q: What are the symptoms and signs of hypothyroidism?

A: The classic symptoms of hypothyroidism include fatigue, weight gain (mild), cold intolerance, constipation, menstrual irregularities, muscle cramps, and slowed mentation. Signs include dry, rough skin; periorbital edema; delayed muscle stretch reflexes (relaxation); and carotenemia (yellowish discoloration of skin) and edema.

Q: Does hypothyroidism cause obesity?

A: No, hypothyroidism does not cause obesity. Hypothyroid patients may experience a very modest weight gain (10 to 20 lb), mostly due to fluid retention. Many hypothyroid patients are in fact thin. Although obese patients may have hypothyroidism, the condition does not go away after treatment.

Q: What is cretinism?

A: **Cretinism** is a condition that occurs in infants with untreated hypothyroidism, resulting in mental retardation, short stature, puffy face and hands, and protuberant abdomen. Congenital hypothyroidism is relatively common, occurring in 1 per 4000 infants. Thyroid agenesis is the typical cause. Mothers with Hashimoto's thyroiditis may transfer TSH-receptor blocking antibody to the fetus, resulting in thyroid agenesis. Inherited defects of thyroid hormone metabolism are rare causes. Pregnant women with hyperthyroidism are not treated with radioiodine, because it results in fetal hypothyroidism when it is given after the 12th week of gestation.

Fortunately, cretinism is very rare in the United States, thanks to mandated thyroid hormone screening in all neonates. Prompt detection and treatment prevents its development.

Q: What are the consequences of hypothyroidism in children?

A: Children with hypothyroidism have delayed growth and mental retardation if their hypothyroidism is untreated. The amount of cognitive dysfunction depends on the age of diagnosis; a 3-year-old child with untreated hypothyroidism would develop more severe deficits than a 10-year-old child.

Children with severe hypothyroidism may develop pituitary enlargement from TRH secretion, which may be mistaken for a tumor with magnetic resonance imaging (MRI). This "pseudotumor" goes away after therapy. Very rarely, isosexual precocity may occur in these patients. TRH, in addition to stimulating TSH secretion, may cause gonadotropin hypersecretion, resulting in early sexual development. After treatment, the sexual precocity regresses.

Q: What is subclinical hypothyroidism?

A: **Subclinical hypothyroidism** is defined as a mildly elevated TSH level with low-normal to normal T_4 levels and an absence of clinical symptoms. Because the treatment is benign if monitored properly, most endocrinologists elect to treat these patients until the TSH is into the normal range. Others elect to follow the patient for signs of symptomatic disease.

Q: How would you differentiate primary from secondary or tertiary hypothyroidism?

A: In primary hypothyroidism, the TSH is always elevated. In secondary or tertiary, the TSH would be inappropriately low for the serum hormone levels.

Q: What is the worst thing that could happen to a patient with untreated hypothyroidism?

A: The end stage of untreated hypothyroidism is **myxedema coma.** Progressive weakness, hypothermia, hypoventilation, stupor, hyponatremia, and cardiovascular failure characterize this disorder. Typically this does not occur with hypothyroidism alone; there is usually a precipitating event such as stroke, sepsis, or myocardial infarction.

The mortality rate is very high even with treatment. Laboratories demonstrate very low T_4 and T_3 levels with elevated TSH (primary) or decreased TSH (secondary). Treatment involves cardiovascular and pulmonary support plus large amounts of intravenous thyroid hormone (T_4 or T_3).

Q: What is the treatment of hypothyroidism?

A: The treatment of choice for hypothyroidism is synthetic L-thyroxine, which is inexpensive and may be taken only once daily due to its long half-life. Older preparations include desiccated thyroid, made from hog and beef thyroids. The latter are not recommended as they are less consistent from batch to batch than is synthetic thyroxine.

In a young, healthy adult with hypothyroidism, it is reasonable to start at a full replacement dose (e.g., 100 μg T_4 daily). Patients with mild hypothyroidism will require lower doses than those who have had total thyroid ablation (after surgery or radioiodine treatment). The latter individuals normally require at least 150–200 μg daily.

Caution must be taken with patients with severe heart disease, as moving from a hypothyroid to a euthyroid state may actually precipitate angina. Hypothyroidism may actually be protective against angina, as it slows the metabolism; in fact, radioiodine (^{131}I) was used long ago to produce hypothyroidism and ameliorate symptoms in angina patients. If the patient has severe coronary disease, it is recommended that this be corrected (via coronary artery bypass graft, angioplasty, or other treatment) before treating the hypothyroidism. If coronary disease persists, the patient should start at a low dose (e.g., 12.5–25 μg T_4 daily); the dose is increased every few weeks as symptoms permit. It may not be possible to restore all such patients to a euthyroid state.

Synthetic T_3 is also available, but it is not recommended for use except in certain circumstances, such as the quick withdrawal of thyroid hormone in thyroid cancer patients. It has a short half-life and must be given two or three times daily.

Q: How is the treatment monitored?

A: In primary hypothyroidism, the dose is titrated until the TSH normalizes. Because the half-life of

T_4 is long (1 week), the levels need not be checked for 6 weeks to 2 months after the dose is changed. In secondary or tertiary hypothyroidism, the TSH will always be low; therefore, a T_4 (free or total) level is monitored.

Q: What is the euthyroid sick syndrome?

A: The **euthyroid sick syndrome** is a common condition occurring in patients with acute or chronic illness. There appears to be an alteration with protein binding due to circulating inhibitors; this leads to decreased protein binding and hence a decreased amount of total T_4 and T_3 proportional to the free amount. These patients almost always have low T_3 levels and may have low T_4 levels in the face of normal TSH (since they are euthyroid). As it is merely an alteration of protein binding, the free hormone levels are normal.

T_4 is normally deiodinated to T_3; in the euthyroid sick syndrome, it is preferentially deiodinated to an isomer, **reverse T_3,** a biologically inactive compound (Fig. 3-7). Reverse T_3 (rT_3) levels may be elevated in this syndrome. These patients are euthyroid, so no treatment is necessary; attempting to treat the condition may actually be harmful.

Q: What is hyperthyroidism?

A: **Hyperthyroidism** is the opposite of hypothyroidism. It is the state in which too much thyroid hormone exists in the blood.

Q: What mechanisms cause hyperthyroidism?

A: Increased thyroid hormone levels may result from three mechanisms: thyroid hormone overproduction, leakage of preformed hormone from the thyroid, and ingestion of excess thyroid hormone.

Q: What are the clinical features of hyperthyroidism?

A: The clinical features of hyperthyroidism include weight loss, tachycardia, hyperphagia, nervousness, increased softness to skin, tremors, disordered mentation, exophthalmos (with Graves' disease only), thyroid "stare," diaphoresis, heat intolerance, and diarrhea.

Q: What are the causes of thyroid hormone overproduction?

A: The three common causes of thyroid hormone overproduction are diffuse toxic goiter (Graves' disease), toxic multinodular goiter, and toxic adenoma. Less common causes of overproduction include struma ovarii (functioning thyroid tissue in ovary), hyperfunctioning thyroid carcinoma, chorionic gonadotropin-secreting tumors (β-hCG has a similar structure to TSH), hydatidiform mole and choriocarcinoma, and hyperemesis gravidarum.

Q: What is Graves' disease?

A: **Graves' disease,** also called **diffuse toxic goiter,** is the most common cause of hyperthyroidism. It is an autoimmune disorder caused by antibody-mediated stimulation of the thyroid gland; thus, it is independent of TSH. Two primary antibodies are involved: **thyroid-stimulating immunoglobulin** (TSIg) and **thyrotropin-blocking antibody** (TRAb). It typically affects young women, 15 to 40 years of age, but may occur in any age group.

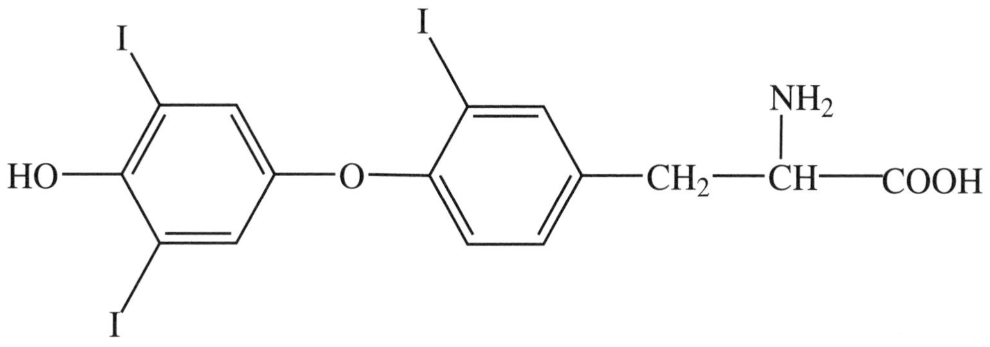

Figure 3-7. Reverse T_3.

The antibodies stimulate the thyroid gland but also may cause other problems, such as **exophthalmos,** the protrusion of eyes due to increased soft tissue infiltration behind the eye (Fig. 3-8).

Q: Do all patients with Graves' disease have exophthalmos?

A: No, exophthalmos is not a requirement for the diagnosis of Graves' disease.

Q: Is it possible to have exophthalmos without hyperthyroidism?

A: Yes, exophthalmos may occur in the absence of hyperthyroidism. Remember that Graves' orbitopathy is caused by the thyroid autoantibodies, not by elevated thyroid hormone levels. So it is possible to have exophthalmos and be euthyroid, hyperthyroid, or even hypothyroid. "Euthyroid Graves' disease" should be considered in patients who have the classic eye signs and normal thyroid studies.

Q: Does exophthalmos improve after treatment of hyperthyroidism?

A: Exophthalmos does not necessarily improve after the treatment of hyperthyroidism. This eye disease can worsen years later, because it is caused by autoantibodies. Thus, patients must have regular eye examinations for the rest of their lives, even if their thyroid disease is well controlled.

Q: Other than hyperthyroidism and exophthalmos, can anything else be caused by the antibodies?

A: The third component of the Graves' disease "clinical triad" is **pretibial myxedema** (PTM): shiny, erythematous to brown plaques, nodules, or non-pitting edema, most commonly affecting the pretibial area (Fig. 3-9). These signs may rarely occur in other body areas, such as the head, neck, pinnae, nose, or preradial area. The pebbly consistency is often described as *peau d'orange* (orange peel). It occurs in about 2% to 4% of patients with Graves' disease. Like exophthalmos, PTM may occur at any stage of Graves' disease, even 20 years after the treatment of hyperthyroidism.

Thyroid acropachy is the rarest manifestation of Graves' disease and results in soft tissue swelling of the extremities, and in clubbing of the digits. Bone histopathology will reveal new, subperiosteal bone formation. This manifestation is usually painless and typically occurs in patients with exophthalmos. Like exophthalmos, it does not necessarily parallel the course of thyroid disease.

Q: What are the differences between Graves' disease, toxic multinodular goiter, and toxic adenoma?

A: Graves' disease, toxic multinodular goiter, and toxic adenoma are all disorders in which thyroid hormone is overproduced. Graves' is an autoimmune disorder caused by antibodies that have TSH-like effects (Fig. 3-10). Toxic multinodular

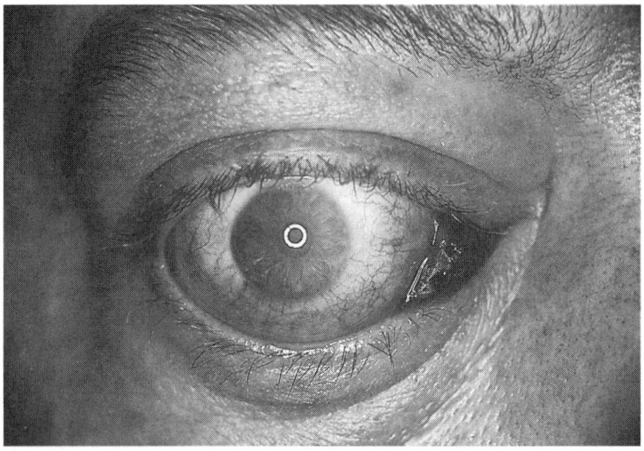

Figure 3-8. Exophthalmos.

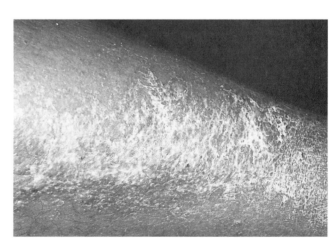

Figure 3-9. Pretibial myxedema.

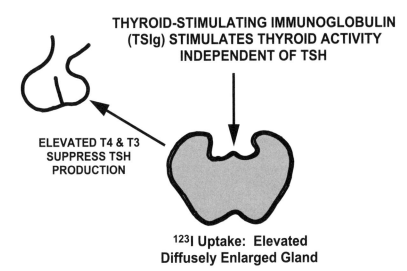

THYROID-STIMULATING IMMUNOGLOBULIN (TSIg) STIMULATES THYROID ACTIVITY INDEPENDENT OF TSH

ELEVATED T4 & T3 SUPPRESS TSH PRODUCTION

^{123}I Uptake: Elevated Diffusely Enlarged Gland

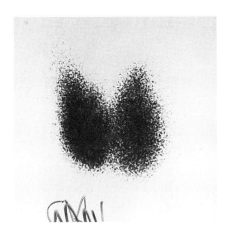

Figure 3-10. Graves' disease.

goiter (Fig. 3-11) and toxic adenoma (Fig. 3-12) are caused by overproduction of T_4 by one nodule (toxic adenoma) or by more than one (toxic multinodular goiter) in abnormal, autonomously functioning thyroid tissue. Exophthalmos and pretibial myxedema are autoimmune phenomena and thus are seen only in Graves' disease.

Q: What is the difference between primary and secondary hyperthyroidism?

A: **Primary hyperthyroidism** is TSH-independent—the thyroid itself secretes too much thyroid hormone, either from overproduction (e.g., Graves' disease), or leakage of preformed thyroid hormone (destructive thyroiditis). **Secondary hyperthyroidism** is very rare and may be caused by a TSH-secreting pituitary tumor. In this case, the thyroid works normally but is responding to an abnormal stimulus.

Q: What laboratory values would be expected in hyperthyroidism?

A: In primary hyperthyroidism, the peripheral hormones T_4 and T_3 are elevated. Usually both the total and free fractions are increased. In Graves' disease, the T_3 is often grossly elevated out of proportion to the T_4 elevation, because of the increased peripheral conversion of T_4 to T_3. The serum T_3 level is usually more useful to follow than T_4, as the former has a much shorter half-life and changes more rapidly in response to therapy. Because these processes are TSH-independent, we would expect feedback inhibition on the pituitary, resulting in decreased or undetectable TSH levels.

In secondary hyperthyroidism, the TSH level would be inappropriately high for the T_4 and T_3 levels. This type of hyperthyroidism is very rare,

**MULTIPLE AUTONOMOUS NODULES FUNCTION
INDEPENDENTLY OF TSH**

**REMAINDER OF GLAND
SUPPRESSED**

**ELEVATED T4 & T3
SUPPRESS TSH
PRODUCTION**

**^{123}I Uptake:
High Normal/High**

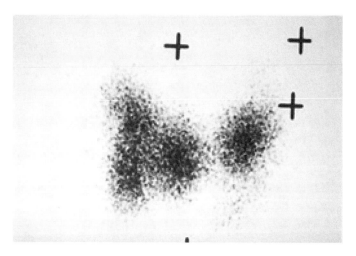

Figure 3-11. Toxic multinodular goiter.

however; for all practical purposes, hyperthyroid patients will have primary hyperthyroidism.

Q: Are there any other causes of secondary hyperthyroidism?

A: **Thyroid hormone resistance** is a rare condition in which either the peripheral cells, the pituitary, or both are resistant to the effects of thyroid hormone (Table 3-3). If the pituitary alone is resistant—pituitary resistance to thyroid hormone (PRTH)—it does not respond to the normal suppressive effect of thyroid hormone, leading to increased (inappropriate) TSH secretion and hyperthyroidism. If the peripheral cells are also resistant—generalized resistance to thyroid hor-

mone (GRTH)—this protects against hyperthyroidism as the increased T_4 and T_3 levels have less effect. GRTH is the most common thyroid hormone resistance syndrome. These patients are usually well compensated, either euthyroid or mildly hypothyroid. Peripheral tissue resistance to thyroid hormone alone (PTRTH) is least common. These patients present with normal T_4 and T_3 levels (due to peripheral resistance) and normal TSH levels (pituitary responsiveness is normal). (Since laboratory studies are usually normal it is often difficult to diagnose.) These patients are always hypothyroid.

Treatment of these disorders is difficult, as conventional parameters (e.g., TSH, T_4) do not accu-

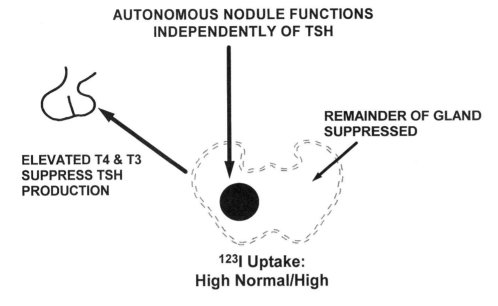

**AUTONOMOUS NODULE FUNCTIONS
INDEPENDENTLY OF TSH**

**REMAINDER OF GLAND
SUPPRESSED**

**ELEVATED T4 & T3
SUPPRESS TSH
PRODUCTION**

**¹²³I Uptake:
High Normal/High**

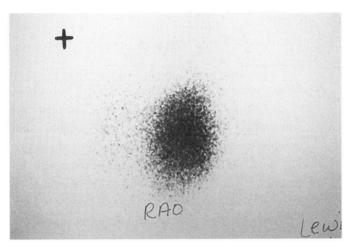

Figure 3-12. Toxic adenoma.

rately reflect hormone action. There are many target organ indices that can be followed to give an estimation of thyroid hormone action, including cholesterol, sex hormone-binding globulin (SHBG), and osteocalcin. Metabolic indices such as basal metabolic rate and heart rate may also be useful.

Q: How can thyroid hormone resistance be distinguished from TSH-secreting tumors?

A: Thyrotropinomas may be visible on MRI or computed tomography (CT) scans. Another way is to measure the alpha subunit (α-SU). The glycoprotein hormones—luteinizing hormone (LH), follicle-stimulating hormone (FSH), TSH, and β-hCG—all share a common alpha subunit, but different beta subunits. In thyroid hormone resistance, the molar ratio of α-SU to TSH is 1; the molar ratio of α-SU to TSH in TSH-secreting tumors is greater than 1.

Q: What is thyrotoxic periodic paralysis?

A: **Thyrotoxic periodic paralysis** (TPP) is a rare complication of hyperthyroidism, typically occurring in males of Asian descent, although it has been described in women and other ethnic groups. TPP is a secondary form of periodic paralysis; a primary, euthyroid, inherited form may also occur. TPP presents with symmetrical muscle weakness, paralysis, and cramping, usually with hypokalemia. There is no sensory deficit, and cognitive processes are usually normal. The

TABLE 3-3.   Thyroid Hormone Resistance Syndromes

SYNDROME	PRESENTATION	TSH	T_4,T_3
Generalized resistance to thyroid hormone (GRTH)	Euthyroid or hypothyroid	Normal, elevated	Elevated
Pituitary resistance to thyroid hormone (PRTH)	Hyperthyroid	Normal, elevated	Elevated
Peripheral tissue resistance to thyroid hormone (PTRTH)	Hypothyroid	Normal	Normal

paralysis typically affects proximal muscles most severely.

The hypokalemia is not due to a true potassium deficit but a transcellular shift of potassium. Thyroid hormone possibly causes increased permeability of skeletal muscle to electrolytes, with influx of potassium into cells. The attacks are often self-limited. If necessary, acute management of the episode includes administration of potassium chloride. After the patient is euthyroid, the condition typically resolves.

Q: How is Graves' disease treated?

A: As we cannot easily treat the cause (autoimmune) of Graves' disease, the treatment is to prevent the end organ (thyroid) from overproducing its product. The three treatments are antithyroid drugs (thionamides), radioactive iodine (^{131}I), and surgery.

Q: What are antithyroid drugs and how do they work?

A: The antithyroid drugs are in a class of compounds known as **thionamides** and are related to several naturally occurring compounds found in foods (such as cabbage). They act by decreasing the synthesis of new thyroid hormone; they are ineffective for T_4 that already has been formed. They do not directly treat the *cause* of Graves' disease (autoimmune), although immune-modifying effects and decreased antibody titers may be seen with therapy. Although they do not permanently cure Graves' disease, they are very effective in controlling hyperthyroidism and are the most rapid method for restoring hormone levels to normal.

The two drugs used in the United States are propylthiouracil (PTU) and methimazole, and both work in the same fashion. PTU also inhibits the peripheral conversion of T_4 to T_3, which is useful in severe hyperthyroidism.

Q: Are there any side effects to the antithyroid medications?

A: Most persons tolerate antithyroid medications well. The most common side effect is rash; less commonly, arthralgias, hepatitis, neuritis, and thrombocytopenia occur. These side effects usually occur in the first few months of treatment and usually resolve after discontinuing the medication. It is important to measure a baseline white cell count before starting thionamides as mild to moderate leukopenia can occur with hyperthyroidism alone.

The most feared side effect is **agranulocytosis** and occurs in 0.1% to 0.2% of individuals. It may manifest as a sudden development of fever or sore throat. It is therefore important to instruct patients to contact their physician if these problems develop so that a white cell count can be measured. The problem usually goes away if detected in time, but can be fatal if the patient continues the medication.

Because of these rare but potential side effects, antithyroid drugs are often not recommended for lifelong therapy. One approach is to give the medication for 6 months to 1 year then withdraw it; approximately 30% of patients will be in remission and remain euthyroid. The remainder will relapse. At this point another trial of antithyroid medication may be considered, or radioiodine or surgery may be elected. Patients who initially are in remission may relapse at a later date.

Q: Is there any method of predicting who will go into remission and who will not?

A: There is no definite way to predict which patients will go into remission. Patients with aggressive hyperthyroidism and large goiters generally have a lower remission rate. Patients with mild hyperthyroidism who can be controlled on small doses of antithyroid medication are better candidates for remission. Measurement of thyroid-stimulating immunoglobulin (TSIg) has some prognostic value, as high levels indicate a lower likelihood of remission. The only sure way to know if remission will occur is to discontinue the medication and check hormone levels afterward.

Q: How is radioiodine (^{131}I) given?

A: Radioiodine is given orally, in capsule or liquid form. Only the thyroid takes up significant amounts; the radiation dose to the rest of the body is minimal, similar to that from other diagnostic tests (e.g., barium enema, CT scan, etc.). The treatment is usually done in the radiology or nuclear medicine department of a hospital on an outpatient basis.

Q: How does ^{131}I therapy work?

A: Tissue destruction occurs with ^{131}I, primarily from β-particle emission. Although the actual radionuclide is gone in a few days, thyroid cell destruction continues for several weeks; gradually thyroid functions return to normal.

Q: What are the side effects of ^{131}I therapy?

A: The only significant side effect of ^{131}I therapy is hypothyroidism, which eventually occurs in most patients. This is treated with L-thyroxine, just like other forms of hypothyroidism. Rarely, radiation thyroiditis occurs, in which patients develop tenderness and swelling around the thyroid. This can usually be controlled by anti-inflammatory agents (e.g., ibuprofen), but steroids may be required. There is no increased incidence of malignancy in those receiving ^{131}I therapy. It has been used ex-

tensively since the late 1940s for the treatment of thyroid disease.

There is some evidence that radioiodine may worsen exophthalmos, possibly as a consequence of the increased thyroid antigen being released into the circulation after treatment. For this reason, it is a common practice to administer corticosteroids (e.g., prednisone) for several weeks after the treatment. This theoretically would diminish any autoimmune response and decrease the potential worsening of orbitopathy. Many endocrinologists do not use radioiodine in patients with severe, progressive eye disease.

Q: Can the newly diagnosed patient with Graves' disease proceed directly to ^{131}I therapy?

A: Most patients require pretreatment with antithyroid medication to reduce hormone levels to normal. Administering ^{131}I to a severely hyperthyroid patient can actually exacerbate the condition and rarely induce the end stage of hyperthyroidism, thyroid storm. Beta-blockade should be given to all patients undergoing ^{131}I therapy. Once hormone levels have been normalized with thionamide drugs, they must be discontinued for several days before the treatment is given, as they interfere with radioiodine uptake.

Q: What are the advantages and disadvantages of surgery?

A: Surgery has few advantages, and thus it is not recommended in most cases. If performed, total thyroidectomy is recommended. Subtotal thyroidectomy is not advised, as the thyroid has tremendous potential for growth and hyperthyroidism often recurs after this procedure. Surgery is the treatment with highest risk, as the Graves' thyroid gland is very large and hypervascular, making the surgery more difficult than removing a normal thyroid. Any major surgery would obviously be more risky than taking a medication. There is a very small risk of hypoparathyroidism due to parathyroid gland damage, which can be treated with expensive vitamin D analogs and requires lifelong blood testing. Rarely, left recurrent laryngeal nerve paralysis may occur.

Q: Would there be any patients in whom thyroidectomy would be the best choice?

A: If the thyroid needs to be removed for another reason (e.g., cancer), then thyroidectomy is the best choice, as there is little additional risk. If a severely hyperthyroid patient is pregnant and cannot take antithyroid medication, then surgery (in the second trimester) is indicated. [131]I is contraindicated in pregnancy because it crosses the placenta and can cause fetal hypothyroidism.

Q: Is any preparation required prior to surgery?

A: As with ^{131}I therapy, the patient should be rendered euthyroid with antithyroid medication prior to surgery. Supersaturated solution of potassium iodide (SSKI) inhibits thyroid hormone release (the Wolff-Chaikoff effect) and can be given if a patient needs to be prepared quickly.

Q: What problems can occur in patients with exophthalmos?

A: Fortunately, most exophthalmos patients do not have vision-threatening problems, although the proptosis can be a cosmetic problem. Proptosis can cause stress on the optic nerve, leading to visual loss. In early stages it may be difficult to detect, so regular eye examinations are always necessary. Corneal irritation may also occur if the eye does not close properly. Extraocular muscle involvement can cause diplopia, which is usually intermittent at first, but may become constant. These problems can permanently impair vision in severe cases, and must certainly be considered among the most serious complications of Graves' disease.

Q: What treatments are available for exophthalmos?

A: In mild cases of proptosis without optic nerve or extraocular muscle impairment, periodic examinations are necessary. In acute flare-ups of inflammatory orbitopathy, glucocorticoids (prednisone) may be useful, although they cannot be continued long term. Lubricants can be applied for corneal irritation.

With optic nerve involvement, the goal is to lessen the pressure on the optic nerve; this can be accomplished by orbital decompression (removing part of the eye socket posteriorly) or with external radiation to the orbits. Extraocular muscle impairment can be corrected with surgery. These latter treatments are all significant undertakings and most ophthalmologists specializing in this disorder follow eye disease conservatively until a significant problem occurs. In severe cases that do not respond to these therapies, plasmapheresis can actually remove the offending antibodies.

Q: How is the pregnant patient with Graves' disease managed?

A: In general, pregnancy has an ameliorating effect on autoimmune diseases, and the pregnant woman with Graves' disease may not require treatment. If the patient is biochemically euthyroid or only minimally hyperthyroid and is asymptomatic, simple follow-up is indicated. If the patient becomes significantly hyperthyroid and symptomatic, then antithyroid drugs are indicated. The goal is to control the patient's symptoms without inducing fetal hypothyroidism. PTU is typically preferred as it crosses the placenta less than methimazole; the latter is often avoided due to the rare incidence of congenital scalp lesions (aplasia cutis). If the woman develops side effects from antithyroid medications, thyroidectomy in the second trimester may be indicated.

Q: Do the mother's elevated thyroid levels affect the fetus?

A: The mother's elevated thyroid levels usually do not affect her fetus to a significant extent. T_4 and T_3 are highly protein bound, and this fraction cannot cross the placenta. The free hormones can cross, but this is such a small amount that it is often insignificant.

Thyroid-stimulating immunoglobulin (TSIg), however, readily crosses the placenta and can induce fetal thyrotoxicosis (fetal or neonatal Graves' disease), a rare condition occurring in 1% of mothers with Graves' disease. In addition to hyperthyroidism, the fetus can develop a large goiter, causing airway difficulties at birth. TSIg should be measured in all pregnant women with Graves' disease in the third trimester, as high levels may indicate the development of neonatal Graves' disease. Even those women who have been treated with radioiodine are at risk, because the antibodies may still be present.

Q: What problems can occur with neonatal Graves' disease?

A: Transient hyperthyroidism can occur in neonatal Graves' disease, lasting 1 to 3 months (due to the long 1-month half-life of TSIg). After this time, the antibodies disappear and recovery occurs. Tracheal obstruction can occur if the goiter is large. Other features can include jaundice, heart failure, tachycardia, hepatosplenomegaly, exophthalmos, hypertension, and thrombocytopenia. Antithyroid drugs may be given if needed.

Q: What is in the differential diagnosis of hyperthyroidism occurring during pregnancy?

A: Graves' disease is always the first consideration with hyperthyroidism during pregnancy. Another possibility is **hyperemesis gravidarum,** which has been associated with mild to moderate hyperthyroidism in pregnancy. The etiology is thought to be β-hCG stimulation of thyroid follicular cells (as β-hCG shares some structural homology with TSH). Subtle thyroid function abnormalities may be seen in up to 50% of patients with hyperemesis. The typical presentation is one of modest elevations of T_4 and T_3 levels with suppressed TSH. There is a positive correlation between the severity of the hyperemesis and the hyperthyroidism. The nausea and thyroid hormone levels tend to diminish by mid-gestation, with amelioration of symptoms.

Treatment is controversial. The main problem is distinguishing this disorder from Graves' disease. Hyperemesis-induced thyroid disease is self-limited and antithyroid therapy is usually not indicated. In selected patients in whom vomiting persists into the second half of gestation, thionamide therapy may be considered.

Other forms of hyperthyroidism, such as toxic adenoma, toxic multinodular goiter, thyroiditis, and thyrotoxicosis factitia may also occur rarely in pregnancy.

Q: What is the differential diagnosis of postpartum hyperthyroidism?

A: Previously undiagnosed Graves' disease must be considered. Autoimmune diseases typically improve during pregnancy and worsen after delivery, and this may cause an exacerbation. **Postpartum thyroiditis** is a type of destructive thyroiditis that occurs in approximately 5% of postpartum women. Hyperthyroidism is usually mild, followed by a hypothyroid phase that is usually transient, but may require therapy in extreme cases. It is self-limited and can be distinguished from Graves' disease by the decreased radioiodine uptake. Other types mentioned above may rarely occur.

Q: What are the clinical features of toxic adenoma?

A: **Toxic adenoma** (Plummer's disease) is an autonomously functioning thyroid nodule not responsive to TSH and not antibody-mediated (see Fig. 3-12). Typically it produces milder hyperthyroidism than Graves' disease and occurs in older patients. The clinical progression is slow over many years. Few patients spontaneously go into remission.

Q: What treatments are available for toxic adenoma?

A: As with other forms of hyperthyroidism, β-blockers are often given for symptomatic control. For correction of the condition, radioiodine (^{131}I) and surgery are the treatments of choice.

^{131}I is generally preferred for older patients who are poor surgical risks, given its ease of administration and lack of side effects. A disadvantage is that ^{131}I can damage the normal thyroid, producing permanent hypothyroidism. Fortunately, this side effect is not common (< 20%), and is easily treated with L-thyroxine if it occurs. ^{131}I treatment has a higher failure rate with toxic adenoma than it does with Graves' disease.

Surgery removes the abnormal tissue while preserving the surrounding thyroid, which should return to normal function. Because surgery practically guarantees a cure without the risk of hypothyroidism, it is often the treatment of choice in younger adults.

Percutaneous ethanol administration is being performed in some centers and appears promising.

The ethanol destroys the hyperfunctioning thyroid tissue while leaving surrounding thyroid tissue intact. It is not in widespread use at this time.

Q: What are the treatments for toxic multinodular goiter?

A: The treatment options for **toxic multinodular goiter** (MNG) (see Fig. 3-11) are similar to those for toxic adenoma. Radioiodine may be less effective due to the larger area of functioning thyroid tissue. Unlike surgery for toxic adenoma which removes only the hyperfunctioning area, surgery for toxic MNG often involves a total thyroidectomy. Thus, after toxic MNG surgery, most patients develop permanent hypothyroidism.

Q: Can antithyroid drugs be used in the treatment of toxic adenoma and toxic MNG?

A: Antithyroid drugs do work, as they decrease thyroid hormone formation; however, with toxic adenoma and MNG they require higher doses than with Graves' disease. These agents are often used short term to prepare patients for surgery and/or radioiodine, but they have no place in the long-term treatment of these disorders. The natural course of these diseases is to progress, and antithyroid drugs do not change their course (this is in contrast to Graves' disease, where some patients will go into remission).

Q: What is destructive thyroiditis?

A: **Destructive thyroiditis** is an inflammation of the thyroid that may cause hyperthyroidism by release of preformed hormone, not by autonomous overproduction of hormone (Fig. 3-13). The thyroid serves as a large storage reservoir for thyroid hormone. If an inflammatory process "punches holes in the tank," the hormone will leak out, causing increased hormone levels (hyperthyroidism). Thyroid hormone production ceases as the TSH decreases in response to the hyperthyroidism. And, because hormone formation is decreased, radioiodine uptake is decreased also—one way of distinguishing destructive thyroiditis from states of hormone overproduction (Graves' disease, toxic adenoma, toxic MNG).

Q: What are the types of destructive thyroiditis?

A: **Subacute thyroiditis** is characterized by painful, tender enlargement of the thyroid. This may follow a viral illness. Hyperthyroidism occurs due to release of preformed hormone. Examination demonstrates an extremely tender thyroid gland and signs of hyperthyroidism. **Silent thyroiditis** is similar except that the thyroid is not painful. **Postpartum thyroiditis** is common (5% of patients) after pregnancy. Patients with Hashimoto's thyroiditis occasionally go through a period of inflammatory hormone release ("Hashitoxicosis").

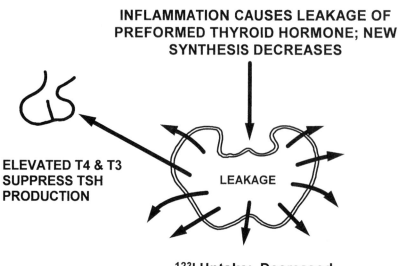

INFLAMMATION CAUSES LEAKAGE OF PREFORMED THYROID HORMONE; NEW SYNTHESIS DECREASES

ELEVATED T4 & T3 SUPPRESS TSH PRODUCTION

LEAKAGE

^{123}I Uptake: Decreased
Thyroglobulin: Increased

Figure 3-13. Destructive thyroiditis.

Q: How can hyperthyroidism occur with decreased radioiodine uptake?

A: Uptake only measures the amount of radioiodine that is trapped and/or organified into thyroid hormone. In destructive thyroiditis, hyperthyroidism is due to the release of preformed hormone, which is unaffected by synthesis of new hormone.

Q: Are there any other forms of hyperthyroidism in which the radioiodine uptake is decreased?

A: In exogenous ingestion of thyroid hormone—**thyrotoxicosis factitia**—the excess thyroid hormone will suppress TSH secretion and hence decrease radioiodine uptake. Iatrogenic hyperthyroidism may also occur if the patient is prescribed too much thyroid hormone; this is usually obvious.

Q: How can I differentiate between destructive thyroiditis and thyrotoxicosis factitia?

A: A history of painful thyroid enlargement with elevated sedimentation rate suggests subacute thyroiditis. The presentation of postpartum thyroiditis is typically straightforward also. When the patient is not being honest, silent thyroiditis may be difficult to distinguish from thyrotoxicosis factitia. Because destructive thyroiditis is due to spillage of thyroid follicular cell contents, the serum thyroglobulin (Tg) is typically elevated; thyroglobulin would be suppressed after ingesting excess thyroid hormone. Table 3-4 illustrates the differential diagnosis of hyperthyroidism.

Q: What is the treatment of destructive thyroiditis?

A: Usually destructive thyroiditis is self-limited, and the hyperthyroidism abates after thyroid hormone stores have been depleted. Beta blockade is indicated for patients with symptoms (tremors, tachycardia, etc.). Patients with pain may require anti-inflammatory agents (e.g., ibuprofen). A short course of corticosteroids may be indicated in some cases. Rarely, the inflammation may be so severe that thyroidectomy is required.

Q: What is the clinical course of destructive thyroiditis?

A: Hyperthyroidism persists until thyroid hormone stores are depleted (usually a few weeks). Then the patient becomes euthyroid and later hypothyroid for a brief period until the TSH elevates and thyroid hormone stores regenerate. Typically the hypothyroidism is mild and self-limited; occasional symptomatic patients may require a brief course of thyroxine therapy. Rarely, the hypothyroidism may be permanent. Compare this to the clinical course of Graves' disease, in which the hyperthyroidism continues to worsen (Fig. 3-14).

Q: What is "apathetic" hyperthyroidism?

A: **"Apathetic" hyperthyroidism** occurs commonly in elderly patients who have a blunted peripheral response to thyroid hormone. Paradoxically, they may be quite hyperthyroid with minimal symptoms, and may even present with depression. Thus, it is important to recognize the possibility of hyperthyroidism in depressed or demented patients.

TABLE 3-4.   Differential Diagnosis of Hyperthyroidism

DISORDER	T$_4$	T$_3$	TSH	RADIOIODINE UPTAKE	THYROGLOBULIN
Graves' disease	↑↑	↑↑↑	↓	↑↑	N/A
Toxic adenoma/toxic multinodular goiter	↑	↑	↓	↑	N/A
Destructive thyroiditis	↑	↑	↓	↓	↑
Thyrotoxicosis factitia	↑	↑	↓	↓	↓
TSH-secreting tumor	↑	↑	↑	↑	N/A

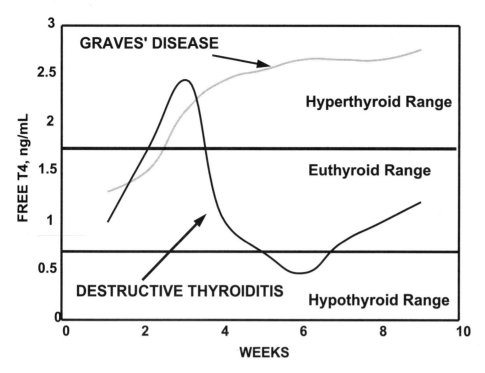

Figure 3-14. T$_4$ levels in destructive thyroiditis and Graves' disease.

Q: What about patients with a low TSH, normal peripheral hormone levels, and no clinical symptoms?

A: A low TSH accompanied by normal peripheral hormone levels and no clinical symptoms indicates **subclinical hyperthyroidism.** The condition may be endogenous (due to Graves' disease, toxic adenoma, etc.) or exogenous (due to excess thyroid hormone).

Q: Should subclinical hyperthyroidism be treated?

A: As exogenous subclinical hyperthyroidism is a well-recognized risk factor for osteoporosis, the dosage of thyroid replacement should be decreased. Treatment of endogenous subclinical hyperthyroidism is not as straightforward. Unlike subclinical hypothyroidism, in which the treatment is fairly benign (small doses of thyroxine), the treatments for endogenous hyperthyroidism have a much greater risk of side effects: thionamides—rash and/or agranulocytosis; radioiodine—permanent hypothyroidism; surgery—hypoparathyroidism or hypothyroidism. In the asymptomatic patient with subclinical hyperthyroidism, watchful waiting may be the best approach. Bone density measurements should be considered to screen for osteopenia.

Q: What is the most severe clinical outcome in a patient with hyperthyroidism?

A: The end stage of untreated hyperthyroidism is **thyrotoxic crisis** or **thyroid storm,** which has a high mortality if untreated. Signs of thyroid storm may include fever, delirium, nausea, vomiting, diarrhea, cardiac arrhythmia, congestive heart failure, and cardiovascular collapse. Often the patient has not sought medical attention because of a fear that he or she has a terminal illness such as cancer.

Q: What are the causes of thyroid storm?

A: Most patients have diffuse toxic goiter (Graves' disease). Other autonomous types of hyperthyroidism (toxic adenoma or multinodular goiter) or destructive thyroiditis rarely cause hormone levels high enough to result in thyroid crisis. Only seldom is thyroid storm caused by factitious ingestion of thyroid hormone, although it may be seen in those who have consumed extremely large amounts (e.g., suicide attempts).

Q: What is the treatment of thyroid storm?

A: Thionamides are the first course of treatment. PTU is preferred over methimazole because of its added effect of inhibiting T$_4$ to T$_3$ conversion. A typical dose is 1200 mg/day (e.g., 200 mg every 4 hours). Although this treatment rapidly decreases the synthesis of new hormone, it has no effect on hormone that is already made (other than decreasing T_4 to T_3 conversion). Inorganic iodide (SSKI) will decrease hormone release and is recommended after starting PTU. Beta blockers are also recommended (e.g., propranolol, orally or intravenously). Glucocorticoids also decrease peripheral T_4 to T_3 conversion and may be helpful. Patients typically require cardiac monitoring in a critical care setting.

Q: What is the perchlorate discharge test?

A: The **perchlorate discharge test** is designed to determine if an organification defect is present. Iodine is first trapped, and then organified. Persons with organification defects have normal trapping but deficient organification. Uptake studies alone cannot distinguish the two processes. If the radioiodine is organified, it is "permanently" inside the thyroid to be incorporated into thyroid hormone. If it is simply trapped and not organified, then it can be "washed out" if another competing substance is given to the patient.

This process is best illustrated by the perchlorate discharge test. Monovalent anions such as perchlorate (ClO_4^-) and pertechnetate (TcO_4^-) are trapped, but not organified by the thyroid. If perchlorate is given to a normal individual (without an organification defect) after radioiodine administration, the uptake will not decrease, because the iodine has already been organified. If the patient has an organification defect, the perchlorate will flush out the trapped (but not organified) radioiodine, resulting in a decrease in uptake from the baseline of at least 20% at 2 hours.

The perchlorate discharge test is occasionally used to evaluate persons suspected of having **Pendred's syndrome,** an inherited disorder presenting with organification defects, goiter, and nerve deafness. Those with this syndrome will have a positive perchlorate discharge test.

Q: What is a thyroid nodule and how does it differ from a "goiter"?

A: **Goiter** is a nonspecific term for any enlargement of the thyroid, so a thyroid nodule is simply a type of goiter. A goiter may be diffuse (Graves' disease, Hashimoto's thyroiditis, "colloid" goiter) or nodular. A **nodule** is a discrete area that is clearly different from the surrounding thyroid tissue. It is usually palpable but may only be seen on ultrasound.

Q: Are most nodules benign or malignant? What are the risk factors for malignancy?

A: Most thyroid nodules are benign. The factors distinguishing benign from malignant nodules are shown in Table 3-5.

Q: What is the difference between a "cold," "warm," and "hot" nodule?

A: "Cold," "warm," and "hot" are terms that relate to the nodule's appearance on radionuclide thyroid scan (Fig. 3.15).

Q: If a nodule is cold, does that mean it is probably malignant?

A: No, most cold nodules are benign (80% to 85%). A cold nodule is more likely to be malignant than is a hot nodule, but the likelihood of malignancy is still low.

Q: Are hot nodules always benign?

A: Hot nodules are usually, but not always, benign. The incidence of malignancy is far less than in cold nodules. Any suspicious, rapidly enlarging lesion should be biopsied.

Q: What is the role of the thyroid scan in evaluating thyroid nodules?

A: A thyroid scan serves little purpose in the euthyroid patient, as benign and malignant thyroid disease cannot reliably be distinguished. Thus, a scan is not recommended as a first-line diagnostic tool. It is useful in the hyperthyroid patient to determine if the hyperthyroidism is due to a toxic nodule or another cause.

Q: Are any other imaging modalities available for evaluating thyroid nodules?

A: Ultrasound is noninvasive and defines anatomy much better than a nuclear scan. Nodules that are cystic in appearance are much less likely to be malignant than those that are solid; however, like

TABLE 3-5.   Differential Diagnosis of Thyroid Nodules

	BENIGN	MALIGNANT
History	Family history of benign goiter	Recent growth of nodule
	Presence for many years	Cough, hoarseness
	Older female	History of neck irradiation
		Young female, male, child
Examination	Multiple nodules	Solitary nodule
	Soft nodule	Firm, hard nodule
		Lymphadenopathy
Thyroid Scan	Hot nodule	Cold nodule*
Fine-Needle Aspiration	Benign	Suspicious/malignant

*a cold nodule increases likelihood for malignancy, but most cold nodules are benign.

thyroid scans, they cannot reliably distinguish benign from malignant lesions.

Q: **What is the best method of distinguishing benign from malignant thyroid nodules?**

A: The procedure of choice for evaluating nodules is fine-needle aspiration (FNA) biopsy. It is minimally invasive, carries minimal risk, and is very accurate (false-negative rate approximately 5%). A skilled pathologist is required to determine the sample adequacy and interpret the results. Many experts recommend a second biopsy to increase predictive value, as there is a small but measurable false-negative rate.

Q: **How are benign thyroid nodules managed?**

A: Suppression with thyroxine has been the traditional therapy for benign nodules; recent investi-

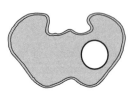

'COLD' NODULE: does not accumulate radioiodine. Photopenic area on scan. 15-20% likelihood of malignancy.

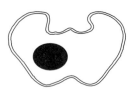

'HOT' NODULE: accumulates radioiodine to greater extent than rest of gland. May be seen in hyperthyroidism. Remainder of gland may be suppressed. Less likely to be malignant than 'cold' nodule.

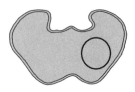

'WARM' NODULE: nodule accumulates radioiodine to same extent as rest of gland.

Figure 3-15.   Thyroid nodules on radionuclide scan.

gations have questioned its efficacy, as many nodules do not respond to therapy. Some will regress somewhat, so T_4 suppression is benign if monitored properly and may be offered to the patient. Inorganic iodide has been used with limited success. If medical therapy is chosen, the patient must understand that complete regression of nodules only rarely occurs. These therapies are now controversial.

If the goiter becomes large enough to obstruct the airway or is a serious cosmetic problem, surgical removal is necessary. Occasionally, benign goiters can grow into the **mediastinum**—mediastinal or substernal goiter. These can cause severe esophageal and tracheal compromise, and often require surgical intervention.

Q: Can radioiodine be used to treat euthyroid nodular goiters?

A: Radioiodine is not routinely used to treat euthyroid nodular goiters. Radioiodine does not rapidly destroy thyroid tissue, so is not useful in someone with airway compromise.

Q: What are the types of thyroid carcinoma?

A: The most common types of thyroid carcinoma are the **thyroid epithelial cell carcinomas,** papillary and follicular. The neuroendocrine medullary thyroid carcinoma is third most common, followed by anaplastic thyroid carcinoma.

Q: What is papillary thyroid carcinoma?

A: **Papillary thyroid carcinoma** is the most common type of thyroid cancer (75%), and the one with the best prognosis. It usually presents as a large, firm, solitary, cold nodule or as the "dominant nodule" in a multinodular goiter. Ten percent of patients present with enlargement of cervical lymph nodes. Pathologically, single layers of thyroid cells with stalk-like papillary projections are seen. Metastases usually occur via local lymph node invasion; they are very slow-growing tumors, and take years to extend beyond the thyroid and local lymph nodes. Death from papillary carcinoma is rare and usually results from local disease (neck tissue invasion). Pulmonary metastases do occasionally occur, but skeletal metastases are uncommon.

Q: How is papillary thyroid cancer treated?

A: The cornerstone of therapy for papillary thyroid cancer is surgical resection. For tumors larger than 1.5 cm, a total thyroidectomy is recommended, except in persons who are poor surgical candidates or who have limited life expectancy from another cause. The prognosis is excellent in patients with localized disease. Those with small "occult" tumors usually only receive a lobectomy and are not treated with radioiodine.

Q: What is the role of radioiodine therapy in papillary thyroid cancer?

A: The primary role of radioiodine is in survey scans to detect metastatic disease, because the papillary tumors concentrate the radioiodine. However, normal thyroid tissue has a far greater affinity for radioiodine than does cancerous tissue, so if even small amounts of normal thyroid tissue are present, a survey scan will be useless. After surgery, small fragments of normal thyroid tissue (remnants) normally remain, but these can be destroyed by a high dose of ^{131}I (higher than in the hyperthyroid patient). This type of high-dose ^{131}I therapy is called **remnant ablation** and is typically done several weeks after surgery to facilitate later ^{131}I scanning. Rarely, residual tissue will not be detected and remnant ablation will not be needed.

The second role of radioiodine therapy is to treat metastatic disease. Six months to one year after remnant ablation, another survey scan is done. If metastatic disease is seen, another high-dose therapy is given. If the results are negative, repeat surveys are done periodically (1 to 5 years).

Q: Are any useful tumor markers available for following these patients?

A: Papillary tumors make no distinctive hormones; because they originate from follicular epithelium, they do make thyroglobulin (Tg), like normal thyroid tissue. Once the normal thyroid tissue has been destroyed by surgery and ^{131}I, serum Tg is a useful marker of tumor burden. Low Tg (< 5 ng/mL) values indicate a good prognosis.

Q: How is a patient prepared for a thyroid cancer survey?

A: The tumor has a relatively low affinity for radioiodine, so the only way to achieve satisfactory uptake is to scan while the TSH is significantly elevated (> 30 μU/mL). The traditional method of achieving a satisfactory TSH elevation is to withdraw the patient from his or her thyroid replacement and induce moderately severe hypothyroidism. The patient normally must be off thyroxine for 4 to 6 weeks. T_3 may be taken up to 2 weeks before the scan; it has a much shorter half-life than T_4 and is rapidly cleared. Thus, patients often feel very poorly at the time of the survey. Synthetic human TSH is now available and obviates the need to induce hypothyroidism in these patients, as TSH is increased artificially. It is given intramuscularly for 2 or 3 days prior to the scan.

Q: How is a high-dose radioiodine treatment performed?

A: A high-dose radioiodine treatment is similar to a hyperthyroidism treatment, except for the higher dose. In the past, U.S. federal regulations required that patients remain in the hospital until their radioactivity levels fell below a certain level. Changes in regulations now allow most of these treatments to be done in an outpatient setting. To avoid radiation contamination, the patient must avoid close contact with others for several days and practice meticulous hygiene.

Q: What is follicular thyroid carcinoma?

A: **Follicular thyroid carcinoma** is a more aggressive form of epithelial thyroid carcinoma, and accounts for 15% to 17% of cases. Follicles of malignant cells form, instead of the papillary projections seen in papillary carcinoma; in some cases, it may be difficult to distinguish the two. The follicular type is more aggressive and may spread by local invasion, lymph node invasion, or hematologic spread. Bone and pulmonary metastases are more common than in papillary carcinoma (Fig. 3-16). Both epithelial tumors rarely are hyperfunctioning and can produce hyperthyroidism (Fig. 3-17).

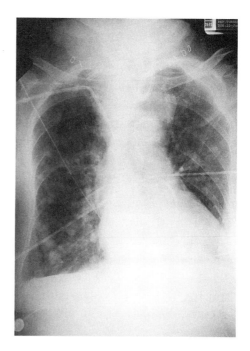

Figure 3-16. Pulmonary metastases in patient with papillary carcinoma.

Q: How is follicular carcinoma treated?

A: The treatment for follicular carcinoma is similar to papillary carcinoma. Surgery is the initial therapy,

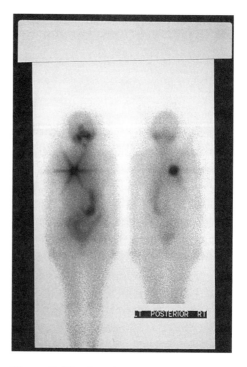

Figure 3-17. Radioiodine scan of patient with pulmonary metastases.

followed by ^{131}I remnant ablation and the treatment of metastases, if present.

Q: Is external radiation therapy used in these types of thyroid cancer?

A: External radiation therapy is not typically used, as ^{131}I is superior at delivering the radiation dose. It may be used in very poorly differentiated tumors that do not concentrate radioiodine.

Q: What is medullary thyroid carcinoma?

A: **Medullary thyroid carcinoma** (MTC) is the third most common type (5%) of thyroid carcinoma. It is a neuroendocrine tumor consisting of sheets of parafollicular (C) cells, which may secrete large amounts of calcitonin. It is more aggressive than epithelial (papillary or follicular) cancer and extends locally to lymph nodes and surrounding structures. Death usually occurs from local invasion. Hypercalcitoninemia may lead to symptoms such as diarrhea or flushing; this may respond to octreotide treatment.

Q: How does the treatment for MTC differ from papillary and follicular cancer treatments?

A: The primary treatment for all these cancers is surgical resection. However, MTC does not concentrate radioiodine, so ^{131}I therapy is typically not useful. External radiotherapy plays a greater role than in the other cancers. Chemotherapy has had limited success. Patients with severe hypercalcitoninemia may have vasomotor side effects (flushing and diarrhea), and treatment with octreotide may be helpful.

Q: Can MTC be inherited?

A: Yes, medullary thyroid carcinoma can be inherited. Although most cases are sporadic, MTC can occur as a familial trait, either by itself or in association with multiple endocrine neoplasia (MEN) IIa and IIb. The familial variety has been linked to chromosome 10, and genetic testing (*ret* proto-oncogene) is available. Genetic testing has largely replaced the pentagastrin-calcium stimulation test that traditionally was required in family members of persons with MTC.

Q: As radioiodine scanning is not useful, how can small metastases be detected?

A: MTC often produces large amounts of calcitonin, and occasionally carcinoembryonic antigen (CEA). Baseline calcitonin levels are usually elevated, but may be normal with small tumors. If basal calcitonin is normal, stimulation with pentagastrin and/or calcium will cause a rise in calcitonin levels if functioning tumor is present.

Q: What precautions should be taken in the patient with MTC before going to surgery?

A: Prior to surgery, the most important step with MTC patients is to exclude pheochromocytoma, which is part of MEN IIa and IIb. This can be done with a 24-hour urinary collection for vanillylmandelic acid (VMA), metanephrines, or catecholamines. Other endocrine disorders associated with MEN IIa/IIb (e.g., hyperparathyroidism) are usually not life threatening.

Q: What is anaplastic thyroid carcinoma?

A: **Anaplastic thyroid carcinoma** is an extremely aggressive and undifferentiated type of thyroid cancer. It presents with rapid development of dysphagia, obstruction, and vocal cord paralysis. There is no effective treatment, and all patients die, usually within months.

BIBLIOGRAPHY

Clark OH. Papillary thyroid carcinoma: rationale for total thyroidectomy. In: Clark OH, Duh QY, eds. Textbook of endocrine surgery. Philadelphia: W.B. Saunders, 1997:90–94.

DeGroot LJ. Thyroid physiology and hypothyroidism. In: Besser GM, Thorner MO, eds. Clinical endocrinology. 2nd ed. St. Louis: Mosby-Wolfe, 1994:15.2–15.15.

Hay ID. Papillary thyroid carcinoma. In: Sheaves R, Jenkins PJ, Wass JAH, eds. Clinical endocrine oncology. Cambridge, MA: Blackwell Science, 1997: 117–121.

Mazzaferri EL, de los Santos ET, Rofagha-Keyhani S.

Solitary thyroid nodule: diagnosis and management. Med Clin North Am 1988;72:1177–1211.

Ridgeway EC. Clinical review 30: clinician's evaluation of a solitary thyroid nodule. J Clin Endocrinol Metab 1992;74:231–235.

Silverberg J, Gharib H. Evaluation and diagnosis of nodular thyroid disease. In: Mazzaferri EL, ed. Endocrine tumors. Cambridge, MA: Blackwell Science, 1994:233–240.

Smith TJ. Localized myxedema and thyroid acropachy. In: Braverman LE, Utiger RD, eds. Werner and Ingbar's the thyroid: a fundamental and clinical text. 6th ed. Philadelphia: Lippincott, 1991:676–680.

REVIEW QUESTIONS

I. SHORT ANSWER

1. The principal secretory product of the thyroid is the hormone _____, with _____ secreted in lesser amounts.

2. The major active thyroid hormone is _____, which is mainly supplied by _____.

3. The trophic hormone for the thyroid is _____, made in the _____. The trophic hormone for this organ is _____.

4. Iodine is transported into the thyroid follicular cell against a gradient by a process called _____. It is transformed into an "activated" form by _____ and then is incorporated onto residues of the amino acid _____ by a process called _____.

5. Thyroid hormone is formed on a protein called _____ in the colloid. The synthesis and release of thyroid hormone is facilitated by the pituitary hormone _____.

6. The principal carrier protein of thyroid hormone is _____. Others include _____ and _____.

7. Name three conditions that can cause increased T_4 levels due to abnormal or increased proteins.

8. Name three conditions that can cause decreased T_4 levels due to abnormal proteins or decreased proteins.

9. An older test used to indirectly quantify the amount of thyroid-binding proteins is called the _____. The product of this value and the serum T_4 is called the _____.

10. The fractional accumulation of a radionuclide into the thyroid after a set time (e.g., 24 hours) is called an _____. The two-dimensional image printed onto x-ray film is called a _____. This test is usually done with the radionuclide _____.

11. A particle-emitting radionuclide with a long half-life used to destroy thyroid tissue is _____. It is typically used in the treatment of _____ and _____.

12. The most common cause of hypothyroidism in the United States is _____.

13. Infants with untreated hypothyroidism may develop _____, with mental retardation and short stature. The most common cause is _____.

14. The most sensitive test in diagnosing hypothyroidism is _____.

15. An 82-year-old woman is brought into the hospital in a coma. She apparently ran out of thyroxine several weeks ago and did not refill it. She is hypothermic (92° F) and has congestive heart failure. Serum T_4 is undetectable, and TSH is elevated. This woman has a complication of hypothyroidism called _____.

16. An 85-year-old chronically ill nursing home resident is brought in for congestive heart failure. Her serum thyroid function studies are as follows:

    Total T_4: 3.1 µg/dL (normal: 4.5–12.0)

    Total T_3: 45 ng/dL (normal: 70–180)

    TSH: 2.23 µU/mL (normal: 0.32–5.00)

    She most likely has _____. In this disorder, T_4 is preferentially deiodinated to _____ instead of T_3.

17. A woman is found to have a mildly elevated TSH on routine laboratory screening. She has no complaints. T_4 level is normal. She is said to have _____.

18. Name three fundamental mechanisms by which hyperthyroidism can occur.

19. The most common cause of thyroid hormone overproduction is _____. The three methods of treating this disorder include _____, _____, and _____. In addition to hyperthyroidism and goiter, a common associated clinical finding is _____.

20. Medications used to blunt the adrenergic symptoms of hyperthyroidism are _____.

21. Two other common forms of hyperthyroidism caused by autonomously functioning abnormal foci of thyroid tissue include _____ and _____. These disorders are treated by _____ and _____. They are somewhat resistant to therapy with _____.

22. Pebbly "orange peel" lesions that occur on the shins of 3% to 4% of patients with Graves' disease are called _____. A rare manifestation resulting in clubbing of the digits is called _____.

23. The major side effect of ^{131}I therapy for hyperthyroidism is _____.

24. A treatment for hyperthyroidism that should never be used in the pregnant patient is _____.

25. Destructive thyroiditis causes hyperthyroidism by _____. A type occurring with pain in the thyroid is called _____. A variant in which there is no pain in the thyroid is called _____. A similar condition that may occur after a pregnancy is called _____.

26. In destructive thyroiditis, the patient is initially _____, then typically becomes _____, and eventually _____. Usually he or she becomes _____ again in a few months.

27. Destructive thyroiditis can be distinguished from Graves' disease with a _____. The value should be _____ in the former and _____ in the latter.

28. A condition caused by surreptitious ingestion of excess thyroid hormone is called _____. It can be distinguished from destructive thyroiditis by measuring serum _____. Levels should be _____ in destructive thyroiditis.

29. An asymptomatic patient with normal T_4 and T_3 levels but with a suppressed TSH is said to have _____.

30. A patient with severe hyperthyroidism, fever, delirium, and tachyarrhythmia is said to have _____.

31. A nonspecific term for any type of thyroid enlargement is _____. This may be either _____ or _____.

32. The best single test for evaluating a thyroid nodule in the euthyroid patient is _____.

33. A test that gives some functional information about a thyroid nodule but which cannot differentiate benign from malignant lesions is _____.

34. A noninvasive test that uses no radiation and gives useful anatomic information about the thyroid is _____.

35. The types of differentiated thyroid epithelial cancers are _____ and _____.

36. A neuroendocrine type of thyroid cancer arising from the parafollicular or C cells is _____. A useful serum tumor marker for this type of cancer is _____.

37. The cornerstone of therapy in thyroid cancer is _____.

38. In epithelial thyroid cancers, microscopic amounts of remaining thyroid tissue are destroyed by _____ in a process called _____.

39. Metastatic epithelial thyroid cancers are treated with _____.

II. MULTIPLE CHOICE

Select the one best answer.

40. A 17-year-old male illicitly uses anabolic steroids to gain strength for football. If he is euthyroid, which one of the following sets of laboratory data might you expect?
    a. normal T_4, T_3, T_3 resin uptake, and TSH
    b. decreased T_4, T_3, and T_3 resin uptake; normal TSH
    c. decreased T_4 and T_3; increased T_3 resin uptake; normal TSH

    d. elevated T_4 and T_3 resin uptake; decreased T_3; increased TSH
    e. decreased T_4 and T_3; increased T_3 resin uptake; elevated TSH

41. The type of thyroid carcinoma with the poorest prognosis is:
    a. follicular
    b. anaplastic
    c. papillary
    d. medullary

42. Risks of thionamide drugs include all but which one of the following?
    a. hepatitis
    b. skin rash
    c. arthralgias
    d. leukocytosis
    e. hypothyroidism

43. The syndrome of silent or painless thyroiditis can best be distinguished from Graves' disease by the finding of:
    a. thyroid enlargement
    b. low radioactive iodine uptake
    c. elevated serum thyroxine levels
    d. low serum TSH levels
    e. low serum triiodothyronine (T_3) levels

44. A 37-year-old woman complains of fatigue, and has a small diffuse goiter on examination. A thyroid uptake/scan is ordered. It shows homogenous uptake with 24-hour value of 47% (normal: 15% to 35%). The diagnosis is:
    a. Graves' disease
    b. toxic adenoma
    c. Hashimoto's thyroiditis
    d. subacute thyroiditis
    e. insufficient information to make a diagnosis

45. A 23-year-old woman complains of heat intolerance, tachycardia, and tremors. She has lost 20 pounds in the last month. Examination reveals a greatly enlarged thyroid gland with bruit, and bilateral exophthalmos. Serum T_4 is 25.6 µg/dL (normal: 4.5–12.0); TSH is undetectable ($<$ 0.03

μU/mL). What further test is needed to establish the diagnosis?

   a. thyroid uptake and scan

   b. thyroid ultrasound

   c. serum thyroid-stimulating antibody (TSIg)

   d. serum triiodothyronine level

   e. no further tests needed to establish the diagnosis

46. A 67-year-old male is admitted to the hospital for myocardial infarction. He complains of fatigue, cold intolerance, and peripheral edema. Serum TSH is elevated at 21.23 μU/mL (normal: 0.32–5.00).

   A. This man has:

     a. euthyroid sick syndrome

     b. TSH-secreting pituitary tumor

     c. primary hypothyroidism

     d. secondary hypothyroidism

     e. toxic multinodular goiter

   B. The best treatment option at this time would be:

     a. start levothyroxine now

     b. start triiodothyronine now

     c. wait until he is stable from a cardiac standpoint, and start T_4 at low doses

     d. treat with radioactive iodine

     e. treat with lithium

47. A 40-year-old man is noted to have a thyroid mass. It is biopsied and findings are consistent with medullary thyroid carcinoma. You tell the patient that another test needs to be done in order to do surgery safely. Which test would this be?

   a. serum insulin level

   b. 24-hour urine for creatinine clearance

   c. 24-hour urine for fractionated catecholamines

   d. serum calcium level

   e. serum TSH

48. Which of the following patients has the highest risk of having or developing a thyroid carcinoma?

   a. 56-year-old female with a diffuse goiter and hypothyroidism

   b. 23-year-old female with goiter, exophthalmos, 20-lb weight loss, resting tremors, palpitations

   c. 56-year-old male with multiple thyroid nodules which have not increased in size over 7 years

   d. 34-year-old male with solitary thyroid nodule and "hot" uptake on radionuclide scan

   e. 22-year-old female with solitary thyroid nodule and "cold" uptake on radionuclide scan

49. A 77-year-old woman complains of fatigue and depression. She is not nearly as active as she was 3 months ago and has lost 10 pounds. A small diffuse goiter is palpable. Laboratory studies demonstrate:

Serum thyroxine: 13.5 μg/dL (normal: 4.5–12.5)

Serum triiodothyronine: 250 ng/dL (normal: 80–200)

Serum TSH: 0.05 μU/mL (normal: 0.25–6.70)

This woman has:

   a. primary hypothyroidism

   b. euthyroid sick syndrome

   c. hypopituitarism

   d. "apathetic" hyperthyroidism

   e. familial dysalbuminemic hyperthyroxinemia

50. A 23-year-old woman who works as a nurses' aide complains of a 2-month history of weight loss, palpitations and tremors, and heat intolerance. Examination reveals a thin woman with absence of goiter or exophthalmos. There is a resting tremor and heart rate is 112. Laboratory studies demonstrate

Serum T_4: 19.7 μg/dL (normal: 4.5–12.0)

T_3 resin uptake: 29% (normal: 22% to 34%)

Serum TSH 0.03 μU/mL (normal: 0.25–5.00)

Radionuclide thyroid scan: 2% uptake at 24 hours (normal: 20% to 35%)

Serum thyroglobulin: 0.4 ng/mL (normal: 2.7–21.9)

This woman likely has:

    a. hypothyroidism

    b. Graves' disease

    c. thyrotoxicosis factitia

    d. silent thyroiditis

    e. euthyroid state with altered TBG binding

51. Correct *acute* management of thyrotoxic crisis might include all but which one of the following?

    a. potassium iodide

    b. radioiodine (^{131}I)

    c. cardiac monitoring

    d. propylthiouracil

    e. propranolol

52. The most common cause of congenital hypothyroidism is:

    a. thyroid dysgenesis

    b. panhypopituitarism

    c. maternal drug use

    d. inherited organification defect

    e. defective thyroglobulin molecule

53. A 30-year-old male takes methimazole for Graves' disease. He calls you on Friday afternoon and complains of a fever (102° F) and sore throat. You saw him in the office 2 weeks ago and his white cell count was normal. You should instruct him to:

    a. continue the methimazole, as he probably just has a viral illness.

    b. stop the methimazole and obtain a white cell count today.

    c. come into the office Monday to get a white cell count.

    d. start on antibiotics; if he still has a fever tomorrow, you will stop the methimazole.

    e. stop methimazole and start propylthiouracil.

54. A 23-year-old woman is 3-weeks postpartum and notices increased nervousness and tachycardia. She has a small goiter but no exophthalmos. Serum T_3 is elevated at 242 ng/dL (normal: 70–180) and TSH is undetectable (< 0.03 μU/mL). Thyroid studies before pregnancy were normal. Radioiodine uptake is 3% at 24 hours (normal: 20% to 38%).

A. This woman most likely has:

    a. Graves' disease

    b. toxic adenoma

    c. thyrotoxicosis factitia

    d. thyroid carcinoma

    e. postpartum thyroiditis

B. Two months from now, she complains of fatigue and dry skin. You would expect which set of thyroid function studies?

    a. high T_3, high T_4, low TSH

    b. high T_3 resin uptake, normal T_4, normal TSH

    c. low T_4, high TSH

    d. low T_4, low TSH

    e. high T_4, high TSH

55. A 42-year-old male presents for a routine examination, and a thyroid profile is measured. Total T_4 is high at 16.2 μg/dL, TSH is normal at 1.12 μU/mL (normal: 0.32–5.00), and free T_4 is normal at 1.2 ng/dL (normal: 0.8-2.0). His examination is normal and he has no complaints. This man likely has:

    a. Graves' disease

    b. euthyroid sick syndrome

    c. hypothyroidism

    d. familial dysalbuminemic hyperthyroxinemia

    e. low serum proteins from illicit androgen use

56. A newborn infant whose mother has Graves' disease has a goiter, exophthalmos, and tachycardia after birth. This problem was caused by:

    a. maternal T_4 and T_3 crossing the placenta

    b. maternal thyroid-stimulating immunoglobulin (TSIg)

    c. fetal thyroid-stimulating immunoglobulin (TSIg)

    d. maternal antimicrosomal (antithyroid peroxidase) antibody

    e. maternal use of propylthiouracil (PTU)

57. The best treatment for primary hypothyroidism is:
    a. synthetic levothyroxine
    b. sheep thyroglobulin
    c. beef/hog thyroid extract
    d. synthetic triiodothyronine
    e. levothyroxine and triiodothyronine

58. Which of the following is true of the thyroid lesion depicted in Figure 3-18?
    a. It is probably malignant.
    b. It concentrates radioiodine as well as the surrounding tissue.
    c. Fine-needle aspiration (FNA) biopsy should be considered.
    d. Suppressive therapy with thyroxine is likely to make it disappear.
    e. It must be removed surgically.

59. A 32-year-old woman received radioiodine therapy 6 weeks ago for hyperthyroidism. She feels very cold and tired and complains of peripheral edema. Deep tendon reflexes are slowed on examination. Laboratory studies demonstrate:

    Total T_4: 1.0 µg/dL (normal: 4.5–12.0)

    Total T_3: 23.9 ng/dL (normal: 75–175)

    TSH: 0.12 µU/mL (normal: 0.32–5.00)

    The next step in treatment would be:

    a. treat again with radioiodine, as she has failed the initial treatment.

    b. send her to a surgeon for thyroidectomy.
    c. start methimazole.
    d. start levothyroxine.
    e. repeat the laboratory studies in 1 month.

60. A 51-year-old woman presents to your office with weight loss, tachycardia, and tremors. Examination reveals a very small thyroid gland and no exophthalmos or pretibial myxedema. She has been taking an unknown medication for weight loss that she obtained from a friend. Thyroid function studies are as follows:

    Serum T_4: < 1.0 µg/dL (normal: 5.0–12.0)

    Serum TSH: < 0.03 µU/mL (normal: 0.32–5.00)

    Radioiodine uptake: < 1% at 24 hours

    This person probably has:

    a. secondary hypothyroidism due to a pituitary tumor
    b. subacute thyroiditis
    c. hyperthyroidism due to triiodothyronine ingestion
    d. tertiary hypothyroidism due to a hypothalamic tumor
    e. pituitary resistance to thyroid hormone

61. A 23-year-old woman with congenital nerve deafness is seen for fatigue and goiter. TSH is elevated at 24.57 µU/mL (normal: 0.32–5.00). Radioiodine uptake increases from 20% to 28% 2 hours after the administration of potassium perchlorate. This woman most likely has:
    a. Hashimoto's thyroiditis
    b. Pendred's syndrome
    c. hypopituitarism
    d. a TSH-secreting tumor
    e. generalized resistance to thyroid hormone

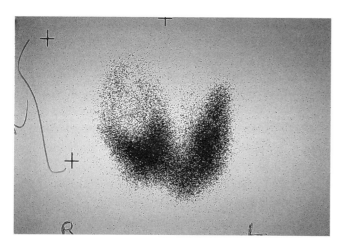

Figure 3-18. Thyroid scan of patient in question 58.

III. TRUE OR FALSE

Answer true or false to each question.

62. Causes of hyperthyroidism resulting in *decreased* radioiodine uptake include:
    ___ a. diffuse toxic goiter (Graves' disease)
    ___ b. postpartum thyroiditis
    ___ c. subacute thyroiditis
    ___ d. toxic multinodular goiter
    ___ e. thyrotoxicosis factitia

63. In thyroid hormone metabolism:
    ___ a. thyroglobulin is the major carrier of thyroid hormones in serum
    ___ b. T_4 is deiodinated to reverse T_3, the active hormone
    ___ c. over 99% of T_4 is protein bound
    ___ d. increased trapping with deficient organification may occur in hypothyroidism due to Hashimoto's thyroiditis, resulting in increased radioiodine uptake
    ___ e. estrogens result in increased thyroid-binding proteins and decreased T_3 resin uptake

64. Regarding Graves' disease:
    ___ a. most patients have pretibial myxedema
    ___ b. antithyroid drugs may have toxic side effects, such as agranulocytosis
    ___ c. all patients have hyperthyroidism
    ___ d. exophthalmos may not improve after treatment of thyroid disease
    ___ e. maternal antibodies may produce neonatal Graves' disease

65. Appropriate treatment of hyperthyroidism caused by subacute thyroiditis may include:
    ___ a. radioactive iodine
    ___ b. anti-inflammatory agents (e.g., ibuprofen)
    ___ c. corticosteroids
    ___ d. β-adrenergic blocking agents
    ___ e. propylthiouracil

66. A 38-year-old woman complains of weight loss, tachycardia, and nervousness. Thyroid function studies done 5 years ago were normal. On examination, she has a diffuse goiter but no exophthalmos. Laboratory studies demonstrate:

    Serum free T_4: 3.5 ng/dL (normal: 0.9–2.0)

    Serum total T_3: 420 ng/dL (normal: 80–180)

    Serum TSH: 12.32 μU/mL (normal: 0.32–5.00)

    A 5-mm pituitary tumor is seen on MRI scan.

    Correct statements about this condition include:
    ___ a. it is probably caused by pituitary resistance to thyroid hormone.
    ___ b. the molar ratio of alpha subunit (α-SU) to TSH is 1.0.
    ___ c. it will likely respond to octreotide therapy.
    ___ d. propylthiouracil will restore T_4 and T_3 levels to normal.
    ___ e. radioiodine is the preferred mode of therapy.

ANSWERS

1. T$_4$ (thyroxine), T$_3$ (triiodothyronine)

2. T$_3$, peripheral deiodination of T$_4$

3. TSH, anterior pituitary; TRH

4. trapping; oxidation, tyrosine, organification

5. thyroglobulin; TSH

6. thyroid-binding globulin (TBG); albumin, thyroxine-binding prealbumin (transthyretin)

7. List three: estrogen therapy, pregnancy, congenital protein abnormalities, acute liver disease, hypothyroidism

8. List three: congenital protein abnormalities, androgen therapy, glucocorticoids, protein malnutrition, nephrotic syndrome, hyperthyroidism

9. T$_3$ resin uptake; free thyroxine index (FT$_4$I)

10. uptake; scan; ^{123}I

11. ^{131}I; hyperthyroidism, thyroid carcinoma

12. Hashimoto's thyroiditis

13. cretinism; thyroid agenesis

14. serum TSH

15. myxedema coma

16. euthyroid sick syndrome; reverse T$_3$ (rT$_3$)

17. subclinical hypothyroidism

18. overproduction by thyroid, spillage of preformed hormone, ingestion of exogenous hormone

19. diffuse toxic goiter (Graves' disease); antithyroid medications (thionamides), radioactive iodine (^{131}I), surgery; exophthalmos

20. β-blockers

21. toxic adenoma, toxic multinodular goiter; surgery, ^{131}I; thionamide drugs

22. pretibial myxedema; thyroid acropachy

23. hypothyroidism

24. radioactive iodine

25. release of preformed thyroid hormone; subacute thyroiditis; painless thyroiditis; postpartum thyroiditis

26. hyperthyroid, euthyroid, hypothyroid; euthyroid

27. radioiodine uptake; low, high

28. thyrotoxicosis factitia; thyroglobulin (Tg); increased

29. subclinical hyperthyroidism

30. thyroid storm or crisis

31. goiter; nodular, diffuse

32. fine-needle aspiration (FNA) biopsy

33. thyroid scan

34. ultrasound

35. papillary, follicular

36. medullary thyroid carcinoma (MTC); calcitonin

37. surgical removal

38. ^{131}I, remnant ablation

39. radioactive iodine (^{131}I)

40. (c). Androgen therapy results in decreased thyroid-binding proteins, with decrease of T$_3$ and T$_4$ levels. The T$_3$ resin uptake is increased, as it is inversely proportional to the amount of binding proteins. TSH is normal since he is euthyroid.

41. (b). Most patients with anaplastic carcinoma die within a few weeks. Medullary is the next most aggressive, followed by follicular and papillary carcinomas.

42. (d). Agranulocytosis, not leukocytosis, is a possible complication. Arthralgias, hepatitis, and skin rash occasionally occur. Hypothyroidism can occur if the dosage is too high.

43. (b). Radioiodine uptake is low in destructive thyroiditis, but high in Graves' disease. T$_4$ levels are high and TSH low in both, if hyperthyroid. Both may present with thyroid enlargement. Neither would have low T$_3$ levels.

44. (e). Thyroid function studies are necessary to make a diagnosis of hyperthyroidism. Radioiodine uptake is a useful adjunct to diagnosis, but cannot be used by itself to establish the diagnosis. Patients with elevated uptake may be euthyroid, hypothyroid, or hyperthyroid. Persons with hypothyroidism caused by Hashimoto's thyroiditis often have enzyme organifica-

tion defects with increased trapping (and radioiodine uptake) but inefficient thyroid hormone synthesis.

45. (e). The clinical presentation of hyperthyroidism, exophthalmos, and diffuse goiter establish a diagnosis of diffuse toxic goiter (Graves' disease). A thyroid uptake/scan is not necessary to confirm it, and would be a waste of money in this case. Thyroid ultrasound would likely confirm a diffuse goiter, but is unnecessary. TSIg and T_3 levels would likely be abnormal but again do not aid in the diagnosis.

46. A. (c). The elevated TSH and clinical symptoms establish a diagnosis of primary hypothyroidism. B. (c). Treatment of hypothyroidism should never be started in a patient with unstable coronary artery disease. Only after the condition has stabilized can replacement be considered. Radioiodine is only indicated for certain types of hyperthyroidism and not for hypothyroidism.

47. (c). Pheochromocytoma should be excluded in all persons with medullary thyroid carcinoma, as both can occur with multiple endocrine neoplasia (MEN) IIa and IIb. Serum calcium may be elevated (hyperparathyroidism), but is not life threatening. Insulinoma (a) is seen in MEN I, not IIa and IIb.

48. (e). Solitary "cold" nodules are more likely to be malignant than are "warm" or "hot" nodules, even though most cold nodules (80% to 85%) are benign. Multinodular goiters are generally less likely to be malignant. Patients with diffuse goiters are not at high risk to develop thyroid cancers. Patients with Hashimoto's thyroiditis rarely can develop thyroid lymphoma. Any suspicious lesion should be biopsied, regardless of its appearance on thyroid scan.

49. (d). Hyperthyroidism often presents with blunted, paradoxical symptoms in the elderly, hence the name "apathetic" hyperthyroidism. Primary hypothyroidism (a) would present with low T_4 and high TSH levels. Euthyroid sick syndrome (b) does not present with high T_4 levels. Patients with hypopituitarism (c) have low TSH and peripheral hormone levels. Persons with familial dysalbuminemic hyper-

thyroxinemia (FDH) are euthyroid and hence have normal TSH levels.

50. (c). The combination of hyperthyroidism, low radioiodine uptake, and low Tg level establish the diagnosis of thyrotoxicosis factitia, which is often seen in health care workers with access to thyroid medication. Tg level should be elevated in destructive thyroiditis. She is not hypothyroid or euthyroid, given the decreased TSH. Radioiodine uptake would be elevated in Graves' disease.

51. (b). Radioiodine should never be given to a severely hyperthyroid patient, as it will induce further spillage of thyroid hormone and worsen the situation—fatalities have been reported. ^{131}I might be considered after a euthyroid state has been achieved. The other choices are appropriate for management.

52. (a). Thyroid dysgenesis is relatively common (1:4000) and is the most common cause of congenital hypothyroidism. Maternal drug-induced hypothyroidism (such as PTU) is uncommon. Congenital organification defects are rare, as are hypopituitarism and thyroglobulin defects. Treatment is lifelong thyroxine replacement.

53. (b). Agranulocytosis is the most feared complication of antithyroid drug therapy and must be investigated in the patient with fever. The white cell count being normal 2 weeks ago is irrelevant, as this problem can present spontaneously. The medication must be stopped *immediately* and a white cell count be checked as soon as possible. It likely is not agranulocytosis, but it must be excluded.

54. A. (e). This is a typical presentation of postpartum thyroiditis. Graves' disease and toxic adenoma would not present with suppressed radioiodine uptake. Thyrotoxicosis factitia cannot be completely ruled out, but is less likely. Hyperfunctioning thyroid cancer is rare. B. (c). She has developed hypothyroidism, which typically follows the hyperthyroid phase of destructive thyroiditis. It usually is self-limited and normalizes after a few months.

55. (d). This man likely has familial dysalbuminemic hyperthyroxinemia (FDH), a benign

disorder in which an abnormal protein has a very high affinity for T_4, leading to high total T_4 levels. He is euthyroid, as free T_4 and TSH are normal.

56. (b). Neonatal Graves' disease is caused by passage of maternal TSIg. The condition is self-limited and abates after the antibody is cleared (about 1 month). Treatment of the neonate with antithyroid medication may be necessary.

57. (a). Synthetic levothyroxine is the treatment of choice. Preparations made from animal thyroids are not recommended as the bioavailability may not be as consistent from batch to batch. As T_3 is made from deiodination of T_4, there is no need to give it orally. T_3 is generally not preferred, given its very short half-life. Its short half-life is exploited in certain circumstances, as with withdrawal of a thyroid cancer patient from thyroid hormone.

58. (c). This is a "cold nodule" and fine-needle aspiration should be done to exclude malignancy. Most cold nodules are benign, not malignant. Removal is not necessary if the biopsy is negative. Suppressive therapy with thyroxine may achieve a small (25%) degree of regression, but the nodule will not disappear. Often there is no change with suppressive therapy.

59. (d). This woman is clinically hypothyroid as a result of ^{131}I therapy, and thyroid hormone replacement should be started. After therapy of hyperthyroidism, the peripheral hormone levels fall much faster than the TSH rises; it is common to see normal or low peripheral (T_4 and T_3) levels with low TSH levels. Left untreated, the TSH will eventually rise to normal and then become elevated. In hyperthyroidism, TSH alone is an inaccurate parameter to follow when monitoring or initiating drug therapy.

60. (c). This woman is clinically hyperthyroid, and has a suppressed TSH. The absence of detectable T_4 suggests that T_3 (triiodothyronine) is the hormone producing the thyrotoxicosis. T_3 is occasionally used (illicitly) for weight loss. T_4 levels are suppressed in this condition due to lack of endogenous formation. Secondary (a) or tertiary (d) hypothyroidism is not consistent with the clinical presentation. Subacute thy-

roiditis (b) is due to leakage of preformed thyroid hormone, so T_4 levels would not be low. Pituitary resistance to thyroid hormone (e) would present with hyperthyroidism but normal or elevated TSH levels.

61. (a). This woman most likely just has Hashimoto's thyroiditis. In Pendred's syndrome (b), the perchlorate test should show discharge of radioiodine and decreased uptake, not increased uptake; the test is therefore negative. Hypopituitarism (c) is ruled out by the high TSH. TSH-secreting tumors and thyroid hormone resistance are extremely rare.

62. True (b, c, e); False (a, d). Postpartum thyroiditis (b) and subacute thyroiditis (c) result in release of preformed thyroid hormone and suppression of radioiodine uptake. Exogenous thyroid hormone (e) has the same effect. If thyroid tissue is stimulated by antibodies (Graves' disease), or is abnormal tissue that functions autonomously without normal feedback inhibition (toxic nodular goiter, toxic adenoma), uptake is increased.

63. True (c, d, e); False (a, b). Thyroid hormones are carried by *thyroid-binding globulin*, not *thyroglobulin* (a). T_4 is primarily deiodinated to T_3, not reverse T_3 (b). Increased radioiodine uptake is common in Hashimoto's thyroiditis (d), despite the presence of hypothyroidism.

64. True (b, d, e); False (a, c). Pretibial myxedema (a) is uncommon. Although most patients have hyperthyroidism (c), it is not a requirement for diagnosis (e.g., "euthyroid" Graves' disease). The clinical course of exophthalmos may be typically different from that of the thyroid disease (e).

65. True (b, c, d); False (a, e). Hyperthyroidism in destructive thyroiditis results in release of formed thyroid hormone. Neither radioiodine (a) nor antithyroid drugs (e) have any effect on thyroid hormone that has already been made. Treatment is aimed at decreasing inflammation with anti-inflammatory agents (b), or with steroids in severe cases (c). Beta-blockade (d) may ameliorate hyperthyroid symptoms.

66. True (c, d); False (a, b, e). This woman likely

has a TSH-secreting pituitary adenoma. This condition is traditionally treated with surgery but also will respond to octreotide therapy (*c*), since somatostatin is a natural inhibitor of TSH. PTU (*d*), although it does not treat the pituitary tumor, will decrease peripheral hormone levels to normal. Neither it nor radioiodine (*e*) is the preferred method of therapy. Hormone levels five years ago were normal, excluding an inherited defect (*a*). In TSH-secreting pituitary tumors, the molar ratio of α-SU to TSH is usually greater than 1.0 (*b*).

CHAPTER 4

ADRENAL GLAND AND ENDOCRINE HYPERTENSION

Q: Where are the adrenal glands?

A: The paired adrenal glands lie in the retroperitoneal cavity above the kidneys. The combined adult weight of these glands is about 10 grams; 90% of the weight is the outer *cortex*, and the remaining 10% is the inner *medulla*.

Q: What is the purpose of the adrenal glands?

A: The outer **cortex** is the site of synthesis for life-sustaining steroids (glucocorticoids and mineralocorticoids). Androgens also are synthesized here, which compliment those made by the gonads. The inner **medulla** is the site of catecholamine synthesis. Although they are not necessary for life, catecholamines are responsible for augmenting many physiological processes.

Q: What are the layers of the adrenal cortex?

A: The adrenal cortex has three layers (Fig. 4-1). The outermost layer, the **zona glomerulosa,** produces mineralocorticoids (primarily aldosterone). The thickest is the middle layer, the **zona fasciculata,** involved in glucocorticoid synthesis. The innermost cortical layer, the **zona reticularis,** synthesizes adrenal sex steroids (primarily androgens), and also glucocorticoids to a small extent.

Q: What are glucocorticoids?

A: Glucocorticoids are steroids and therefore interact with a nuclear receptor rather than a second messenger. **Glucocorticoids** or **corticosteroids** are potent hormones that inhibit DNA and RNA synthesis and accelerate protein catabolism in peripheral tissues. The name "glucocorticoid" is derived from their ability to increase glucose concentrations via increased gluconeogenesis and decreased peripheral glucose uptake. Glucocorticoids in normal amounts are necessary for life, but excess leads to numerous deleterious effects (Table 4-1).

Q: How are steroids synthesized?

A: Steroids are synthesized in the adrenal cortex from cholesterol (Fig. 4-2). Most of the steroidogenic enzymes are part of the cytochrome P450 oxy-

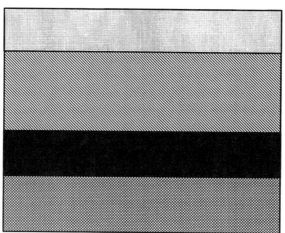

OUTER

ZONA GLOMERULOSA
Mineralocorticoids

ZONA FASCICULATA
Glucocorticoids

ZONA RETICULARIS
Sex steroids

MEDULLA
Catecholamines

INNER

Figure 4-1.   Layers of the adrenal gland.

genase enzymes. The zona glomerulosa and inner layers (zonae fasciculata and reticularis) function as two separate units, and contain different enzymes. For example, the inner layers lack the enzymes necessary to convert 11-deoxycorticosterone to aldosterone, and the glomerulosa lacks the 17α-hydroxylase activity necessary for synthesis of cortisol and sex steroids.

The inner layers depend on ACTH for normal steroid secretion. The glomerulosa, while stimulated by ACTH, does not require it for viability; it is controlled primarily by the **renin-angiotensin system** (RAS).

Steroids are made of four rings (A, B, C, and D), numbered sequentially; there are 17 carbon atoms in all. Additional carbon groups are numbered 18 to 21. Each has a "common" name (e.g., aldosterone, estradiol), and an official chemical name. Steroids are also denoted by the groups attached to the steroid nucleus; for example, progesterone has a methyl group at C_{21} and is thus called a C_{21} steroid (Fig. 4-3). Androstenedione has a ketone group at C_{17} and is thus a 17-ketosteroid.

Q: What is the major glucocorticoid?

A: **Cortisol** (hydrocortisone), a 17-hydroxysteroid, is the major glucocorticoid (Fig. 4-4). Like other steroids, it circulates highly bound to a carrier protein; the one for cortisol is **corticosteroid-binding globulin** (CBG, transcortin), which binds 95% of the total hormone. It is necessary for life.

TABLE 4-1.   Effects of Glucocorticoid Excess in Humans

BONE	INHIBIT FORMATION, INCREASE BONE-RESORBING CELLS
Connective tissue	Collagen loss, fibroblast inhibition
Liver	Increased gluconeogenesis, lipolysis; decreased glucose uptake in periphery
Adipose tissue	Lipolysis, release of free fatty acids
Cardiovascular	Increase cardiac output, vascular tone, augment responsiveness of adrenergic receptors
Calcium metabolism	Decrease calcium balance; increased vitamin D synthesis; calciuria
Brain	Alteration of behavior and cognitive function
Immunologic	Decreased inflammation

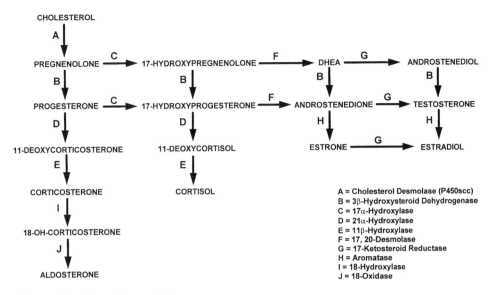

Figure 4-2. Steroid biosynthesis.

Q: What are the trophic and inhibitory hormones for the zona fasciculata?

A: The trophic hormones for the zona fasciculata are adrenocorticotrophic hormone (ACTH, corticotropin), secreted by the corticotrophs of the anterior pituitary gland, and corticotropin-releasing hormone (CRH), secreted by the hypothalamus (Fig. 4-5). ACTH infusion results in a rapid increase in cortisol levels within minutes. It is secreted in a diurnal rhythm (levels highest in morning, lowest in evening). Without ACTH, the zona reticularis atrophies and cortisol secretion diminishes. There is no specific inhibitory hormone.

Increased glucocorticoids (cortisol or synthetic derivatives) suppress ACTH secretion.

Q: What physiological processes increase cortisol secretion?

A: Glucocorticoids are "stress" hormones, their purpose being to increase fuel availability (glucose and other products of catabolism). Therefore, stressors such as illness, surgery, fever, pain or fear increase cortisol secretion.

Q: What is Cushing's syndrome?

A: **Cushing's syndrome** (CS) is a state of chronic glucocorticoid excess. It may either be *endogenous*—a result of the body's own overproduction

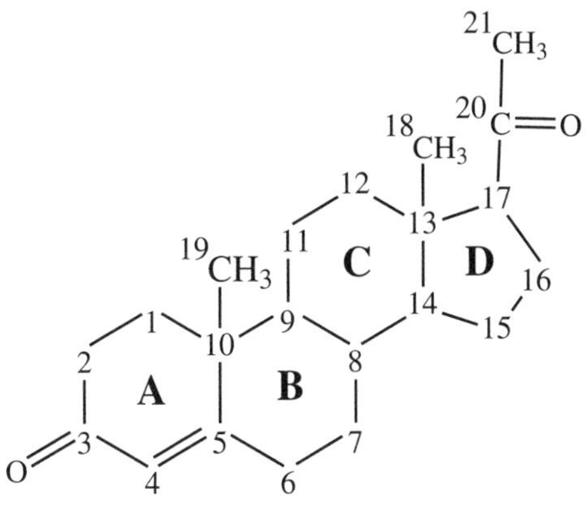

Progesterone (4-Pregnene-3,20-dione), a C_{21} steroid

Figure 4-3. Steroid nomenclature.

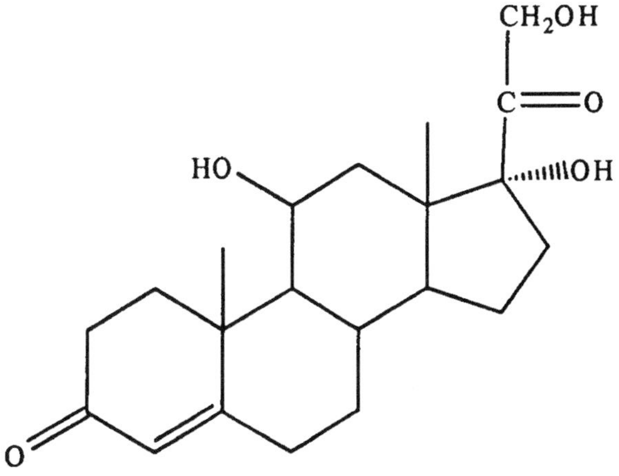

Figure 4-4. Cortisol.

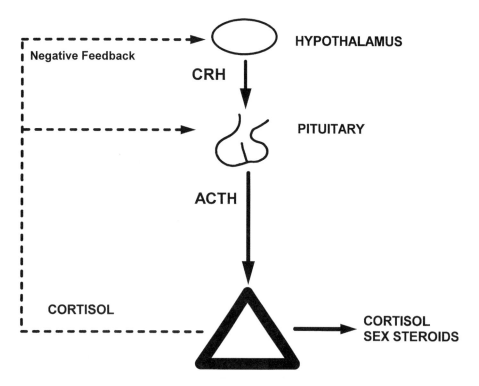

Figure 4-5. Normal adrenal function.

of cortisol, or *exogenous*—the result of excess glucocorticoid ingestion.

Q: What are the causes of endogenous Cushing's syndrome?

A: Endogenous CS may be grouped into ACTH-dependent and ACTH-independent causes:

ACTH-dependent
- Cushing's disease—ACTH-secreting pituitary tumor (Fig. 4-6)
- Ectopic ACTH syndrome: ACTH-secreting peripheral tumors (Fig. 4-7), CRH-secreting tumors (rare)

ACTH-independent:
- glucocorticoid-secreting adrenal tumors (adenomas or carcinomas) (Fig. 4-8)

Q: What is the most common cause of Cushing's syndrome?

A: By far the most common cause of CS is iatrogenic, due to the chronic use of glucocorticoids (as in pulmonary or rheumatologic disease). The most common causes of endogenous CS are Cushing's disease (65%), ectopic ACTH syndrome (20%),

adrenocortical adenoma (10%), and adrenocortical carcinoma (5%).

Q: What are the clinical features of Cushing's syndrome?

A: The clinical features of CS are the symptoms related to the chronic glucocorticoid excess: obesity, facial plethora, hirsutism, menstrual irregularity, hypertension, muscle weakness, osteoporosis, and pigmented abdominal striae (Fig. 4-9).

Q: Why do women with Cushing's syndrome often have hirsutism?

A: In the ACTH-dependent forms, ACTH excess also stimulates adrenal androgen secretion, resulting in increased levels. Corticosteroid-secreting tumors often secrete other steroids, such as androgens.

Q: How is the patient screened for Cushing's syndrome?

A: There are two typical screening tests for CS: the overnight or "standard" dexamethasone suppression test (DST) and the 24-hour urinary free cortisol. Note that a random cortisol measurement is

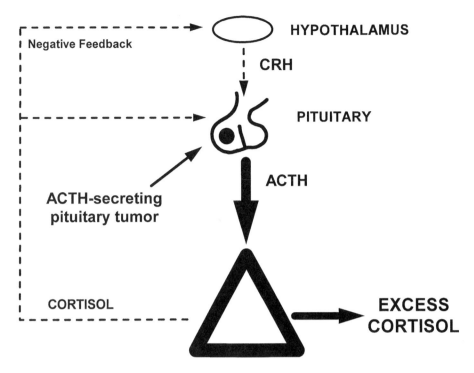

Figure 4-6. Cushing's disease.

not useful in screening, as a baseline level may be elevated in normal individuals.

Q: How is the overnight dexamethasone suppression test performed?

A: For the **overnight dexamethasone suppression test,** 1 mg dexamethasone is given at 11 PM and a serum cortisol is drawn the next morning. A normal response is suppression to less than 5 μg/dL. False positives can occur in patients with obesity, depression, and alcohol abuse, and in those taking certain medications (anticonvulsants). It is standard practice to obtain a serum dexamethasone level to make sure that it is in the acceptable range. If the dexamethasone level is low, the test is invalid, as the patient may not have taken it, or may be a rapid metabolizer of dexamethasone.

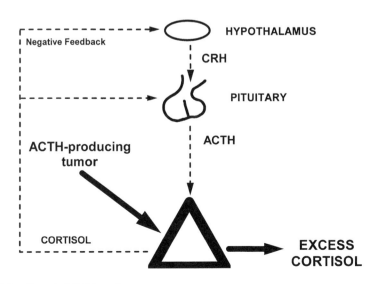

Figure 4-7. Ectopic ACTH syndrome.

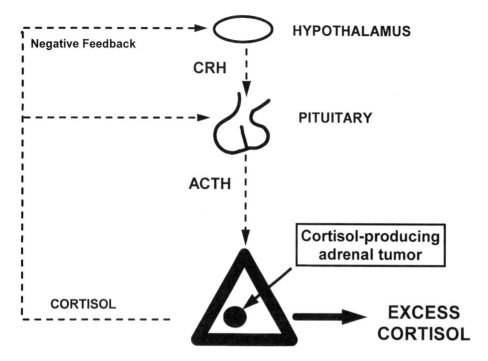

Figure 4-8.   Cushing's syndrome due to adrenal tumor.

Q: How is the 24-hour urinary cortisol test done?

A: For the **24-hour urinary cortisol test,** the patient is sent home with a container and must collect all of the urine for a 24-hour period. The sample is then assayed for free cortisol (which helps eliminate the problems associated with abnormal protein binding). A normal value is typically less than 50 μg for 24 hours. This test produces fewer false positives than the overnight DST.

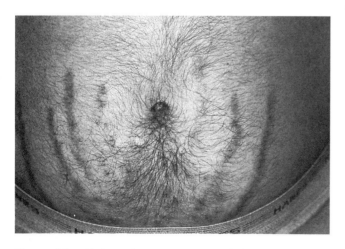

Figure 4-9.   Abdominal striae in patient with Cushing's disease.

Q: If either the overnight DST or the 24-hour urine free cortisol is abnormal, does it mean the patient has Cushing's syndrome?

A: No, these are only screening tests, so they do not yield a definitive diagnosis. Although a very abnormal value (e.g., urine free cortisol of 800 μg/24 hour) is highly suggestive of CS, further testing is typically done.

Q: What is the low-dose dexamethasone suppression test (DST)?

A: The **low-dose DST** is a confirmatory test for CS, designed to sort those who truly have CS from false positives and from those with "pseudo-Cushing's" states. **Pseudo-Cushing's syndrome,** characterized by a mild excess cortisol secretion due to increased CRH, occurs commonly in patients with depression, obesity, and alcoholism.

In the low-dose DST, 0.5 mg of dexamethasone is given orally every 6 hours for a total of 8 doses. A baseline 24-hour urinary free cortisol (UFC) is done beforehand, and is done again on the second day of dexamethasone. A normal result is suppression of UFC by more than 90% of baseline. The 24-hour excretion of 17-hydroxysteroids may also be measured; suppression to over 70% of baseline is normal. Serum cortisol is also measured at baseline, at 24 hours, and at 48 hours after the dexamethasone doses have been started; a normal result is suppression to less than 5 μg/dL.

A recently developed test, the **CRH test,** may be of use in distinguishing true Cushing's from pseudo-Cushing's states. It is possible to distinguish between these patients by performing a CRH test immediately following a standard low-dose DST. The last dose of dexamethasone is given at 6 AM, followed by an 8 AM injection of CRH. Those with true Cushing's have suppressed CRH levels, and the corticotroph cells are therefore very sensitive to exogenous CRH; levels of cortisol typically rise to more than 20% of baseline at 30 and 45 minutes after CRH infusion. Patients with pseudo-Cushing's simply have higher than normal CRH levels, and their levels of cortisol do not rise as much (< 20%). Levels of ACTH also rise higher in those with Cushing's disease, to over 35% of baseline at 15 and 30 minutes after CRH infusion.

Q: Does the low-dose DST distinguish among the different causes of Cushing's syndrome?

A: No, the low-dose DST cannot reveal the causes of CS. Further testing is required.

Q: Is there a DST designed to help distinguish among the various causes of Cushing's syndrome?

A: The **high-dose dexamethasone test** helps distinguish Cushing's disease from ectopic ACTH syndrome, as ACTH levels are high in both. CS from adrenal tumors is usually easily separated from these two disorders, as the ACTH level is suppressed. The rationale behind the high-dose DST is that ACTH-secreting pituitary tumors maintain some normal feedback mechanisms, so high levels of steroid will cause some fall in cortisol levels. This does not happen in the ectopic ACTH syndrome, and cortisol levels do not suppress.

In the high-dose DST, 2 mg dexamethasone is given every 6 hours for a total of 8 doses (four times the low-dose regimen). Urine free cortisol and/or 17-hydroxycorticosteroids are measured;

UFC in typical patients with Cushing's disease will suppress by 90%, and 17-OH steroids by 70%. Plasma cortisol also suppresses to less than 5 μg/dL. Patients with ectopic ACTH syndrome traditionally do not suppress.

Again, these are not perfect tests—some patients with Cushing's disease will not suppress, while some with ectopic ACTH syndrome will (e.g., those with branchial carcinoids). In many cases, further testing is needed. The exact number of tests needed to establish the diagnosis of CS may vary from patient to patient.

Q: Do the various dexamethasone suppression tests always yield the correct answer?

A: Like any test, the DSTs are imperfect, but they remain very useful in establishing the diagnosis. In the future, they may be replaced by better tests.

Q: Is there a better way to distinguish ectopic ACTH syndrome from Cushing's disease?

A: The gold standard test is **petrosal sinus sampling,** in which venous catheters are advanced from the groin to the left and right petrosal sinuses, which drain the pituitary gland. By comparing the petrosal sinus ACTH to peripheral ACTH, the site of ACTH excess can be pinpointed (Table 4-2). The accuracy of this test is improved by administering CRH (corticotropin-releasing hormone).

In Cushing's disease, petrosal sinus ACTH should be higher than peripheral ACTH. In ectopic ACTH syndrome, the petrosal sinus ACTH should be equal to or less than that in the peripheral blood. If the ACTH levels are higher on one side than the other, this procedure also allows the surgeon to predict which side the tumor is on, which may improve the patient's outcome.

Q: How are patients with steroid-secreting tumors distinguished from those with either Cushing's disease or ectopic ACTH syndrome?

A: Patients with corticosteroid-secreting neoplasms should have suppressed ACTH levels. The ACTH levels are usually quite high in the ectopic ACTH syndrome, and are also elevated (potentially only minimally) in Cushing's disease. Patients with ectopic ACTH syndrome often have very aggressive

TABLE 4-2.   Differential Diagnosis of Cushing's Syndrome

DISORDER	ACTH	SUPPRESS: LOW-DOSE DST	SUPPRESS: HIGH-DOSE DST	PETROSAL SINUS ACTH VERSUS PERIPHERAL
Cushing's disease	↑	–	+	↑
Adrenocortical tumor	↓	–	–	N/A
Ectopic ACTH	↑↑	–	–	equal or ↓
Iatrogenic	↓	N/A	N/A	N/A

disease; hypertension and hyperkalemia are usually the presenting complaints, as the obesity, facial plethora, or striae may take months to develop.

Q: What is the metyrapone test?

A: Metyrapone, as an inhibitor of 11β-hydroxylase, inhibits the conversion of 11-deoxycortisol (compound S) to cortisol, and 11-deoxycorticosterone to corticosterone (the precursor of aldosterone). Thus, the **metyrapone test** is another means occasionally used to distinguish ectopic ACTH syndrome from Cushing's disease. Administration of metyrapone to patients with Cushing's disease results in increased ACTH levels due to decreased feedback inhibition (remember that these pituitary tumors still are inhibited slightly by high cortisol levels); the levels of serum 11-deoxycortisol and urine 17-hydroxysteroids typically increase by 50%. Ectopic tumors that secrete ACTH do not increase secretion, because no feedback inhibition is present; the levels of 11-deoxycortisol and 17-OH steroids do not increase. The same is the case in patients with functioning adrenal tumors. Because it is a somewhat cumbersome test to perform, it is not often done.

The metyrapone test also has been used to test ACTH reserve in those with adrenal insufficiency. Patients with secondary or tertiary adrenal insufficiency lack ACTH reserve and cannot increase levels in response to metyrapone, which blocks cortisol synthesis. This test is rarely done for this purpose, because it can be quite hazardous and may provoke adrenal insufficiency.

Q: What types of adrenocortical tumors cause Cushing's syndrome?

A: Most adrenocortical tumors are benign adenomas, usually unilateral. Adrenocortical carcinomas are very aggressive and often fatal. They may secrete a variety of other adrenal steroids, such as testosterone. Macronodular hyperplasia (either ACTH-dependent or independent) is a rare cause of Cushing's syndrome.

Q: What is the treatment of Cushing's disease?

A: Tumor removal is the mainstay of CS therapy. The prognosis is better in patients with smaller tumors (< 1 cm). Radiation therapy to the pituitary may be used in patients with residual disease after surgery, but it carries a substantial risk of later hypopituitarism, and works slowly.

Q: What is Nelson's syndrome?

A: **Nelson's syndrome** occurs in patients with Cushing's disease who have had bilateral adrenalectomy instead of pituitary tumor resection. As the high cortisol levels have some small suppressive effect (remember the high-dose dexamethasone suppression test), removing the adrenal steroid excess may cause the tumor to grow even more, leading to even higher ACTH levels and subsequent hyperpigmentation. Fortunately, this complication is not seen often today with the advent of pituitary microsurgery.

Q: What is the treatment of Cushing's syndrome when caused by a cortisol-secreting tumor?

A: The treatment of choice for a cortisol-secreting tumor is surgical resection of the involved adrenal gland. Because the remaining gland is suppressed, maintenance steroids must be given and gradually weaned off as the gland recovers. This process may take over a year. Mineralocorticoids are not needed, as the renin-aldosterone axis is intact.

Q: What is the treatment of ectopic ACTH syndrome?

A: With ectopic ACTH syndrome, treatment of the primary tumor (commonly small-cell lung carcinoma) is recommended. Distant metastases are often present, so inhibitors of adrenal steroid synthesis may be required. Ketoconazole is commonly used for this purpose. Mitotane and aminoglutethimide can be used in severe cases.

Q: What is the treatment for iatrogenic Cushing's syndrome?

A: For iatrogenic Cushing's syndrome, decreasing or stopping the steroids is the best treatment, if this is possible. This may not be feasible, however, if the primary disease does not permit it. It may take over a year to completely wean a person who has been on steroids for years. One approach is to give a steroid with a relatively short duration (e.g., hydrocortisone) once in the morning. This supplies the patient with steroid during the day but allows the hypothalamus-pituitary axis (HPA) to recover at night, thus hastening overall recovery.

Q: What is "periodic" Cushing's syndrome?

A: **Periodic** or **cyclic Cushing's syndrome** has been described in persons with both Cushing's disease and ectopic ACTH syndrome. These persons have episodic ACTH secretion—periods of obvious hormonal excess with normal hormonal secretion in between.

Q: Are there any very rare causes of endogenous Cushing's syndrome?

A: **Macronodular adrenal hyperplasia** is an uncommon form of CS associated with multiple bilateral adrenal nodules. These may be ACTH-independent, in which case the nodules behave like multiple autonomous adrenal adenomas. Bilateral adrenalectomy is curative. Macronodular hyperplasia may also be ACTH-dependent, due to an ACTH-secreting pituitary tumor (Cushing's dis-

ease); these persons are best treated with pituitary surgery.

In **food-dependent hypercortisolism,** large increases in cortisol occur after eating, resulting in macronodular adrenal hyperplasia. **Primary pigmented nodular adrenal hyperplasia** (PPNAD) is another rare form of CS that typically occurs in the second decade of life; this form of CS may be inherited. Treatment is bilateral adrenalectomy. The rare association of PPNAD and cardiac myxomas is called Carney's syndrome.

Q: What are the types of adrenocortical insufficiency?

A: Primary adrenocortical insufficiency (also called Addison's disease) is caused by the destruction of or inability of the adrenal gland to produce adequate amounts of cortical steroids. In secondary adrenocortical insufficiency, the adrenal is intact but there is insufficient ACTH to stimulate it.

Q: What is Addison's disease, and what causes it?

A: **Addison's disease** refers to primary adrenal insufficiency, caused by the destruction of the adrenal glands. It is most commonly caused by autoimmune destruction (80%). Tuberculosis accounts for approximately 18% of cases. Less common causes include adrenal hemorrhage, fungal destruction, adrenoleukodystrophy, sarcoidosis, hemochromatosis, AIDS, inborn adrenal synthetic defects, and metastatic tumor.

Q: How does AIDS cause adrenal insufficiency?

A: Adrenal insufficiency occurs in at least 10% of patients with AIDS. It appears to be caused by cytomegalovirus infection, resulting in adrenalitis. Histoplasmosis rarely can cause adrenal insufficiency.

Q: Does metastatic cancer often cause adrenal insufficiency?

A: Cancer frequently metastasizes to the adrenals; if enough adrenal tissue is destroyed, adrenal insufficiency may result. Approximately 20% of those with adrenal metastases have a suboptimal cortisol response to ACTH, although full-blown adrenal crises are uncommon. Those persons with extensive adrenal metastases should always be tested for insufficiency. Those with decreased reserve should receive supplemental steroids.

Q: What is adrenoleukodystrophy?

A: **Adrenoleukodystrophy** (ALD) is an X-linked disorder occurring in 1 in 25,000 males. There are two types. **Cerebral adrenoleukodystrophy** occurs in childhood and presents with behavioral dysfunction, mental retardation, and neurologic disturbances. Adrenal insufficiency often presents before the neurologic abnormalities; young males with adrenal insufficiency should be screened for adrenoleukodystrophy.

Adrenomyeloneuropathy is a milder form and typically presents in young adulthood. These patients may present with spinal cord symptoms, cognitive impairment, and impotence.

Both disorders result from defects in fatty acid metabolism; persons may be screened by measuring urinary excretion of very long-chain fatty acids (VLCFA); high levels are suggestive of ALD. Genetic testing is also available, and genetic counseling is indicated for affected males. There is no effective medical treatment.

Q: What are the clinical features of primary adrenal cortical insufficiency?

A: The clinical features of Addison's disease include weakness, fatigue, anorexia, weight loss, hyperpigmentation, hypotension, nausea/vomiting, salt craving, and depression.

Q: Why do patients with Addison's disease have hyperpigmentation?

A: When the primary organ (adrenal) fails, the trophic hormone (ACTH) increases, often to 100 times normal or more. ACTH has biologic homology to melanocyte-stimulating hormone (MSH), which stimulates melanin deposition in melanocytes. (MSH has negligible importance in humans, but is important in lower animals.) Increased ACTH therefore results in increased skin pigmentation. It usually improves after treatment, but may not completely regress.

Q: What are the laboratory findings in Addison's disease?

A: Some or all of the following finding may be present with Addison's disease:

Hyperkalemia (due to aldosterone deficiency)

Hyponatremia (due to cortisol deficiency)

Anemia

Hypoglycemia (due to cortisol deficiency)

Elevated blood urea nitrogen (BUN) and creatinine (due to dehydration)

Hypercalcemia (due to dehydration and increased gastrointestinal calcium absorption).

Q: How is Addison's disease diagnosed?

A: Random cortisol levels are not useful in establishing either hyper- or hypocortisolism, as there is significant diurnal variation in secretion. What is necessary is a *stimulatory* test of the adrenal reserve.

The standard test is the **rapid ACTH test,** in which 0.25 mg cosyntropin (a synthetic ACTH derivative) is given intravenously or intramuscularly; serum cortisol is measured at baseline, at 30 minutes, and at 60 minutes. An increase in serum cortisol to over 18 μg/dL or by over 7μg/dL from baseline excludes adrenal insufficiency. The ACTH level should also be elevated in Addison's disease.

Q: What is secondary adrenal insufficiency?

A: **Secondary adrenal insufficiency** occurs when the organ (adrenal) is intact, but the trophic hormone (ACTH) is deficient. The most common cause is **iatrogenic**—chronic steroid administration—which results in atrophy of the zonae fasciculata and reticularis due to low ACTH levels. (The zona glomerulosa is only minimally affected by ACTH deficiency, as the renin-angiotensin system provides the primary stimulus.) A similar scenario occurs after treatment of Cushing's syndrome caused by adrenocortical tumors; the chronic steroid excess leads to atrophy of the other gland due to suppressed ACTH.

ACTH deficiency also can occur in states of hypothalamic or pituitary disease (e.g., tumors, trauma). Again, only glucocorticoid secretion is affected, as ACTH is not required for mineralocorticoid secretion. Other signs of pituitary/hypothalamic failure are usually present, such as hypogonadism, diabetes insipidus, hypothyroidism, or short stature (in children). See Chapter 2 for further discussion of the diagnosis of secondary adrenal insufficiency.

Q: What differences in clinical features exist between primary and secondary adrenal insufficiency?

A: Hyperpigmentation is absent in secondary deficiency, because ACTH secretion is low. Mineralocorticoid secretion is normal in secondary adrenal insufficiency, so hyperkalemia does not occur. Hyponatremia and hypoglycemia may occur in both conditions, as they are related to cortisol deficiency.

Q: What is the treatment of adrenal insufficiency?

A: In patients with adrenal insufficiency, oral glucocorticoids are required to sustain life. The most commonly used are the naturally occurring **hydrocortisone** (cortisol) and **cortisone.** These are typically given in divided doses totaling 30 mg and 37.5 mg per day, respectively. Cortisone itself is inactive but is rapidly converted to cortisol in the liver. Synthetic glucocorticoids, although used widely for other conditions, are not commonly used for the treatment of adrenal insufficiency.

As seen in Table 4-3, cortisol and cortisone are relatively weak compared to their synthetic counterparts. They also possess some mineralocorticoid activity, which the synthetic ones lack. Although hydrocortisone and cortisone have some mineralocorticoid activity, it is not enough for some patients; these patients require the synthetic oral mineralocorticoid **fludrocortisone**, 0.05–0.2 mg daily. (Aldosterone is not effective when given orally.) Patients with secondary adrenal insufficiency do not require a mineralocorticoid, as aldosterone secretion is intact. In the treatment of non-endocrine disease, a lack of mineralocorticoid activity is desirable in a steroid, as only the glucocorticoid properties are required.

Q: How is the dosage of medication monitored?

A: Unlike certain other endocrine diseases (e.g., hypothyroidism), there is no simple biochemical parameter to follow in treatment of adrenal insufficiency. The traditional method has been to follow clinical symptoms, but this is not always accurate. The long-term concern is not that patients receive too little steroid (adrenal crisis is rare in patients who take their medication faithfully), but rather that patients may be overmedicated, which in time can lead to deleterious effects such as osteoporosis. A 24-hour urine free cortisol assay is useful in determining whether the dosage is correct; this test, of course, requires that the patient take cortisone or hydrocortisone, and not a synthetic steroid. Adequacy of mineralocorticoid replacement can be estimated by checking electrolytes and renin levels—potassium and renin are elevated with inadequate replacement.

Q: What should patients do when they get sick?

A: All patients should have a wallet card or wear jewelry that identifies them as having adrenal in-

TABLE 4-3.   Relative Potencies of Commonly Used Glucocorticoids

GLUCOCORTICOID	NATURALLY OCCURRING	RELATIVE POTENCY (TO CORTISOL)	REPLACEMENT DOSE (mg/day)
Hydrocortisone (cortisol)	Yes	1	20–30
Cortisone*	Yes	0.8	25–37.5
Prednisone*	No	4	5–7.5
Methylprednisolone	No	5	4–6
Dexamethasone	No	30	0.75–1

*Cortisone and prednisone are themselves inactive but are converted to the active cortisol and prednisolone, respectively, in the liver.

sufficiency so that emergency medical personnel will be immediately aware of their condition. Patients need to double their dose in cases of illness (fever, nausea, vomiting) and should be able to inject hydrocortisone when it cannot be taken orally. The patient should *not* double the dose for a minor illness such as a cold or sore throat, even if he/she feels badly. The steroid may make them feel better (just as we would feel better if we took extra glucocorticoids), but is not needed—and chronic use exposes them to the risks of steroid excess.

Q: What is cortisol resistance?

A: Individuals with **cortisol resistance** have genetic mutations in the cortisol receptor, resulting in decreased cortisol effect despite elevated levels. Because the pituitary is also resistant to cortisol, ACTH levels rise; this results in increased mineralocorticoid and androgen synthesis, which in turn results in hyperaldosteronism, virilization, and precocious puberty. There is no definite treatment at this time.

Q: What is adrenal crisis?

A: **Adrenal crisis,** the end stage of adrenal insufficiency, is characterized by shock, hypotension, hyperkalemia, hyponatremia, and death, if untreated. It only rarely occurs in patients who faithfully take their medication and increase it as needed. A dangerous scenario may result when a patient on chronic steroids for another condition (such as an organ transplant) is sent to surgery without adequate steroid coverage. All patients with adrenal insufficiency require "stress steroids" in times of severe illness or stress, including surgery.

Q: What is the treatment of adrenal crisis?

A: For adrenal crisis, initially the fluid volume should be restored with large amounts of normal (0.9%) saline. If the diagnosis of adrenal insufficiency is in doubt, a random cortisol level can be sent off and treatment can then begin. This would be an occasion when a random level is useful: hypotension and shock is an adequate stimulus for steroid secretion, and any such person with a cortisol level *not* exceeding 20 μg/dL should be assumed to have adrenal insufficiency. Alternatively, dexamethasone (which does not interfere with the cortisol assay) can be started, and the cosyntropin test can then be performed. This allows for diagnosis without delaying treatment.

Hydrocortisone is the glucocorticoid of choice, typically given at a dosage of 100 mg intravenously every 6 to 8 hours. In such high doses, it has adequate mineralocorticoid activity, and mineralocorticoid supplementation is not necessary. The dosage is gradually tapered to a maintenance dose (30 mg/day) as the crisis subsides. Aggravating conditions such as infection or myocardial infarction should also be treated. Oral fludrocortisone may be required in primary adrenal insufficiency.

Q: What are "stress steroid" doses?

A: In a **stress steroid** dose, extra steroids are given to patients with adrenal insufficiency, either primary or secondary (commonly due to exogenous steroids). For major surgery, hydrocortisone, 100 mg every 6 to 8 hours, is given. For minor surgery, doubling the oral dose should be sufficient.

Q: What are mineralocorticoids?

A: **Mineralocorticoids** are steroids made in the zona glomerulosa whose primary purpose is to promote sodium retention, potassium excretion, and a positive water balance. The primary mineralocorticoid is **aldosterone** (Fig. 4-10).

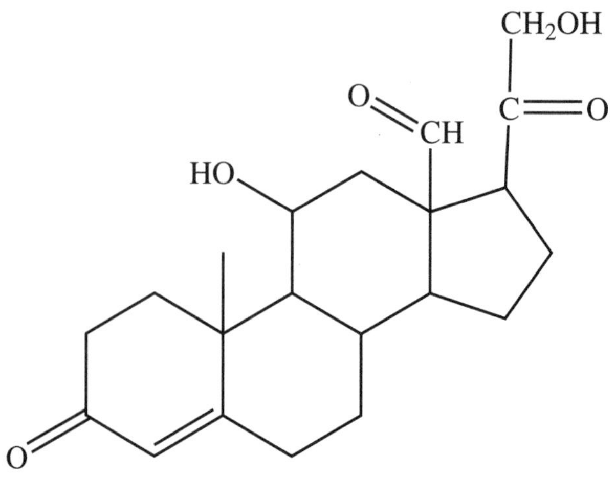

Figure 4-10. Aldosterone.

Q: How is the secretion of aldosterone regulated?

A: The secretion of aldosterone is mediated by the renin-angiotensin system (Fig. 4-11). Unlike cortisol, aldosterone secretion is not dependent on ACTH; ACTH does result in a rise in aldosterone levels, but it is not required for normal levels.

The stimulus for aldosterone secretion is primarily a decrease in blood pressure, hyperosmolarity, and decreased intravascular volume. This is sensed by the **juxtaglomerular cells** in the kidney, which then secrete the peptide hormone **renin.** Renin then acts upon the protein **angiotensinogen** (produced by the liver) to produce angiotensin I. Angiotensin is then converted to the active protein **angiotensin II** by the angiotensin-converting enzyme (ACE). Angiotensin II itself has potent vasoconstrictive effects and helps return the blood pressure to normal. It also stimulates the zona glomerulosa of the adrenal gland to secrete aldosterone, which has the effect of increasing sodium reabsorption, enhancing potassium excretion, and increasing fluid volume.

Arginine vasopressin (ADH) is also a potent stimulator of aldosterone production by the zona glomerulosa cells. This appears to exert a protective effect in states of free-water excess.

Q: Do any hormones promote sodium excretion?

A: A peptide hormone, **atrial natriuretic peptide** (ANP), is secreted by cardiac atrial cells. Volume overload causes atrial distention, resulting in release of ANP. The primary effect of ANP is on the kidney, where it results in natriuresis, increased glomerular filtration rate, and decreased renin secretion. It also inhibits adrenal cortical aldosterone production.

Q: What is hyperaldosteronism?

A: **Hyperaldosteronism** is a clinical state that results from aldosterone excess, typically due to adrenal gland hypersecretion (primary aldosteronism). It may also be a secondary condition, as in the case of renin-secreting tumors or renovascular hypertension.

Q: What are the causes of hyperaldosteronism?

A: The most common cause of hyperaldosteronism is **Conn's syndrome** (75% of cases), an aldosterone-secreting adenoma that is usually unilateral. Approximately 25% of cases are due to **bilateral adrenal hyperplasia** (also known as **idiopathic hyperaldosteronism**). Some experts feel that hyperplasia may be more common than previously thought; the hyperaldosteronism caused by hyper-

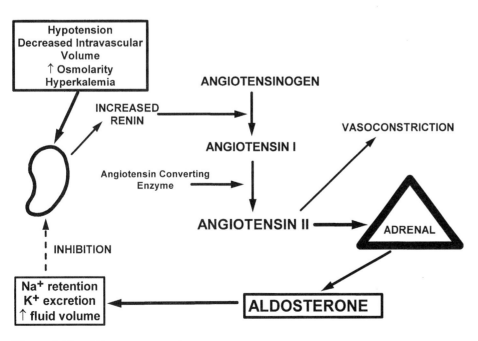

Figure 4-11. Aldosterone secretion.

plasia is typically milder than that from adenomas, so some patients may be escaping detection.

Q: What are the clinical features of hyperaldosteronism?

A: Most patients present with spontaneous hypokalemia (i.e., not due to drugs such as diuretics). K$^+$ levels may be quite low, often below 2.5 mEq/L (normal: 3.5–5.3). Symptoms related to this include fatigue and weakness. With severe depletion, paresthesias may be present. Na$^+$ levels are typically not elevated unless the patient is dehydrated. Polyuria is often present due to the increased potassium excretion (which causes renal resistance to vasopressin). Headaches are common. Hypertension is typically present and may range from mild to severe. Malignant hypertension (hypertension associated with renal and/or cardiovascular disease) may be seen in severe cases.

Q: How is primary hyperaldosteronism diagnosed?

A: A simple screening test for hyperaldosteronism is to obtain a random plasma aldosterone and renin level simultaneously. Because aldosterone secretion is regulated by renin, the ratio is usually consistent in most physiologic states. Aldosterone secretion is autonomous, so renin is suppressed. An aldosterone/renin ratio of over 25 (aldosterone expressed in ng/mL, renin in ng/mL/hour) is suggestive of hyperaldosteronism.

Other tests include measurement of 24-hour urinary aldosterone and the saline suppression test. The saline test is done by giving the patient 2 liters of normal (0.9%) saline over 4 hours, and measuring aldosterone before and after. Normally, aldosterone should fall below 10 ng/dL, but it remains elevated in primary aldosteronism.

Q: If the laboratory tests clearly suggest primary aldosteronism, what is the next step?

A: Most cases of primary aldosteronism are caused by functioning adrenal tumors, so computed tomography (CT) or magnetic resonance imaging (MRI) of the adrenals is a reasonable next step. In patients with very high aldosterone levels, a solitary tumor is usually the cause. For milder cases, it may be prudent to prove that a tumor is the cause of aldosterone excess, as nonfunctioning adrenal tumors are common (around 3%) in the general population.

Confirmation is done by **adrenal venous sampling,** in which aldosterone levels are measured from each adrenal gland (Table 4-4). If the aldosterone level is much higher on one side than the other, this suggests a functioning adrenal tumor. If the levels are similar, bilateral hyperplasia is suggested. Aldosterone and cortisol samples are simultaneously sampled. An infusion of ACTH is usually given to stimulate cortisol secretion by the adrenals; elevated cortisol levels verify that the samples are of adrenal origin. If the cortisol level is not elevated in the adrenal gland sample, it means that the operator did not successfully cannulate the adrenal, and was likely in the vena cava instead.

Q: What is the treatment of primary hyperaldosteronism?

A: After preparation with spironolactone (a diuretic that is an aldosterone antagonist), patients with

TABLE 4-4.   Venous Sampling Data in Patient with Left-Sided Aldosteronoma

SITE	ALDOSTERONE (ng/dL)	CORTISOL (μg/dL)	A/C RATIO
Left adrenal	22,660	846.5	26.80
Right adrenal	86	796.5	0.18
Inferior vena cava below adrenals	100	51.4	1.95
Inferior vena cava below adrenals	125	50.2	2.49

adrenal tumors undergo resection. The remaining adrenal is sufficient for life, and aldosterone and potassium levels should return to normal. Hypertension may still persist, although it should be much easier to control.

Patients with bilateral hyperplasia are treated with medical therapy (spironolactone). Surgery is not effective, as hypertension may still persist even after removal of both adrenal glands.

Q: Do other causes of hyperaldosteronism exist?

A: The other causes of hyperaldosteronism are extremely rare. **Dexamethasone-suppressible hyperaldosteronism** is a rare disorder in which levels of aldosterone are suppressed to normal after administration of dexamethasone. The 11- and 17-hydroxylase deficiency forms of **congenital adrenal hyperplasia** result in increased mineralocorticoid levels and secondary hyperaldosteronism. Ingestion of **glycyrrhizic acid** (an inhibitor of 11-hydroxylase) also results in secondary hyperaldosteronism by the same mechanism as inherited 11-hydroxylase deficiency; this substance is found in certain kinds of licorice and chewing tobacco, and individuals who use large amounts may develop hypertension.

Another rare disorder that may mimic hyperaldosteronism is 11β-hydroxysteroid dehydrogenase deficiency. This enzyme is present in the kidney and normally metabolizes cortisol to the inactive cortisone, which is excreted in the urine. In this disorder, too much cortisol binds to the mineralocorticoid receptor, and is also called **apparent mineralocorticoid excess syndrome**. It may produce hypertension and hypokalemia. Genetic analysis or identifying an increased urinary cortisol:cortisone ratio can identify these patients.

Q: What is renovascular hypertension?

A: **Renovascular hypertension** is the most common cause of surgically reversible hypertension (5% of all hypertensive patients). Etiologies include atherosclerosis and fibromuscular hyperplasia. The stenotic kidney sees too little blood flow, and secretes excess renin, which in turn results in excess angiotensin II, a potent vasoconstrictor (Fig. 4-12). Aldosterone secretion is increased, although this plays a minor role in the hypertension in most cases.

Q: What are some clues that might suggest renovascular hypertension?

A: Renovascular hypertension is suggested by signs of secondary hypertension: rapidly worsening hypertension, onset of hypertension before age 25 or after age 55, and diastolic renal bruit on examination.

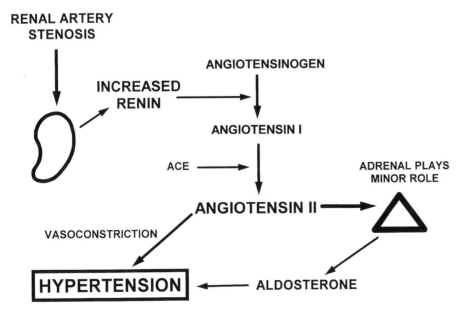

Figure 4-12. Renovascular hypertension.

Q: How is renovascular hypertension diagnosed?

A: The gold standard test for renovascular hypertension is the **renal arteriogram.** As this is an invasive procedure, a less invasive screening test may be desirable. **Renal vein renin sampling** is a functional test, that can show a large "step-up" of renin levels in the involved kidney.

A relatively new test with high sensitivity and specificity is the **ACE inhibitor nuclear renogram.** In patients with a stenotic kidney, ACE inhibitors result in markedly decreased blood flow. This property can be exploited to improve the accuracy of a nuclear renogram: renal flow is measured before and after ACE inhibitor administration. The affected kidney demonstrates markedly decreased blood flow and retention of the tracer after the ACE inhibitor. In a patient with known left renal artery stenosis (as illustrated by Figs. 4-13 and 4-14), the renograms (which estimate blood flow) are similar prior to the ACE inhibitor, although the left side does show some delayed uptake. After the ACE inhibitor, however, the results are dramatic; there is much less blood flow into the stenotic kidney and prolonged retention when compared to the normal side. The ACE inhibitor nuclear renogram is now the screening test of choice in many institutions because of its ease and lack of invasiveness.

Renal duplex ultrasound provides both a functional and anatomic assessment of renal arteries. Renal vein renin sampling may aid in localization; renin levels are higher in the stenotic kidney. **High-resolution spiral CT** and MRI also have high sensitivity and specificity.

Q: Are laboratory studies useful in diagnosing renovascular hypertension?

A: Typically, laboratory studies have no role in renovascular hypertension diagnosis. Aldosterone and renin levels are generally not helpful, although they both may be elevated in severe cases. Hypokalemia is usually not present.

Q: What is the treatment of renovascular hypertension?

A: There are two methods of correcting the stenotic lesion. The first is **percutaneous angioplasty,** in which a balloon catheter is advanced and expanded to dilate the stenosis. This procedure is less invasive, but the lesion may recur in a minority of cases. The second method is surgical correction, which is more invasive than angioplasty and may be required when angioplasty fails. Renovascular hypertension may also be treated medically in those patients who are unable to tolerate the invasive procedures.

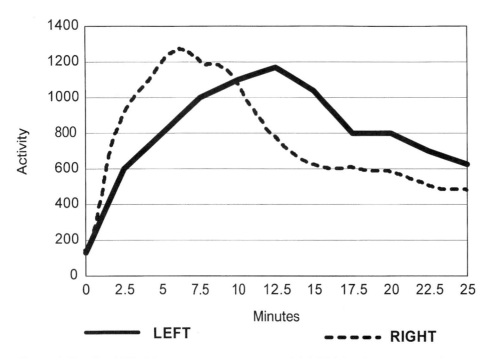

Figure 4-13. Pre-ACE inhibitor renogram in patient with left RAS (renal artery stenosis).

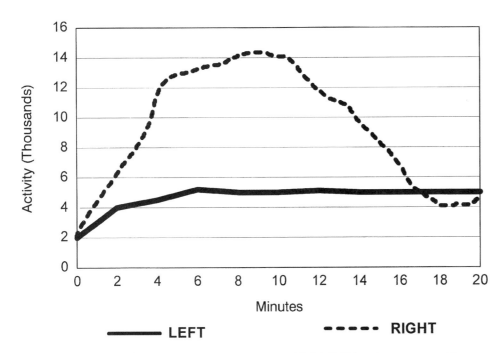

Figure 4-14. Post-ACE inhibitor renogram in patient with left RAS (renal artery stenosis).

Q: What is congenital adrenal hyperplasia?

A: The **congenital adrenal hyperplasias** (CAH) are a group of autosomal recessive disorders of steroid biosynthesis. There are several different types, depending on the enzymatic block. The common element in each is that an end product is not made, leading to increase in ACTH and hence adrenal hyperplasia.

Q: What clinical findings can be seen in CAH?

A: The clinical findings in CAH depend on the enzyme defect and the precursor that accumulates. Problems seen include virilization, feminization, adrenal insufficiency, and/or hypertension.

Q: What is the most common type of CAH?

A: **P450c21-hydroxylase deficiency** is the most common type of CAH. The defect is localized to a gene abnormality on chromosome 6, and occurs in several different forms. Each has in common a variable defect in this enzyme, resulting in deficient cortisol and aldosterone synthesis, and increased ACTH and androgen levels. The **classic** form is divided into salt-wasting and non-salt wasting forms. In the **salt-wasting** form, inadequate aldosterone and cortisol production leads to adrenal crisis and shock shortly after birth, if untreated. In

the **non-salt wasting** form, adequate steroid synthesis exists to sustain life, but is not enough for times of stress. These patients may develop adrenal crisis during severe illness.

The secondary problem is the vicious cycle that occurs in all forms of CAH. In this case, the inadequate formation of the end product (cortisol) leads to increased ACTH and accumulation of androgenic steroids, as cortisol and aldosterone are not made adequately (Fig. 4-15; see also Fig. 4-14). In girls, the increased androgen results in virilization, ambiguous genitalia, and female pseudohermaphrodism (male appearance in a genetic female). It is the most common cause of ambiguous genitalia in the female. In boys, the increased androgen results in virilization at an early age, causing severe psychological and developmental problems. In both sexes, early excess of sex steroids results in **precocious puberty,** with initial increase in growth velocity and eventual short stature due to early fusion of the epiphyseal plates (from androgen excess). Thus, the goals of treatment are

1. Prevent adrenal crisis and death.

2. Recognize the condition early in the female so that she can be reared as the correct sex.

TABLE 4-5.   Clinical Features of Congenital Adrenal Hyperplasia

ENZYME DEFICIENCY	MAJOR ACCUMULATED PRECURSORS	HYPERTENSION	VIRILIZATION (FEMALES)	FEMINIZATION (MALES)
21α-hydroxylase	17-hydroxyprogesterone, progesterone	–	+	–
3β-hydroxysteroid dehydrogenase	17-hydroxypregnenolone, pregnenolone	–	+	–
11β-hydroxylase	11-deoxycortisol, 11-deoxycorticosterone	+	+	–
17α-hydroxylase	Pregnenolone, progesterone	+	–	+

3. Treat the condition early in both sexes to prevent precocious puberty and the resultant short adult stature and psychological problems.

Q: Do milder forms of 21-hydroxylase deficiency exist?

A: **Nonclassic** or **"cryptic" 21-hydroxylase deficiency** is the most common form of 21-hydroxylase deficiency. This is one of the most common inherited disorders, with a frequency of 1:100 in certain populations. The defect is mild, so adrenal crisis and severe virilization do not occur. However, it can result in hirsutism (male pattern hair) in girls as well as infertility. It is an important condition to recognize because of its relatively frequent occurrence.

Q: How is 21-hydroxylase deficiency diagnosed?

A: In the classic forms of 21-hydroxylase deficiency, 17-hydroxyprogesterone (17-OHP) is grossly elevated, as is serum renin. ACTH-stimulated serum cortisol may be low. In the nonclassic form, baseline 17-OHP may be normal. After stimulation with synthetic ACTH (cosyntropin, 0.25 mg IV or IM), levels increase by five- to tenfold in those with nonclassic 21-hydroxylase deficiency.

Q: How is 21-hydroxylase deficiency treated?

A: Treatment is to replace the end product (i.e., cortisol) that is not being made (Fig. 4-16). Patients may be treated with "natural" steroids (cortisone, hydrocortisone) or synthetic ones (dexametha-

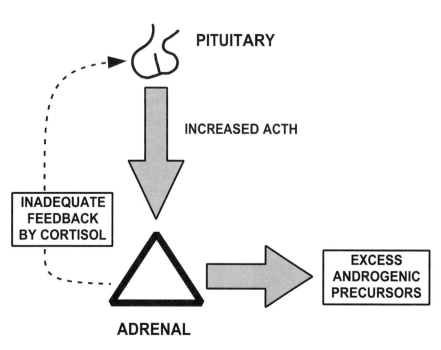

Figure 4-15.   Untreated 21-hydroxylase deficiency.

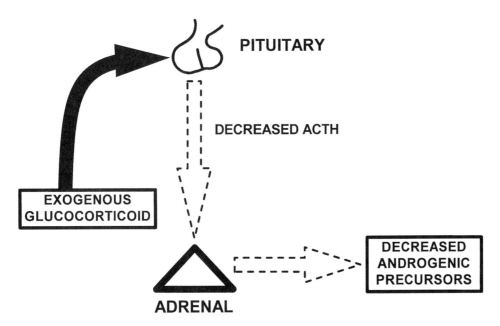

Figure 4-16. Treated 21-hydroxylase deficiency.

sone). This serves to prevent adrenal crisis (in those with classic CAH), and reduce androgen levels to prevent virilization and precocious puberty in classic CAH and hirsutism/infertility in nonclassic CAH. Mineralocorticoids (fludrocortisone) may also be required.

Q: What are some of the other forms of CAH?

A: **3β-Hydroxysteroid dehydrogenase** (3β-HSD) deficiency (see Fig. 4-2) also causes buildup of androgenic precursors and presents in classic and nonclassic forms. This can result in salt-wasting crisis, male pseudohermaphrodism, hirsutism, and infertility. The intermediates pregnenolone, 17-OH pregnenolone, and DHEA accumulate in this disorder. It is treated in the same fashion as 21-hydroxylase deficiency.

Another severe form of CAH is **cholesterol side-chain cleavage deficiency** (P450scc deficiency) (see Fig. 4-2). This defect is the first step of steroid biosynthesis, and therefore results in decreased levels of all steroid hormones; commonly, it results in male pseudohermaphrodism and adrenal insufficiency. This disorder has been associated with a mutation in **steroidogenic acute regulatory protein (StAR)**, which is necessary for transport of cholesterol from outer to inner mitochondrial

membranes. Treatment is glucocorticoid and mineralocorticoid replacement.

P450 aromatase deficiency (see Fig. 4-2) results in female pseudohermaphrodism due to defective conversion of C_{19} steroids to estrogens, resulting in increased androgen levels.

Q: Can any of the forms of CAH produce hypertension?

A: Yes, hypertension can result from P450c11β-hydroxylase deficiency and P450c17α-hydroxylase deficiency. **11-Hydroxylase deficiency** results in deficient conversion of 11-deoxycortisol into cortisol and 11-deoxycorticosterone into corticosterone, resulting in accumulation of 11-deoxycorticosterone (DOC), 11-deoxycortisol (compound S), and excess androgen (see Fig. 4-2); this in turn leads to hypertension and virilization. Plasma renin levels are suppressed. Treatment is glucocorticoid administration.

17-Hydroxylase deficiency leads to deficient conversion of pregnenolone into 17-hydroxypregnenolone, and progesterone into 17-hydroxyprogesterone. This leads to cortisol and androgen deficiency, and the accumulation of mineralocorticoids (see Fig. 4-2), resulting in hypertension and male pseudohermaphrodism. Females have sexual

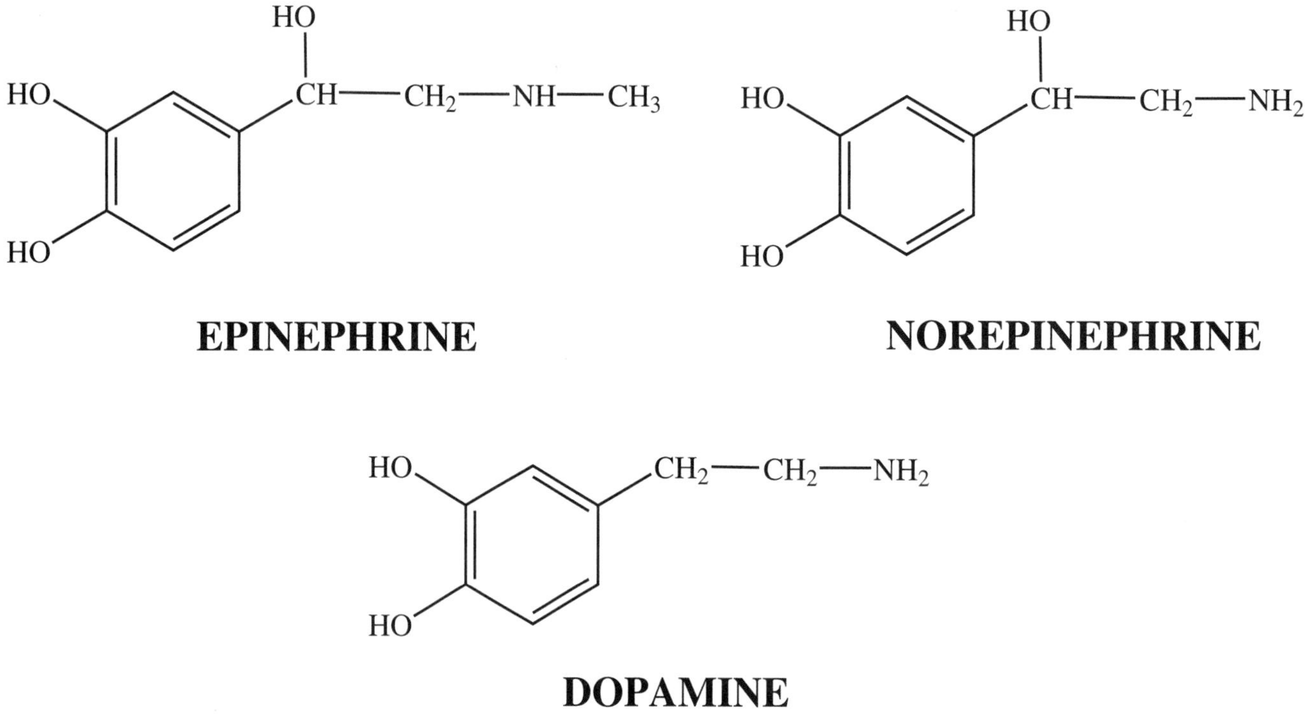

EPINEPHRINE

NOREPINEPHRINE

DOPAMINE

Figure 4-17. Major catecholamines.

infantilism due to diminished estrogen synthesis. Treatment is glucocorticoid administration.

Q: What is the function of the adrenal medulla?

A: The adrenal medulla is a highly specialized part of the sympathetic nervous system and the major site of catecholamine synthesis (Fig. 4-17). Its major product, **epinephrine,** is important in response to stress. While epinephrine is found mainly in the adrenal medulla, **norepinephrine** is found in the central nervous system and in the sympathetic chain. The precursor to norepinephrine, **dopamine,** is also found in the medulla and sympathetic system. The catecholamines are synthesized from the amino acid tyrosine.

Q: What is the stimulus for adrenal medullary catecholamine secretion?

A: Catecholamine secretion is stimulated by stress, including exercise, surgery, sepsis, myocardial infarction, or hypoglycemia—essentially any physical stressor on the body. This secretion is the well-described "fight or flight" response, and usually is accompanied by increase in some other hormones, notably cortisol and growth hormone.

Q: Are there any disorders of adrenal medullary hypersecretion?

A: **Pheochromocytoma** is a neuroendocrine tumor that produces excess catecholamines. It is an uncommon condition, accounting for 0.1% of patients with diastolic hypertension. Most of these tumors are benign (90%) and occur in the adrenal gland (90%); 10%, however, are extra-adrenal. These tumors may occur wherever neuroendocrine tissue is found (e.g., the sympathetic chain); 10% are bilateral, and 10% are malignant.

Q: What are the clinical features of pheochromocytoma?

A: Most patients with pheochromocytoma have some symptoms all of the time, but usually the symptoms wax and wane in paroxysmal fashion. Typical symptoms include headache (most common symptom), diaphoresis, tachycardia, anxiety, fear of "impending doom," abdominal or chest pain, nausea and vomiting, tremors, hypertension, and pallor. Flushing is actually rare in pheochromocytomas, which usually cause vasoconstriction. Paroxysms may be induced by drugs such as opiates, glucagon, guanethidine, and tricyclic antidepressants.

Q: What is the outcome of a patient with untreated pheochromocytoma?

A: Possible outcomes of untreated pheochromocytomas include myocardial infarction, stroke, cardiac arrhythmias, shock, renal failure, dissecting aortic aneurysm, and death.

Q: How is pheochromocytoma diagnosed?

A: The traditional diagnostic method is to measure the catecholamines or their breakdown products in the urine by a 24-hour collection. Patients with pheochromocytoma excrete extremely large amounts of the catecholamines or their metabolites. Those with large tumors may excrete disproportionately large amounts of metabolites, so metanephrines or VMA (vanillylmandelic acid) are often measured in addition to total and fractionated catecholamines. Measurement of plasma catecholamines during a paroxysm is very sensitive, but this often difficult to accomplish.

Q: What imaging studies are useful in the management of patients with suspected pheochromocytoma?

A: After a biochemical diagnosis has been established, adrenal CT or MRI should be performed, as 90% of these tumors are in the adrenals. Other tests include radioiodine-labeled metaiodobenzylguanidine (MIBG), which is taken up by adrenal medullary tissue and is useful for localization of pheochromocytoma. The ^{111}In-labeled somatostatin analogue octreotide has also been useful in localizing a variety of neuroendocrine tumors, including pheochromocytomas.

Q: What is the treatment for pheochromocytoma?

A: Surgery is the definitive treatment, after the patient has been properly prepared. Initially, α-adrenergic blockade (phenoxybenzamine) is given to control hypertension. After adequate α-blockade has been established, β-blockade (propranolol) may be required to control tachycardia. Instituting β-blockade alone in a patient with pheochromocytoma is hazardous and may actually worsen symptoms, so it should never be started until adequate α-blockade has been achieved. Inhibition of catecholamine synthesis by use of the drug α-methyltyrosine may be used in severe cases.

Q: Are any other endocrine problems associated with pheochromocytoma?

A: Pheochromocytoma may be associated with the multiple endocrine neoplasia syndromes (MEN) type IIa and IIb:

> IIa: pheochromocytoma, medullary thyroid carcinoma, hyperparathyroidism
>
> IIb: pheochromocytoma, medullary thyroid carcinoma, mucosal neuromas, Marfanoid habitus.

Pheochromocytoma may also be associated with neurofibromatosis and Von Hippel-Lindau disease.

Q: What is an "incidental" adrenal mass?

A: An **incidental mass** is one discovered while doing imaging procedures for another problem. They are quite common, affecting approximately 3% of the general population.

Q: What are the concerns in persons with incidental adrenal masses?

A: Incidental adrenal masses should be evaluated to make sure that they are neither biochemically functional nor malignant. Tumors greater than 6 cm in diameter are likely to be malignant. Those 3 to 6 cm are less likely to be malignant but should be watched closely. If they enlarge in size, they should be removed. Biochemical disorders (Cushing's syndrome, hyperaldosteronism, pheochromocytoma, and virilizing tumors) should be excluded, and functioning adrenal tumors should be removed. CT or MRI should be repeated in 6 months, 1 year, and 2 years. Biochemistries should be repeated if endocrine symptoms are suspected.

BIBLIOGRAPHY

Cook DM, Loriaux DL. Cushing's: medical approach. In: Bardin CW, ed. Current therapy in endocrinology and metabolism. 6th ed. St. Louis: Mosby, 1997:59–63.

Dluhy RG, Williams GH. Endocrine hypertension. In: Wilson, JD, Foster DW, Kronenberg HM, Larsen PR, eds. Williams' textbook of endocrinology. 9th ed. Philadelphia: W.B. Saunders, 1998:729–744.

Ehrhart-Bornstein M, Hinson JP, Bornstein SR, Scherbaum WA, Vinson FP. Intraadrenal interactions in the regulation of adrenocortical steroidogenesis. Endocr Rev 1998;19:101–143.

Findling JS, Aron DC, Tyrrell JB. Glucocorticoids and adrenal androgens. In: Greenspan FS, Strewler GJ, eds. Basic and clinical endocrinology. 2nd ed. Stamford, CT: Appleton & Lange, 1997:317–352.

Manger WM, Gifford RW. Clinical manifestations. In: Manger WM, Gifford RW, eds. Clinical and experimental pheochromocytoma. 2nd ed. Cambridge, MA: Blackwell Science, 1996:89–149.

Orth DN, Kovacs WJ. The adrenal cortex. In: Wilson JD, Foster DW, Kronenberg HM, Larsen PR, eds. Williams' textbook of endocrinology. 9th ed. Philadelphia: W.B. Saunders, 1999:517–660.

Tsigos C, Kamilaris TC, Chrousos GP. Adrenal diseases. In: Moore WT, Eastman TC, eds. Diagnostic endocrinology. 2nd ed. St. Louis: Mosby, 1996: 125–419.

Yanovski JA, Cutler BG, Chrousos GP, Nieman LK. Corticotropin-releasing hormone stimulation following low-dose dexamethasone administration. JAMA 1993;269:2232–2238.

REVIEW QUESTIONS

I. SHORT ANSWER

1. The adrenal glands are paired organs that lie above the kidneys; 90% of their weight is in the outer _____, and 10% is in the inner _____.

2. The adrenal cortex is responsible for synthesizing three types of steroids: _____, _____, and _____. The adrenal medulla is responsible for synthesizing _____

   c outermost cortical layer, the _____, synthesizes _____. The middle and thickest layer is the _____, which synthesizes _____. The innermost layer, the _____, synthesizes _____.

4. The layers _____ and _____ are stimulated by the trophic hormone _____, located in the pituitary. Secretion of this pituitary hormone is enhanced by the hypothalamic hormone _____.

5. The major glucocorticoid is _____, which largely circulates as a protein-bound (inactive) form, attached to the protein _____.

6. Name three physiologic stimuli that increase cortisol secretion.

7. The state of chronic glucocorticoid excess is called _____. The most common cause of this condition is _____. The most common endogenous cause is a _____,

more specifically called _____, followed by _____, _____, and _____.

8. Name five clinical features of Cushing's syndrome.

9. Two commonly used screening tests for Cushing's syndrome (CS) include _____ and _____.

10. A confirmatory test for Cushing's syndrome is the _____. After a diagnosis of Cushing's syndrome has been firmly established, another helpful laboratory test is measurement of serum _____. A perturbation study to help distinguish Cushing's disease from ectopic ACTH syndrome is the _____. Another, invasive test to help separate those with Cushing's disease from those with ectopic ACTH syndrome is _____.

11. Patients with glucocorticoid-secreting adrenal tumors can usually be separated from those with Cushing's disease and ectopic ACTH syndrome by measurement of _____. This level should be _____ with adrenal tumors, and _____ with the other two causes.

12. The most common adrenal tumor causing Cushing's syndrome is _____. A less common cause is _____, which may be very aggressive and fatal.

13. The first line of treatment for Cushing's disease is _____. Removal of both adrenal glands in a patient with Cushing's disease may result in a hyperpigmented condition known as

_____. The treatment of steroid-secreting adrenal tumors is _____. Treatment of ectopic ACTH syndrome is _____. In cases of Cushing's syndrome not responsive to conventional therapy, _____ may be required.

14. Primary adrenal insufficiency is called _____. The most common cause is _____, followed by _____.

15. Name six clinical features of Addison's disease.

16. Because of elevated _____ levels, persons with Addison's disease develop _____. Because of _____, they commonly have _____ potassium levels. Other common laboratory findings include (list three) _____, _____, _____.

17. A stimulatory test to test adrenal reserve is the _____ test. It is done by giving _____ and measuring serum cortisol levels at _____. A normal response is _____ or _____, _____, _____.

18. The most common cause of secondary adrenal insufficiency is _____. Other causes include _____. ACTH levels should be _____ in this disorder, therefore the patient should not have _____.

19. Treatment of primary adrenal insufficiency always includes _____. The most commonly used medications are _____ and _____. Many patients also require _____; the one commonly used is _____. Patients with secondary adrenal insufficiency do not require _____.

20. Patients with adrenal insufficiency should _____ their glucocorticoid when they are ill. If they cannot take the medication by mouth, they should _____.

21. Patients with adrenal insufficiency who present with shock, hypotension, and dehydration are said to have _____. This life-threatening condition should be treated with _____ and _____.

22. The primary mineralocorticoid in humans is _____, which is secreted by the _____ of the adrenal gland. The hormone _____ is secreted by the kidney in response to hypotension and increased serum osmolality. This hormone serves to help convert the hepatic peptide _____ into _____, which in turn is converted by the enzyme _____ into _____.

23. In addition to having potent vasoconstrictive activity, the latter compound in question 22 acts on the _____ to increase _____ production.

24. The condition of aldosterone excess is called _____, and is usually primary in origin. The most common cause is _____ followed by _____.

25. The most common laboratory finding with the condition featured in question 24 is _____.

26. List three clinical features of this disorder.

27. A simple screening test for hyperaldosteronism is the simultaneous measurement of _____ and _____. In patients with hyperaldosteronism, levels of _____ should be high, and levels of _____ should be low.

28. A _____ can help determine if an adrenal tumor is present; however, a functional test may be needed as approximately 3% of normal persons have _____.

29. A functional test designed to determine the cause of hyperaldosteronism is _____. Levels that are much higher on one side suggest _____, whereas levels that are similar suggest _____.

30. The most common cause of surgically reversible hypertension is _____; causes include _____ and _____. Increased secretion of _____ by the kidney eventually results in excess of the potent vasoconstrictor _____. This substance also increases secretion of _____ from the adrenal gland, although the latter usually plays a minor role in this disorder.

31. Some clues that suggest the presence of secondary hypertension include _____, _____, and _____.

32. The gold standard test for diagnosing RVH is _____. Less invasive tests include _____, _____, _____, _____, and _____.

33. The three treatments for RVH are _____, _____, and _____.

34. A group of steroid biosynthetic defects resulting in accumulation of various intermediates is called _____. They are inherited in _____ fashion.

35. The most common form of CAH is _____, which occurs in several different forms. The classic form is divided into _____ and _____ forms. The accumulation of _____ leads to _____ and _____ in young males and females. Females develop _____. A useful biochemical marker is the steroid intermediate _____. Treatment is _____.

36. A less severe form of CAH, the _____ form, is the most common form of 21-hydroxylase deficiency and one of the most common inherited disorders. It can result in _____ and _____ in young women if not treated.

37. Another form of CAH that can result in salt-wasting, male and female pseudohermaphrodism (appearance opposite that of the genetic sex), and infertility is _____.

38. Two types of CAH that can cause hypertension are _____ and _____. _____ leads to androgen accumulation and virilization, whereas _____ leads to inadequate androgen production and feminization of genetic males.

39. The major secretory product of the adrenal medulla in humans is _____. This and the other catecholamines are synthesized from the amino acid _____.

40. List three stimuli for adrenal medullary secretion.

41. A neuroendocrine tumor resulting in catecholamine excess is _____. _____% occur in the adrenal gland, whereas _____% are extra-adrenal in origin. _____% are benign.

42. List five clinical features of the condition in question 41.

43. The traditional method of diagnosing pheochromocytoma is to measure _____. Measurement of _____ during an attack is also useful.

44. List three imaging studies that are useful in the localization of pheochromocytoma.

45. Initial treatment of pheochromocytoma includes administration of _____ until the hypertension is controlled. Later, _____ may be required to control tachycardia. The definitive treatment is _____. For patients with metastatic or unresectable disease, the inhibitor of catecholamine synthesis _____ may be required.

II. MULTIPLE CHOICE

Select the one best answer.

46. A 54-year-old man presents with a 6-month history of gradual weight gain, muscle weakness, central obesity, and hypertension. On examination he is noted to have marked truncal obesity, moon facies, purple striae, and numerous ecchymoses. His blood pressure is 176/115. Laboratory studies demonstrate:

    Serum K$^+$: 2.9 mEq/L (normal: 3.5–5.0)

    Urinary free cortisol: 332 μg/24 hours (normal: 15–55)

    Serum cortisol after overnight dexamethasone suppression 23.4 μg/dL (normal: 5)

    Serum ACTH (peripheral blood): 3478 pg/mL (normal: 20–100)

    Serum ACTH from left inferior petrosal sinus: 3342 pg/mL; right 3122 pg/mL (normal: 20–100)

    Which is the most likely diagnosis?

    a. primary aldosteronism
    b. exogenous steroid ingestion
    c. Cushing's disease
    d. cortisol-producing adrenal cortical adenoma
    e. ectopic ACTH syndrome

47. A 52-year-old white female presents with a 5-year history of hypertension. Her blood pressure is 175/95. A 10-mm right adrenal tumor is noted on CT scan of the abdomen. Laboratory studies demonstrate:

    Serum K$^+$: 3.2 mEq/L (normal: 3.5–5.0)

    Serum Na$^+$: 142 mEq/L (normal: 135–145)

Plasma renin activity (supine): 0.2 ng/mL/hr (normal: 0.3–2.0)

Plasma aldosterone (supine): 21 ng/dL (normal: 2–6)

Adrenal vein sampling (with ACTH stimulation) for aldosterone demonstrates:

SAMPLING SITE	ALDOSTERONE (ng/dL)	CORTISOL (μg/dL)
Left adrenal	1340 ng/mL	433.2
Right adrenal	1410 ng/mL	378.5
Inferior vena cava below adrenals	45 ng/mL	43.2
Inferior vena cava above adrenals	72 ng/mL	37.8

A. This woman most likely has:

    a. renovascular hypertension
    b. primary aldosteronism due to right adrenal adenoma
    c. primary aldosteronism due to bilateral hyperplasia
    d. primary aldosteronism due to left adrenal adenoma
    e. diabetes insipidus

B. The best treatment would be:

    a. medical therapy
    b. right adrenalectomy
    c. left adrenalectomy
    d. bilateral adrenalectomy
    e. renal artery angioplasty

48. Of the following, which one is the most common cause of reversible hypertension?
    a. renovascular hypertension
    b. Cushing's disease
    c. pheochromocytoma
    d. ingestion of oral contraceptives
    e. primary aldosteronism

49. Which one of the following is not an effect of cortisol excess?
    a. diminished bone mass
    b. increased muscle mass

c. glucose intolerance

d. increased neutrophil count

e. sodium and water retention

50. Which finding might you see in persons with Addison's disease but not secondary adrenal insufficiency?

    a. hyponatremia

    b. hypoglycemia

    c. weakness

    d. hypotension

    e. hyperkalemia

51. A 39-year-old woman presents with truncal obesity, hypertension, moon facies, and new onset diabetes. Multiple purplish abdominal striae are present. The 24-hour urinary cortisol is several times normal. Urine free cortisol suppresses by > 80% (of baseline) on high-dose dexamethasone testing, but not on low-dose. Her ACTH level is three times normal. Sellar MRI demonstrates a 10-mm pituitary tumor. This patient most likely has:

    a. Cushing's syndrome due to adrenocortical carcinoma

    b. Cushing's disease

    c. iatrogenic steroid excess

    d. hyperaldosteronism

    e. ectopic ACTH syndrome

52. The technique of petrosal sinus sampling is designed to:

    a. establish the diagnosis of Cushing's syndrome.

    b. distinguish between adrenal adenomas and adrenal carcinomas.

    c. distinguish between adrenal adenomas and ectopic ACTH syndrome.

    d. distinguish between Cushing's disease and ectopic ACTH syndrome.

    e. distinguish between Cushing's disease and adrenal adenomas.

53. A 46-year-old woman notes the recent onset of increased body hair. Examination shows increased facial hair and body hair, male pattern baldness, clitoral hypertrophy, and a deep voice. Blood pressure is 190/100, and serum potassium is low. There is a palpable abdominal mass in the left upper quadrant. The most likely diagnosis is:

    a. congenital adrenal hyperplasia

    b. polycystic ovarian syndrome

    c. Cushing's disease

    d. virilizing adrenal carcinoma

    e. idiopathic hirsutism

54. A 45-year-old man is seen for hypertension that is refractory to several medicines. Laboratory studies, including 24-hour urine catecholamines, electrolytes, aldosterone, and renin levels, are normal. Physical examination is unremarkable except for hypertension. He undergoes a nuclear renogram before and after enalapril (an angiotensin-converting enzyme inhibitor). This shows no significant difference in uptake between the right and left kidneys. The results of these tests are most consistent with:

    a. renovascular hypertension

    b. hyperaldosteronism

    c. "essential" hypertension

    d. pheochromocytoma

    e. Cushing's syndrome

55. The *initial* treatment of a patient with pheochromocytoma should be:

    a. propranolol

    b. surgery

    c. radiation therapy

    d. phenoxybenzamine

    e. chemotherapy

56. A patient with neurofibromatosis has a higher incidence of developing:

    a. Cushing's disease

    b. ectopic ACTH syndrome

    c. pheochromocytoma

    d. hyperaldosteronism

    e. Addison's disease

57. A 37-year-old male presents with weakness and fatigue. He was quite large and muscular

as a young child but stopped growing before age 10, resulting in adult short stature. Examination demonstrates a short, stocky man with male pattern baldness. He has a small penis but no testes. Serum testosterone is in the upper normal limits for a male, and serum ACTH is elevated. This man's problem is the result of:

    a. autonomous adrenal production of steroids with low ACTH

    b. autonomous pituitary production of ACTH

    c. failure to produce an adrenal product necessary to cause negative feedback on pituitary ACTH secretion

    d. excessive conversion of estradiol to testosterone in the periphery

    e. excessive cortisol production from an ectopic source

58. A 13-year-old girl noticed amenorrhea, weight gain, and striae 3 months ago. She states that the symptoms are better now and that she has lost some weight. Examination shows slight facial plethora and ecchymoses; blood pressure is 140/80. Urine free cortisol and ACTH levels are normal. Three months later she presents with worsening symptoms, and urine free cortisol is elevated at 245 μg/24 hours (normal: < 50). ACTH level is approximately twice normal. This girl probably has:

    a. factitious Cushing's syndrome due to illicit steroid use

    b. cyclic or "periodic" Cushing's syndrome

    c. Cushing's syndrome due to adrenal adenoma

    d. Cushing's syndrome due to adrenocortical carcinoma

    e. pheochromocytoma

59. A 68-year-old woman presents to your office complaining of peripheral visual loss. She was diagnosed with Cushing's disease in 1964 and underwent bilateral adrenalectomy. Her medications include hydrocortisone, fludrocortisone, estrogen, and a diuretic (for hypertension). Physical examination reveals a dark-skinned Caucasian woman with increased melanin pigment in her skin folds. She has bitemporal hemianopsia on visual field testing. This woman's problem is due to:

    a. Addison's disease

    b. recurrent Cushing's disease

    c. hemochromatosis

    d. Nelson's syndrome

    e. acromegaly

60. A 10-year-old boy, who has known primary adrenal insufficiency, is having increasing cognitive dysfunction and emotional lability, and has developed a dystaxic gait. He most likely has:

    a. adrenomyeloneuropathy

    b. 17-hydroxylase deficiency

    c. adrenoleukodystrophy

    d. P450 aromatase deficiency

    e. StAR deficiency

III. TRUE OR FALSE

61. Glucocorticoids synthetically modified to have decreased mineralocorticoid activity include:

    ___ a. methylprednisolone

    ___ b. cortisone

    ___ c. prednisone

    ___ d. dexamethasone

    ___ e. hydrocortisone.

62. Adrenocortical carcinomas can cause:

    ___ a. hyperaldosteronism

    ___ b. catecholamine excess

    ___ c. Cushing's syndrome

    ___ d. virilization

    ___ e. feminization

63. Figure 4-18 shows an abdominal CT scan taken to evaluate a patient's abdominal pain. Correct management at this time might include:

    ___ a. surgical removal

    ___ b. biochemical evaluation for hyperfunction

    ___ c. repeat CT scan in 6 months

    ___ d. biopsy

    ___ e. MRI scan

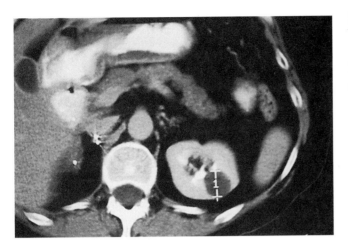

Figure 4-18. Abdominal CT of patient in question 63.

64. The oral metyrapone test

____ a. increases levels of 11-deoxycortisol in patients with ectopic ACTH syndrome.

____ b. should be used with caution in patients with suspected adrenal insufficiency.

____ c. decreases levels of cortisol in patients with Cushing's disease.

____ d. increases corticosterone levels in patients with Cushing's disease.

____ e. does not change the levels of 11-deoxycortisol in patients with functioning adrenal tumors

IV. MATCHING

Match each item with the appropriate answer. Each may be used only once.

65. Each of the three patients below presents to the emergency room.
    Match each patient with the appropriate clinical disorder.

____ A. 34-year-old man has central obesity, moon facies, purple striae; he is comatose but wears a bracelet that says "Renal Transplant Patient."

____ B. A 23-year-old woman has a 6-month history of increased pigmentation, weight loss, anorexia, weakness, and vitiligo.

____ C. A 45-year-old man has a history of weakness, anorexia, loss of libido, and loss of hair on his body. His skin is normal in color but dry and scaly.

____ D. A 34-year-old male has short stature, but is well virilized. His was very tall as a young child. He ran out of all medications.

a. Addison's disease

b. secondary adrenal insufficiency

c. 21-hydroxylase deficiency

d. hypopituitarism

66. Match the adrenal enzyme defect with the metabolite(s) that accumulate.

____ A. 21α-hydroxylase deficiency

____ B. 11β-hydroxylase deficiency

____ C. 3β-hydroxysteroid dehydrogenase deficiency

____ D. 17α-hydroxylase deficiency

a. 17-hydroxypregnenolone

b. pregnenolone, progesterone

c. 17-hydroxyprogesterone, progesterone

d. 11-deoxycortisol

ANSWERS

1. cortex, medulla

2. glucocorticoids, mineralocorticoids, sex steroids; catecholamines

3. zona glomerulosa, aldosterone; zona fasciculata, cortisol (glucocorticoids); zona reticularis, sex steroids

4. zona fasciculata, zona reticularis; ACTH (adrenocorticotrophic hormone); CRH (corticotropin-releasing hormone)

5. cortisol (hydrocortisone), transcortin (corticosteroid-binding globulin)

6. List three: illness, fever, pain, hypoglycemia, shock (severe stresses on the body)

7. Cushing's syndrome; iatrogenic; ACTH-secreting pituitary tumor, Cushing's disease, ectopic ACTH syndrome, adrenocortical adenoma, adrenocortical carcinoma

8. List five: obesity, facial plethora, hirsutism, menstrual irregularity, hypertension, muscle weakness, osteoporosis, pigmented abdominal striae

9. overnight (1 mg) dexamethasone suppression test (DST), 24-hour urinary free cortisol

10. low-dose DST; ACTH level; high-dose DST; petrosal sinus sampling

11. serum ACTH level; suppressed, elevated

12. adrenocortical adenoma; adrenocortical carcinoma

13. removal of pituitary tumor; Nelson's syndrome; surgical resection; treatment of primary tumor; inhibitors of glucocorticoid synthesis (e.g., ketoconazole)

14. Addison's disease; autoimmune, tuberculosis

15. List six: weakness, fatigue, anorexia, weight loss, hyperpigmentation, hypotension, nausea/vomiting, salt craving, depression

16. ACTH, hyperpigmentation; decreased aldosterone levels, elevated. List three: hyponatremia, anemia, hypoglycemia, elevated BUN/creatinine, hypercalcemia

17. cosyntropin (ACTH) stimulation test; cosyntropin 0.25 mg IV or IM; baseline, 30 minutes, and 60 minutes; peak serum cortisol > 18 μg/dL, increase from baseline > 7 μg/dL

18. iatrogenic steroid excess; pituitary or hypothalamic disease; decreased; hyperpigmentation

19. glucocorticoids; cortisone acetate, hydrocortisone; mineralocorticoids; fludrocortisone; mineralocorticoids

20. increase; take injectable steroids (hydrocortisone)

21. adrenal crisis; intravenous hydrocortisone, intravenous fluids (normal saline)

22. aldosterone, zona glomerulosa; renin; angiotensinogen, angiotensin I, angiotensin-converting enzyme, angiotensin II

23. adrenal gland (zona glomerulosa), aldosterone

24. hyperaldosteronism; adrenal adenoma, bilateral hyperplasia (idiopathic)

25. hypokalemia

26. List three: hypertension, edema, fatigue, weakness, paresthesias, polyuria, headaches

27. serum renin, aldosterone; aldosterone, renin

28. CT or MRI scan; incidental adrenal masses

29. adrenal vein sampling for aldosterone; adrenal adenoma, bilateral hyperplasia

30. renovascular hypertension; atherosclerosis, fibromuscular hyperplasia; renin, angiotensin II; aldosterone

31. rapidly worsening hypertension, onset of hypertension before age 25 or after age 55, diastolic renal bruit on physical examination

32. renal arteriogram; renal vein renin sampling, ACE inhibitor renogram, high-resolution (spiral) CT, duplex ultrasound, MRI.

33. surgical correction, percutaneous angioplasty, medical

34. congenital adrenal hyperplasia (CAH); autosomal recessive

35. 21-hydroxylase deficiency; salt-wasting, non-salt wasting; androgens, virilization, precocious puberty; pseudohermaphrodism; 17-hydroxyprogesterone; glucocorticoid (and possibly mineralocorticoid) replacement

36. nonclassic or "cryptic"; hirsutism, infertility

37. 3β-hydroxysteroid dehydrogenase (3β-HSD) deficiency

38. 17-hydroxylase deficiency, 11-hydroxylase deficiency; 11-hydroxylase deficiency, 17-hydroxylase deficiency

39. epinephrine; tyrosine

40. List three stressors: exercise, surgery, sepsis, myocardial infarction, hypoglycemia, trauma

41. pheochromocytoma; 90%; 10%; 90%

42. List five: headache, diaphoresis, tachycardia, anxiety, abdominal or chest pain, nausea/vomiting, tremors, hypertension

43. 24-hour urinary collection for catecholamines or metabolites (metanephrines or vanillylmandelic acid); plasma catecholamines

44. List three: CT scan, MRI scan, radioiodine-labeled MIBG scan, ^{111}In-octreotide scan

45. α-blockade (phenoxybenzamine); β-blockade (propranolol); surgery; α-methyltyrosine

46. (e). This man obviously has Cushing's syndrome; the rapid onset of symptoms is typical of ectopic ACTH syndrome. The peripheral ACTH is equal to or greater than petrosal sinus ACTH, suggesting an ectopic rather than a pituitary source of ACTH.

47. A (c). This woman has hypertension with elevated aldosterone and suppressed renin levels, suggestive of primary aldosteronism. Venous sampling demonstrates similar values from both adrenals, suggestive of bilateral hyperplasia rather than an adenoma. The right-sided lesion on CT scan is thus incidental, nonfunctioning, and not the source of hyperaldosteronism. Sampling from an adenoma would have demonstrated much higher values on one side. The cortisol levels are elevated in both adrenal gland samples, verifying that the operator did successfully sample the adrenal veins instead of adjacent structures. B (a). Hyperplasia is treated medically, not surgically.

48. (d). Oral-contraceptive-induced hypertension is the most common cause of reversible hypertension.

49. (b). Cortisol is primarily a catabolic hormone that *decreases* muscle mass.

50. (e). Hyperkalemia is only seen in cases of mineralocorticoid deficiency (primary adrenal insufficiency only). The other findings can be seen with glucocorticoid deficiency.

51. (b). Clinical findings suggest Cushing's syndrome, and biochemical studies confirm the diagnosis. Suppression on high-dose but not low-dose dexamethasone is classic for Cushing's disease. The elevated ACTH and large pituitary tumor strongly suggest the diagnosis. If there is any doubt, petrosal sinus sampling could be done.

52. (d). This technique allows for sampling the petrosal sinuses, which drain blood directly from the pituitary. It provides a more accurate way of differentiating Cushing's disease from ectopic ACTH syndrome than the high-dose dexamethasone suppression test. With Cushing's disease, petrosal sinus ACTH should be higher than peripheral ACTH. Petrosal sinus ACTH is equal to or less than peripheral ACTH in the ectopic ACTH syndrome.

53. (d). Rapid onset of virilization with a palpable abdominal mass suggests adrenocortical carcinoma. Cushing's disease (c) can cause virilization but usually not this rapidly. The other conditions are chronic disorders.

54. (c). Normal laboratory studies usually exclude pheochromocytoma, hyperaldosteronism, and Cushing's syndrome. The nuclear renogram shows similar renal flow in each side before and after the ACE inhibitor, ruling against renal artery stenosis. The patient likely has essential hypertension.

55. (d). Alpha blockade (phenoxybenzamine) should always be started first. Beta blockers (propranolol) should *never* be started until adequate alpha blockade has been achieved. Surgery should only be done after hypertension is well controlled. Radiation and chemotherapy may be of use in unresectable or metastatic disease.

56. (c). Neurofibromatosis is associated with a higher incidence of pheochromocytoma.

57. (*c*). This phenotypic male is likely a female pseudohermaphrodite with classic, non-salt wasting 21-hydroxylase deficiency. The testosterone is almost entirely adrenal in origin. Failure to make cortisol (end product) results in ACTH hypersecretion and adrenal precursor accumulation, with virilization in childhood and premature fusion of the epiphyses, hence the short stature.

58. (*b*). Waxing and waning of symptoms is a classic presentation of cyclic or periodic Cushing's syndrome. It may occur in those with Cushing's disease or ectopic ACTH syndrome. Biochemical testing may be normal in the "off" cycle, so clinicians must be careful not to dismiss complaints of persons with typical clinical findings but normal laboratory values. Cushing's syndrome due to exogenous steroids (*a*) or adrenal tumors (*c, d*) would result in low ACTH levels. Pheochromocytoma (*e*) does not cause these symptoms.

59. (*d*). Nelson's syndrome occurs in those with ACTH-secreting pituitary tumors who have undergone adrenalectomy. This surgery was commonly done in the past before the advent of CT, MRI, and pituitary microsurgery. Without cortisol suppression from the adrenal glands, the tumor enlarges, and may produce mass effects such as bitemporal hemianopsia. The skin may be dark due to increased ACTH levels. The treatment is removal of the pituitary mass.

60. (*c*). The history of adrenal insufficiency and progressive neurologic deficits in a young male suggests adrenoleukodystrophy, an X-linked disorder occurring in approximately 1 in 25,000 males. A milder form, adrenomyeloneuropathy, occurs in later life. 17-Hydroxylase deficiency, P450 aromatase deficiency, and StAR (steroidogenic acute regulatory protein) deficiency are all congenital enzyme defects resulting in congenital adrenal hyperplasia. They may cause adrenal insufficiency but not these neurologic findings.

61. True (*a, c, d*); False (*b, e*). Hydrocortisone (cortisol) is a naturally occurring glucocorticoid with inherent mineralocorticoid activity. The naturally occurring cortisone is easily converted to cortisol by 11β-hydroxysteroid dehydrogenase. The others are synthetically modified to have more potent glucocorticoid activity while minimizing mineralocorticoid activity. This is beneficial when the salt-retaining properties are not desired, as for treatment of patients with chronic pulmonary or rheumatologic disease.

62. True (*a, c, d, e*); False (*b*). Cortical tumors can hypersecrete any hormone normally made there (i.e., aldosterone, corticosteroids, sex steroids). Catecholamines are made in the medulla and are therefore not secreted by pure cortical tumors.

63. True (*b, c*); False (*a, d, e*). This is an "incidental" left adrenal mass that was discovered while looking for other pathology. Because it is small (about 2 cm) it is not likely to be malignant. Biochemical evaluation for hyperfunction should be done. If the result is negative, a repeat CT in 6 months, 1 year, and 2 years is indicated. Biopsy and surgical removal are not indicated. An MRI scan would provide no short additional information.

64. True (*b, c, e*); False (*a, d*). Metyrapone inhibits 11β-hydroxylase and decreases cortisol synthesis in all patients. Those with a partially intact feedback loop (Cushing's disease) respond with increased ACTH levels and increased 11-deoxycortisol and 11-deoxycorticosterone levels. ACTH levels do not increase further in those with ectopic ACTH syndrome (*a*). Metyrapone must be used cautiously in those with suspected adrenal insufficiency (*b*). Corticosterone levels (*d*) decrease in all patients. Those with functioning adrenal tumors (*e*) have no increase in 11-deoxycortisol or 11-deoxycorticosterone levels.

65. A (*b*); B (*a*); C (*d*); D (*c*)

66. A (*c*); B (*d*); C (*a*); D (*b*)

CHAPTER 5

GLUCOSE METABOLISM

Q: What is diabetes mellitus?

A: **Diabetes mellitus** is a disease of glucose metabolism. The name is derived from the Greek words *diabetes* (siphon) and *mellitus* (sweet), and it was first described in an Egyptian papyrus dated 1500 BC. The ancients noted that ants were attracted to urine of diabetics because of the high glucose content. They also made a distinction between two types of diabetes. The first form was noted to occur in children and young adults who were thin. These persons essentially "wasted away" and had a dismal future, with death occurring in 1 to 2 years. This type of diabetes, now referred to as **type 1 diabetes,** results from **absence** or **deficiency of insulin.** Another form was described in older, overweight individuals; this form, now known as **type 2 diabetes**, is caused by **impaired insulin action** or **insulin resistance.** These persons typically lived for many years.

Q: How common is diabetes?

A: Diabetes is an extremely common disorder, affecting approximately 5% of the U.S. population. Type 2 is the most common form, accounting for 90% of those with diabetes. The prevalence of type 2 has increased as obesity and sedentary lifestyles have become more common. The remaining 10% have type 1 diabetes; the highest incidence occurs in northern European nations (e.g., Sweden, Finland). Diabetes is an enormous economic problem; one out of every seven health care dollars is spent on diabetes and its complications.

Q: What are the symptoms of diabetes?

A: The typical triad of diabetes symptoms, often called the "polys," includes **polydipsia** (excessive thirst), **polyphagia** (excessive eating), and **polyuria** (excessive urination). Weight loss and fatigue are also typical.

Q: How is diabetes diagnosed?

A: There are three accepted ways of diagnosing diabetes:

1. Two fasting blood glucose (serum) levels $\geq$ 126 mg/dL (7.0 mmol/L).

2. Typical signs and symptoms of diabetes, with a random blood glucose ≥ 200 mg/dL (11.1 mmol/L).

3. A 2-hour **glucose tolerance test** (GTT) with 75-gram glucose load; 2-hour glucose ≥ 200 mg/dL.

Diabetes should be diagnosed only with serum glucose levels; glucometer readings should not be used.

Q: Should diabetes be diagnosed in ill or hospitalized patients?

A: The three usual criteria (with the exception of the second) are generally intended for stable outpatients. A patient with new onset diabetic ketoacidosis obviously has diabetes. Other patients with impaired glucose tolerance may exhibit "stress hyperglycemia" when confronted with a serious illness (such as sepsis or myocardial infarction). Normoglycemia may return after the illness abates. Truly *normal* persons do not develop stress hyperglycemia; there must be some component of impaired insulin reserve and/or insulin insensitivity for the condition to occur. If the person is hyperglycemic, he or she must be treated with whatever means necessary (insulin, oral agents, etc.); whether the label "diabetes" is given is a matter of semantics, and treatment must be individualized. These patients must be monitored closely after discharge, as they most certainly have impaired glucose tolerance and are likely to develop diabetes in the future.

Q: What is impaired glucose tolerance?

A: Impaired glucose tolerance (IGT) occurs in individuals with mild hyperglycemia who do not meet the criteria for diabetes. They fall in a gray area, and should be followed closely for development of overt diabetes. IGT is diagnosed with a 2-hour (75-gram) oral glucose tolerance test (OGTT) (75-gram glucose load); a 2-hour glucose level ≥ 140 mg/dL (7.8 mmol/L); but 200 mg/dL (11.1 mmol/L) with any intermediate value ≥ 200 mg/dL is diagnostic.

Another category of impaired glucose tolerance, impaired fasting glucose (IFG), applies to persons with fasting glucose ≥ 110 mg/dL (6.1 mmol/L) but < 126 mg/dL.

Q: Do patients with impaired glucose intolerance develop diabetes?

A: Approximately 30% of those with IGT develop type 2 diabetes over a 10-year period. Fifty percent continue to have IGT, while the remaining persons revert to normal after several years. Those with type 2 diabetes may also convert to IGT if they lose weight or if a secondary cause (e.g., corticosteroid therapy) is removed.

Q: What is insulin?

A: Insulin is a peptide hormone produced in the β cells of the pancreas. Insulin starts as the precursor molecule **preproinsulin,** which is then cleaved to proinsulin in the endoplasmic reticulum (Fig. 5-1). **Proinsulin** is a single 86-amino acid peptide consisting of A and B chains (connected at two places by disulfide bridges) and a C chain. In the Golgi apparatus, proinsulin is then converted to the 51-amino acid insulin molecule, four amino acid residues, and a 31-amino acid residue, **C-peptide.** C-peptide is secreted with insulin in equimolar amounts; it appears to have no biological activity. Other, inactive cleavage products exist at lower concentrations.

Q: What is the function of insulin?

A: Insulin is an anabolic hormone that promotes energy storage. It promotes glycogen synthesis and triglyceride storage, and inhibits glycogenolysis, hepatic ketogenesis, and gluconeogenesis. Insulin increases glucose transport across cell membranes by means of glucose transporters (GLUT). So far, five different glucose transporter proteins have been identified.

Insulin is secreted in response to hyperglycemia. Inhibitors include hypoglycemia and the pancreatic hormone somatostatin (also a hypothalamic hormone). Drugs such as sulfonylureas and repaglinide stimulate insulin release.

Q: What is glucagon?

A: Glucagon is a 29-amino acid peptide made in the α-cells of the pancreas. Its function is mainly **catabolic** (to provide energy for cells), in contrast to

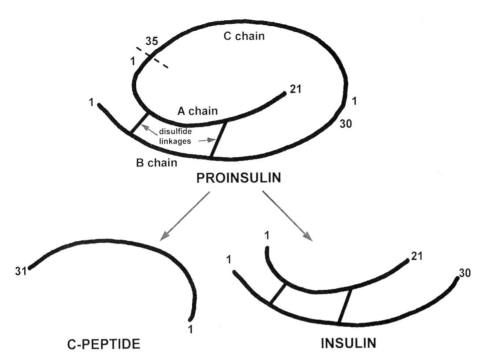

Figure 5-1.   Proinsulin and cleavage products.

insulin, which is anabolic in nature. Secretion is inhibited by high glucose and fatty acid levels, and is stimulated by hypoglycemia. Glucagon is important in recovery from hypoglycemia; type 1 diabetics eventually lose their glucagon response to hypoglycemia.

Q: What is type 1 diabetes?

A: Type 1 diabetes, also called **insulin-dependent diabetes mellitus** (IDDM), results from the absence or deficiency of insulin. Type 1 is typically an autoimmune disease, resulting in destruction of **pancreatic islet cells** by **anti-islet cell antibodies** (Fig. 5-2). Deficiency of insulin results in hyperglycemia, ketoacidosis, and death if untreated. Type 1 may also result from destruction of islet cells by other diseases (e.g., pancreatitis), or if the pancreas is removed.

Q: How is type 1 diabetes (IDDM) inherited?

A: Like many other autoimmune endocrine diseases, predisposition for IDDM is carried by HLA haplotypes on chromosome 6. HLA-DR3 and DR4 are associated with type 1 diabetes; HLA-DR2 is protective. However, having the genetic predisposition alone is not enough; for IDDM to occur there must be some triggering of the autoimmune process by a stimulus (possibly exposure to an environmental antigen or virus). The concordance rate for identical twins is only about 50% to 60%, versus nearly 100% for type 2 diabetes.

Q: What causes type 1 diabetes?

A: Islet cell antibodies (ICA) result in inflammation and destruction of the islet cells, with preservation of exocrine cells. There are subclasses of islet cell antibodies, such as those produced against the islet cell surface, against insulin (autoantibodies to insulin), cytotoxic islet cell antibodies, and antibodies to glutamic acid decarboxylase (GAD). About 70% of new-onset type 1 diabetics have positive islet cell antibodies at the time of diagnosis. Levels may be detected several years before clinical diabetes results. Eventually, antibody levels diminish in most patients.

Q: Are all type 1 diabetics young when diagnosed?

A: Although the onset of IDDM is most common in children and young adults, IDDM may occur at any age, even in adults in their 40s, 50s, or 60s. The distinction is important, as patients with IDDM have an absolute requirement for insulin to prevent ketoacidosis and death.

TYPE I (INSULIN-DEPENDENT) DIABETES

PATHOGENESIS: DESTRUCTION OF PANCREAS
IMMUNOLOGIC: MOST COMMON CAUSE (ANTI-ISLET CELL ANTIBODIES)

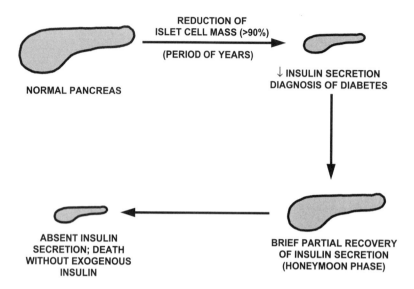

NORMAL PANCREAS

REDUCTION OF
ISLET CELL MASS (>90%)

(PERIOD OF YEARS)

↓ INSULIN SECRETION
DIAGNOSIS OF DIABETES

ABSENT INSULIN
SECRETION; DEATH
WITHOUT EXOGENOUS
INSULIN

BRIEF PARTIAL RECOVERY
OF INSULIN SECRETION
(HONEYMOON PHASE)

Figure 5-2. Type I diabetes.

Q: What is the honeymoon period of type I diabetes?

A: At the time they are first diagnosed, type 1 diabetics typically still have a substantial insulin reserve. Because of this reserve, a brief state of "remission" may occur after treatment begins, in which symptoms and glucose levels normalize. This **honeymoon phase** is short lived (typically several months), and is followed by absolute dependence on exogenous insulin. Aggressive treatment with insulin during this period is recommended, as it appears to preserve the insulin reserve.

Q: What is type 2 diabetes?

A: Unlike type 1, which is a state of insulin deficiency, **type 2 diabetes** is a state of **insulin resistance**, in which insulin receptors lose their sensitivity to insulin (Fig. 5.3), hence the term **non-insulin-dependent diabetes mellitus** (NIDDM). Insulin secretion initially is normal; in fact, insulin levels are often elevated early in the disorder, leading to **hyperinsulinism**. In time, impaired glucose tolerance (IGT) occurs, followed by overt hyperglycemia and development of diabetes mellitus. Most patients with type 2 are asymptomatic at the time of diagnosis and are diagnosed by routine screening, since only 25% present with typical signs and symptoms. Type 2 is far more common than type 1, accounting for 90% of persons with diabetes. It is more common in certain ethnic groups (African Americans, Hispanic Americans, and Native Americans).

Q: Are all persons with type 2 diabetes obese?

A: Type 2 diabetes is a very heterogeneous disorder, affecting patients of all body shapes and sizes. The majority of patients (85%) are overweight, however, which contributes to insulin resistance and hyperglycemia.

Q: How is type 2 diabetes (NIDDM) inherited?

A: NIDDM is a heterogeneous disorder, with multifactorial inheritance. Penetrance is quite high; if one identical twin has NIDDM, the chance that the other will have it approaches 100% (in contrast to IDDM, in which the likelihood of a second twin being affected is only about 50% to 60%).

NIDDM may rarely be inherited in autosomal dominant fashion; this occurs in the maturity-onset diabetes of the young (MODY) syndrome. These are individuals with early onset of ketosis-resistant diabetes that may be controlled with oral

TYPE 2 (NON-INSULIN DEPENDENT) DIABETES

PATHOGENESIS: INEFFECTIVE USE OF ENDOGENOUS INSULIN
EVENTUAL DECREASE OF BETA CELL MASS OVER YEARS

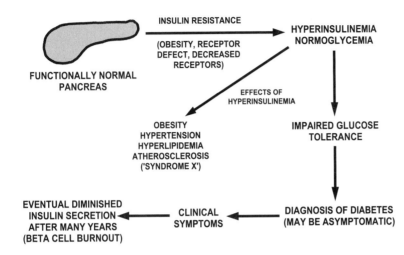

Figure 5-3. Type 2 diabetes.

agents, although some patients will require insulin. The patient typically has several first-degree relatives with the same disorder.

Q: What is glucose toxicity?

A: **Glucose toxicity** is a phenomenon occurring in type 2 diabetics in which hyperglycemia impairs insulin secretion, resulting in low insulin and C-peptide levels. Restoration of normoglycemia may improve insulin secretion, and patients who in-

itially required large doses of insulin may be controllable on oral agents or even diet.

Q: What is "syndrome X"?

A: **Syndrome X** refers to the constellation of metabolic problems that results from chronic obesity, insulin resistance, and hyperinsulinism: atherosclerotic disease, glucose intolerance, hypertension, and hyperlipidemia (predominantly hypertriglyceridemia) (Fig. 5-4). These problems may not present at

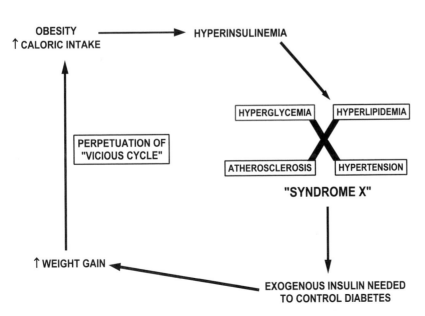

Figure 5-4. Hyperinsulinism and syndrome X.

the same time; for example, a patient may experience hypertension and hypertriglyceridemia years before developing diabetes mellitus.

Q: **What is the mechanism of insulin resistance in type 2 diabetes?**

A: The most common reason for insulin resistance is obesity, which results in a reversible decrease in receptors and receptor binding. Not all diabetics with this type of resistance are obese, however (15%). Excess growth hormone (acromegaly) and glucocorticoids (Cushing's syndrome) produce similar defects in susceptible persons.

Two uncommon forms of insulin resistance occur, both with acanthosis nigricans. The first is seen in young women with hyperinsulinism and hyperandrogenism, with associated features of the latter (polycystic ovaries, hirsutism, amenorrhea). These women, who have **type A insulin resistance,** appear to have either deficient or mutant receptors. **Type B insulin resistance** occurs in older women who have insulin receptor antibodies that decrease insulin activity. They often have high titers of other autoantibodies, evidence of other systemic autoimmune disease, and absence of androgenic features.

Q: **What are some ways to distinguish type 1 from type 2 diabetes?**

A: The two types of diabetes are usually not difficult to distinguish (Table 5-1). For example, a teenager with the ketoacidosis of type 1 diabetes is easily distinguished from an obese middle-aged individual with type 2 diabetes. A strong family history is also more suggestive of type 2 diabetes. Not all type 2 patients are obese, however. The distinction becomes less clear in the middle-aged adult who is thin, as there are exceptions to the general rules. Type 2 diabetes may occur in thin individuals and in teenagers or young adults (as with maturity-onset diabetes of the young, MODY), and type 1 diabetes may occur in overweight or older individuals. Serum insulin and C-peptide levels are typically elevated in newly diagnosed type 2 patients.

Generally, patients with type 1 diabetes require relatively low doses of insulin (0.4–0.7 U/kg/day) as compared to those with type 2, and are often prone to unexplained swings of hyper- and hypoglycemia. Patients with type 2, however, often require larger insulin doses (>1 U/kg/day) and are less prone to hypoglycemia. After many years, those with type 2 lose insulin reserve and may behave like type 1 diabetics.

Q: **Why is the fasting glucose often high in those with type 2 diabetes?**

A: Much of the phenomenon of elevated fasting glucose in type 2 diabetics is related to increased hepatic gluconeogenesis at night. Increased growth hormone secretion at night (the *dawn phenomenon*) also increases insulin resistance and contributes to fasting hyperglycemia.

TABLE 5-1.   Typical Features of Type 1 and Type 2 Diabetes

	TYPE 2 DIABETES	TYPE 1 DIABETES
Age at onset	Middle age	Child or young adult
Body habitus	Overweight (85%)	Thin
Insulin and C-peptide levels	Increased initially; decreased after many years	Decreased
Islet cell autoantibody	Negative	Positive in 70%
Ketosis	Resistant	Develops without insulin
Response to oral agent	Usually good; insulin may be needed eventually	Poor
Insulin requirements	Often high	Relatively lower
Hypoglycemia	Less common (early)	Often frequent

Q: What is the euglycemic clamp?

A: The **euglycemic clamp** is a technique used to measure insulin kinetics and sensitivity. The patient is connected to an "artificial pancreas" in which insulin is infused intravenously at a constant rate. Glucose is then infused automatically by the apparatus to keep the glucose at a steady state (e.g., 100 mg/dL). This is accomplished by means of an intravenous glucose sensor that provides feedback to the device. The amount of glucose needed for a given insulin infusion rate is recorded.

This is an elegant method of measuring insulin effects in vivo in humans. Those who are very insulin resistant (i.e., type 2 diabetics) require relatively little glucose to maintain normoglycemia when compared to normal individuals. Those who are more sensitive to insulin require more glucose for a given insulin infusion rate. This tool has done much to further the investigation of insulin resistance and type 2 diabetes.

Q: What is MODY?

A: **Maturity-onset diabetes of the young** (MODY) is an atypical form of type 2 diabetes occurring in teenagers or young adults. In contrast to the more common form of type 2 diabetes, which is multifactorial in inheritance, MODY is inherited in autosomal dominant fashion. There are several distinct genetic defects that have been described. The patient typically has several first-degree relatives with ketosis-resistant diabetes that developed at a young age. Most MODY patients can be controlled on oral agents, although insulin may be required.

These patients are ketosis-resistant, relatively resistant to complications, and most are not obese. MODY is an uncommon disorder in Caucasians with diabetes; its incidence is much higher in diabetics of other ethnic groups (such as African Americans, Hispanic Americans). MODY patients lack the HLA-DR3/DR4 association with type 1 diabetes and do not have anti-islet cell antibodies.

Q: What is secondary diabetes?

A: **Secondary diabetes** is diabetes due to another condition. Diabetes may occur after repeated episodes of pancreatitis, because of reduction in β-cell mass; approximately 80% of islet mass must be destroyed for clinical hyperglycemia to occur. Pancreatectomy obviously results in insulin deficiency and insulin-dependent diabetes.

Infiltrative diseases may result in pancreatic destruction and hyperglycemia. The most common cause is **hemochromatosis**, which results in excessive iron accumulation in visceral organs and pancreatic destruction. This condition is also called "bronze diabetes" because of the dark skin pigmentation that results from iron accumulation.

Many drugs can induce hyperglycemia. Individuals taking long-term glucocorticoids can develop "steroid diabetes." Thiazide diuretics, octreotide, and phenytoin may impair insulin secretion and cause hyperglycemia. These persons typically have an underlying predisposition to glucose intolerance.

Q: What is gestational diabetes mellitus?

A: **Gestational diabetes mellitus** (GDM) develops during pregnancy, as opposed to preexisting forms of diabetes (type 1 or 2). Usually, the term is applied to a state of glucose intolerance that occurs in the late second trimester of pregnancy in about 3% of pregnant women. Its diagnosis precludes a previous diagnosis of diabetes. As the growing fetoplacental unit increases in size, substances such as human placental lactogen (hPL) and human placental growth hormone (GH) are secreted in large amounts, increasing insulin resistance. Progesterone and cortisol also may increase insulin resistance. In susceptible individuals, gestational diabetes will result. Risk factors include obesity, family history of type 2 diabetes, and advanced maternal age. Gestational diabetes usually resolves after delivery. Type 1 or 2 diabetes can also develop during pregnancy; these diseases will persist for life.

Q: How is gestational diabetes diagnosed?

A: A screening test for diabetes is done in all women at 24 to 26 weeks of gestational age by giving a 50-gram glucose load and measuring serum glucose 1 hour afterward. A value of ≥ 140 mg/dL (7.8 mmol/L) necessitates a 3-hour OGTT. These are the American Diabetes Association criteria;

others have recommended a cutoff of 130 mg/dL (7.2 mmol/L). The most commonly used criteria for diagnosis of GDM with the 3-hour, 100-gram OGTT are those of the National Diabetes Data Group (NDDG):

Fasting ≥ 105 mg/dL (5.8 mmol/L)

1-hour ≥ 190 mg/dL (10.5 mmol/L)

2-hour ≥ 165 mg/dL (9.1 mmol/L)

3-hour ≥ 145 mg/dL (8.0 mmol/L)

If two or more of the values are met or exceeded, GDM is present. These are based on serum measurements; the levels are lower if whole blood is used.

Women with a previous diagnosis of GDM or those at very high risk (morbid obesity, strong family history of diabetes) should be tested as soon as pregnancy is discovered.

Q: What are the goals of treating diabetes in pregnancy?

A: Good control of diabetes during pregnancy is important to prevent complications. The desired values, which are lower than those for non-pregnant diabetics, are based on the measurement of serum glucose levels in normal pregnant women:

Fasting 60–90 mg/dL (3.3–5.0 mmol/L)

Before meals 60–105 mg/dL (3.3–5.8 mmol/L)

2 hours after meals 120 mg/dL (6.7 mmol/L)

Q: What are the consequences of poorly controlled diabetes during pregnancy?

A: The rate of spontaneous abortion is increased in poorly controlled diabetics. Poor control during organ development results in a fourfold increase in congenital abnormalities, primarily neural tube and cardiac defects. Organ malformations occur in women with preexisting diabetes (type 1 or 2); they typically do not occur in women with gestational diabetes, because the organs are already formed by the time the glucose abnormalities occur (24 to 26 weeks of gestation).

Poor glucose control late in pregnancy can lead to **macrosomia,** an abnormally large fetus. Delivery of a large infant may be difficult and can lead to complications. Infants of poorly controlled dia-

betic mothers experience hyperglycemia during pregnancy, which can result in fetal β-cell hyperplasia to compensate. After delivery, the source of hyperglycemia (the mother's blood) is gone, and the hyperinsulinemic state leads to **neonatal hypoglycemia,** which can be severe, cause seizures, and require prolonged intravenous administration of glucose. Neonatal respiratory distress syndrome is also increased in infants of poorly controlled diabetics in the third trimester.

Patients with preexisting diabetes must have excellent control before considering pregnancy. Adequate contraceptive measures are necessary in those without optimal control.

Q: How are glucose levels monitored?

A: The best method of monitoring glucose levels is **self-monitoring of blood glucose** (SMBG) by means of a small glucose meter (Fig. 5-5). Early meters were quite cumbersome and required "wiping" the blood from the strip; newer meters are much smaller and use a non-wipe technique in which a drop of capillary blood is placed onto the test strip. The patient pricks his or her finger with an automated lancing device to obtain the blood. Newer laser lancing devices are now available. Many meters have a memory chip that stores glucose values so that the patient or physician may download the readings into a computer for easy viewing and storage. Most meters report values as whole blood values, which are 10% to 15% lower than serum (plasma) levels. Some newer meters report glucose as plasma levels.

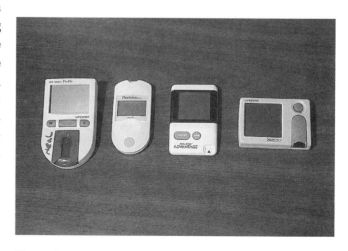

Figure 5-5. Glucose meters.

SMBG is advantageous as it provides immediate feedback of blood glucose levels. There is a direct correlation between the amount of monitoring and effective diabetes control; in one study, those who checked most often had lower glycohemoglobin levels.

The disadvantages of SMBG include inconvenience (interrupting normal daily activities) and pain (pricking the finger). Noninvasive monitoring devices are being studied, but these are still experimental. One of the major obstacles to good diabetes care is the patient who is unwilling to do SMBG. Unless patients are willing to provide information to their physician, changes in the diabetes regimen cannot be done competently.

Monitoring of urine glucose is not recommended routinely because of its inaccuracy, as the renal threshold for glucose varies among individuals. It may be used in patients who are unwilling to do SMBG.

Q: What are the goals for treatment of diabetes?

A: Treatment goals depend on the individual, and it is often useful to outline for the patient what is considered "ideal," "acceptable," and "poor" (Table 5-2). In most cases, the provider and patient should strive for the best possible control.

Q: What is the Diabetes Control and Complications Trial?

A: The Diabetes Control and Complications Trial (DCCT), completed in 1993, studied approximately 1500 patients with type 1 diabetes. Patients were randomized to receive either standard therapy (one or two injections per day) or intensive therapy (multiple daily injections or insulin infusion pump). It was shown that intensively treated patients had a lower incidence of microvascular disease (retinopathy, neuropathy, and nephropathy) than those in the standard group. It is estimated that the benefits in intensively treated patients translate into 15 extra years of life without complications.

The DCCT did not study macrovascular complications (such as coronary artery disease or peripheral vascular disease) or those with type 2 diabetes. The United Kingdom Prospective Diabetes Study (UKPDS), another major trial, studied approximately 5000 type 2 diabetics over a 20-year period. The results of this recently completed trial demonstrated that tight glucose control reduces microvascular complications in type 2 diabetics. The data regarding macrovascular disease were inconclusive. Improved blood pressure control did reduce incidence of stroke in the UKPDS.

Q: Should all patients be intensively treated?

A: Not all patients are good candidates for intensive therapy. Patients in the intensive treatment arm of the DCCT had a threefold incidence of hypoglycemia when compared to the standard treatment group. In certain patients, hypoglycemia is extremely hazardous and may cause serious morbidity or even death. This group includes elderly patients with unsteady gait and/or physical disabilities (who may suffer severe consequences if they fall down), those with severe cardiovascular disease, and those who do not recognize hypoglycemia (hypoglycemia unawareness). The latter group is especially at risk while asleep or when performing a task demanding mental and physical coordination (such as driving an automobile or using heavy machinery).

The physician must always weigh the benefits of intensive therapy against the risks of increased hypoglycemia. What is acceptable in a young, healthy adult may not be appropriate in an older individual with cardiovascular disease and unawareness of hypoglycemia.

TABLE 5-2.   Target Glucose Values (mg/dL) in Patients with Diabetes

TIME	IDEAL	ACCEPTABLE	POOR
Pre-meal	70–120	< 140	> 200
2 hours after meal	< 140	< 180	< 240

Q: What is glycated hemoglobin?

A: **Glycated** or **glycosylated hemoglobin,** a useful index of long-term diabetic control, is formed by a reaction between glucose and the *N*-terminus of the β-chains of normal hemoglobin (Hgb A). Sugar attachment to hemoglobin A results in hemoglobin A_1, totaling about 7% of hemoglobin in normal individuals. The minor forms are Hgb A_{1a} and A_{1b}, each comprising about 1% of the total hemoglobin. The most important moiety is hemoglobin A_{1c}, which totals about 5% in normal persons and thus is the major constituent of the A_1 group. It is relatively specific for glucose and thus is the most important constituent. The glucose residues make the molecules migrate faster in chromatographic or electrophoretic techniques, allowing for their separation; diabetics have more "fast" hemoglobins than their nondiabetic counterparts.

The reaction between glucose and hemoglobin is slow, irreversible, and not mediated by an enzyme. Therefore, Hgb A_1 is a time-integrated measure of the glucose concentration to which the red cell has been exposed (red cell life span is about 120 days); therefore, we should expect the glycated Hgb to reflect blood glucose over about one-half the life span of the cells (6 to 8 weeks).

Glycated hemoglobin is proportional to fasting plasma glucose concentrations in the majority of circumstances. At this point, however, the test cannot be recommended as a diagnostic test for diabetes mellitus. In most patients, the less expensive A_1 is as useful as the more expensive Hgb A_{1c}; the goal is to achieve levels of less than 8.5% for Hgb A_1 (6.5% for Hgb A_{1c}).

Q: Are there persons in whom glycohemoglobin is not accurate?

A: Normal hemoglobin must be present for the glycohemoglobin test to accurately reflect long-term glucose levels (Table 5-3). Those with hemoglobinopathies (e.g., sickle cell disease) have abnormal values. In addition, conditions that alter red cell survival will affect glycohemoglobin.

Q: Should a glycohemoglobin be used to diagnose diabetes?

A: Glycohemoglobin currently is not recommended for diagnosing diabetes. It should only be used for those persons with established disease. It is not a diagnostic test, just as cancer tumor markers should not be used to diagnose cancer.

Q: What is fructosamine?

A: **Fructosamine** is an estimate of glycated albumin and gives an estimate of serum glucose over the previous 2 weeks. It is not affected by abnormal hemoglobin and may be useful in patients in whom a glycohemoglobin is inaccurate.

Q: What are the complications of diabetes?

A: The complications of diabetes may be divided into three types:

1. Macrovascular disease (affecting the large vessels) includes coronary artery disease (angina pectoris and myocardial infarction),

TABLE 5-3.   Conditions Affecting Glycohemoglobin Values

FALSELY LOW VALUES	FALSELY HIGH VALUES
Hgb S (sickle cell)	Thalassemia
Hgb C	Uremia
Hgb SC	Hypertriglyceridemia
Conditions reducing red cell survival (hemolytic anemia, bleeding); venesection for patients with hemochromatosis.	Lead poisoning
	Hemoglobin J, K, I, H, Bart's syndrome
	Prolonged survival of red cells (e.g., splenectomy)

cerebrovascular disease (stroke), and peripheral vascular disease.

2. Microvascular disease (affecting small vessels) refers to diabetic *retinopathy* (eye disease) and *nephropathy* (renal disease).

3. Neuropathy, including peripheral nerve (somatic) and autonomic neuropathies.

Q: How do complications of diabetes occur?

A: Evidence indicates that many diabetic complications are not caused by glucose itself but by advanced glycation endproducts (AGEs). Long-term hyperglycemia causes glycation of many proteins. These products themselves may cause protein dysfunction, or may activate specific AGE receptors on the cell, causing production of deleterious products such as tumor necrosis factor and interleukins. Some AGEs appear to bind to the cell membrane, resulting in alterations (e.g., increased permeability to albumin). Experimental agents that inhibit AGE formation (e.g., aminoguanidine) are being studied in clinical trials.

Another substance implicated in the development of neuropathy is sorbitol. Glucose is converted to sorbitol by aldose reductase; excess sorbitol may contribute to diabetic neuropathy. Aldose reductase inhibitors such as tolrestat and zopolrestat inhibit sorbitol production and theoretically would improve this condition. Thus far, results with these drugs have been inconclusive.

Q: What is diabetic neuropathy?

A: **Neuropathy,** a common complication of diabetes that can result in significant morbidity, is divided into peripheral nerve (somatic) neuropathies and autonomic neuropathies (Table 5-4). The most common form of neuropathy is a **distal extremity sensory neuropathy,** resulting in chronic distal numbness in a "stocking" distribution. A common form of autonomic neuropathy is **hypoglycemia unawareness,** in which the patient is unaware when his or her glucose is low. This condition may have devastating consequences, as the person may suffer a seizure, wreck a motor vehicle, or even die without the intervention by another person.

TABLE 5-4.   Diabetic Neuropathy

I. PERIPHERAL (SOMATIC) NEUROPATHIES

Diffuse motor neuropathy
  Rare; unrelated to hyperglycemia
  Severe muscle weakness and wasting
  Minimal sensory loss

Proximal motor myopathy (amyotrophy)
  Moderate to severe pain
  Severe muscle weakness and wasting
  May present with autonomic neuropathy
  May present with hyperglycemia
  Little or no sensory loss

Chronic sensory neuropathy (most common)
  Sensory loss in a 'stocking' distribution
  Symmetrical
  Minimal to moderate muscle weakness

Acute painful neuropathy
  Rare; present with severe pain
  Minimal sensory loss

Focal nerve palsies
  Pressure: Ulnar, common peroneal
  Vascular: CN III, IV, VI, thoracoabdominal, phrenic

II. AUTONOMIC NEUROPATHIES

Orthostatic hypotension

Hypoglycemia unawareness

Sudomotor abnormalities
  Gustatory sweating

Gastrointestinal motility disorders
  Gastroparesis
  Colonic atony
  Diarrhea

Urinary retention

Pupillary dysfunction

Heart rate abnormalities
  Fixed tachycardia

Pain may occur with diabetic neuropathy, and may be very difficult to treat. The most severe form of neuropathy is called **diabetic neuropathic cachexia,** in which severe pain and muscle wasting occur. These patients often appear as if they have advanced malignancy or other severe chronic disease.

Q: What is the treatment of diabetic neuropathy?

A: Neuropathy is often difficult and frustrating to treat. The first goal must be the attainment of euglycemia, which can dramatically improve the symptoms. Narcotics should be avoided if possible, because they are addicting and generally not helpful in the long term. Non-narcotic analgesics such as ibuprofen may be useful but should be used with caution in patients with renal disease. Tricyclic antidepressants (e.g., amitriptyline) and anticonvulsants (e.g., gabapentin, carbamazepine) may be useful. Topical capsaicin cream may help alleviate painful symptoms.

Q: What is diabetic gastroparesis?

A: **Gastroparesis** is a form of diabetic autonomic neuropathy that causes delayed gastric emptying. Because stomach contents are delayed, nausea, vomiting, and early satiety (feeling full before the entire meal is eaten) may occur. Because food is absorbed erratically, poor diabetes control often develops.

Gastroparesis can be diagnosed by performing a solid-phase **gastric-emptying study.** This is a nuclear medicine procedure in which food labeled with ^{99m}Tc-sulfur colloid is administered so that the transit time through the stomach can be measured. Those with gastroparesis have a markedly delayed gastric-emptying time. Gastroparesis can also be diagnosed with direct endoscopy, which will reveal a distended stomach and retained gastric contents.

Treatment of gastropathy includes prokinetic agents. The dopamine antagonists cisapride, metoclopramide, and domperidone are useful. The macrolide antibiotic erythromycin is also prokinetic.

Other types of diabetic gastropathy include diabetic diarrhea and colonic atony, for which antidiarrheal agents (for diarrhea) and bulk-forming agents (for colonic atony) may be helpful.

Q: What is "brittle" diabetes?

A: **Brittle diabetes** is characterized by extremely erratic glucose control (unpredictable highs and lows) despite intensive therapy, which causes significant disruption of the patient's lifestyle.

This condition is common in those with autonomic neuropathy and defective counterregulatory mechanisms.

Often, the poor control can be attributed to psychosocial factors, such as family disturbances, behavior problems, depression, or anxiety. Some patients are noncompliant on purpose in order to achieve a secondary gain (absence from work, school, or home responsibilities). Eating disorders (anorexia and bulimia) should be considered in patients with weight loss. Concurrent endocrine disease (hypothyroidism, hypoadrenalism) should be excluded. Physiologic causes such as gastroparesis should also be considered. In many cases, no cause can be found. Pump therapy may benefit such patients.

Q: What foot problems do diabetics develop?

A: Patients with well-controlled diabetes without neuropathy are no more likely to develop problems than the general population. Those with neuropathy and/or peripheral vascular disease are at risk for developing foot ulceration and infection. The physician should look at the patient's feet at every visit, inspecting closely for breaks in the skin and ulceration. Peripheral pulses should be tested, and the feet should be examined for neuropathy. Many specialists use a monofilament calibrated to bend at a certain pressure level; patients unable to detect the pressure of the monofilament have neuropathy and are at risk for foot ulceration. They should be referred to a podiatrist and/or pedorthist for custom shoes. Patients with chronic foot ulcerations should be seen by a surgeon or podiatrist for further evaluation and wound care.

Foot ulcerations may require debridement and assessment of vascular status; improvement in blood supply may aid in healing. Osteomyelitis should be suspected in patients with chronic penetrating wound infections. Culture of a diabetic foot ulcer is generally unsatisfactory, as it yields mixed organisms. Osteomyelitis is best diagnosed with a bone biopsy. A three-phase bone scan may be helpful. Plain x-rays are often of little use, given the chronic changes associated with the diabetic foot. The infected diabetic foot should be treated with antibiotics with emphasis on gram-positive and anaerobic microorganisms (e.g., ampicillin or ticarcillin with clavulanic acid). Those with severe peripheral vascular disease and non-healing ulcers may require amputation. Genetically engineered platelet-derived growth factor (becaplermin), a topical gel that increases the healing of diabetic foot ulcers, may be used in refractory cases.

Q: What skin disorders are seen in diabetes?

A: The most common skin disorder is **diabetic dermopathy,** pigmented pretibial patches usually less than 1 cm in diameter. These lesions are of little clinical significance. **Necrobiosis lipoidica diabeticorum** is rare and appears as oval, erythematous, waxy plaques also on the anterior shins. Histologically, necrobiosis of collagen and inflammation around blood vessels are seen. These areas often wax and wane with the control of diabetes and may be quite friable and bleed easily.

Lipoatrophy is the atrophy of subcutaneous tissue at the site of insulin injections. It is typically autoimmune in nature. **Lipohypertrophy,** the buildup of subcutaneous tissue at the injection site, is more common. As it usually results from repeated injections in the same area, rotating injection sites may help.

Acanthosis nigricans, a grayish-brown hyperpigmentation and hyperkeratosis of the skin seen in the epidermis, is most commonly found in skin folds of the neck and axillae (Fig. 5-6). It has been associated with malignancy (especially gastrointestinal neoplasms). It also can be associated with a variety of endocrinologic disorders, the most common being insulin resistance and glucose intolerance. It may also be associated with obesity, hirsutism, polycystic ovaries, hyperandrogenemia, acromegaly, and Cushing's syndrome.

Diabetic bullae are tense blisters that appear suddenly on apparently normal skin, usually on the extremities, without evidence of trauma. These usually resolve spontaneously unless they become infected. **Eruptive xanthomas** are pustular lesions that occur on the buttocks and extensor areas (e.g.,

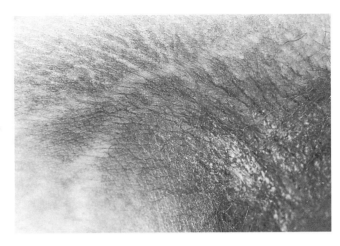

Figure 5-6.   Acanthosis nigricans.

elbows). They are seen in persons with severe hypertriglyceridemia.

Scleredema is a rare condition resulting in thickening of dermal collagen and deposition of mucopolysaccharides between collagen bundles. Broad areas of nonpitting edema and hardening of the skin on the face, neck, and upper trunk are seen.

A variety of secondary skin disorders are more common in diabetics, including *Candida albicans* infections, cutaneous bacterial infections (especially from *Staphylococcus aureus*), and opportunistic fungal infections (*Mucor, Rhizopus*). **Rhinocerebral mucormycosis** presents with facial invasion and block drainage and is fatal unless treated. **Malignant otitis externa** presents with purulent drainage and granulation tissue in the auditory canal. It may be fatal if untreated.

Q: What is diabetic retinopathy?

A: **Retinopathy,** a devastating complication of diabetes, is one of the leading causes of blindness (Table 5-5). Many patients after years of diabetes have **nonproliferative** or **"background" retinopathy,** which in and of itself does not cause visual loss. If it does not progress, it is of minimal clinical significance in the peripheral visual field. If exudates occur in the central (macular) area, **macular edema,** the swelling of the macula, may occur. This is more common in older patients and may lead to diminished vision.

TABLE 5-5.   Diabetic Retinopathy

NONPROLIFERATIVE (BACKGROUND)
Venous dilatation
Microaneurysms
Flame hemorrhages (superficial)
Dot-blot hemorrhages (deep)
Hard exudates

PREPROLIFERATIVE
Cotton-wool spots
Venous abnormalities (loops, beading)
Arterial abnormalities (segmental narrowing or occlusion)

PROLIFERATIVE
Neovascularization
    on disc
    elsewhere (NVE)
Preretinal hemorrhage
Vitreous hemorrhage
Retinal detachment

MACULAR EDEMA

Proliferative retinopathy is much more ominous than the nonproliferative type. It leads to neovascularization (new formation) of blood vessels and possible vitreous hemorrhage and retinal detachment, with resulting visual loss and blindness.

Q: How is diabetic retinopathy treated?

A: The best treatment for diabetic retinopathy is prevention. All patients should undergo a dilated eye examination yearly by an optometrist or ophthalmologist who has expertise in diabetic eye disease. If complications occur, referral to a retinal specialist is indicated.

Nonproliferative retinopathy should be followed closely for signs of progression. If significant proliferative retinopathy is present, laser treatment or **photocoagulation** may be advised. A microscopic laser beam is focused on the abnormal blood vessels in the peripheral visual field (the fovea is avoided), destroying the abnormal areas. This lessens the likelihood of hemorrhage and retinal detachment, but does not affect central vision. As most rods are in the peripheral visual field, night vision may be decreased after laser treatment. Macular edema is also treated with photocoagulation.

Vitreous hemorrhage is treated with **vitrectomy,** in which a small suction probe is placed into the eye to remove the blood. Vision may be restored by this procedure. A detached retina may be reattached.

Q: What is diabetic nephropathy?

A: Like retinopathy, **nephropathy** is a microvascular (small vessel) disease (Table 5-6). The very first manifestation is hyperfiltration (increased creatinine clearance, stage I); transient microalbuminuria may also occur. The nephropathy then progresses to a clinically silent stage (stage II) followed by microalbuminuria (stage III). Microalbuminuria appears to be reversible in type 1 patients with intensive treatment. Stage IV nephropathy, heralded by overt proteinuria ($>$ 500 mg per day), develops eventually in 30% to 40% of type 1 diabetics. Those with end-stage nephropathy (stage V) have renal failure and azotemia, and require dialysis. Life expectancy is typically less than 2

TABLE 5-6.   Diabetic Nephropathy

Stage I (hyperfiltration-hypertrophy stage)	Increased GFR (30% to 40%), hypertrophy of the kidneys. Microalbuminuria may occur. Potentially reversible with intensive treatment.
Stage II (silent stage)	Normal microalbumin excretion and, in many cases, normalization of GFR. Around 30% to 50% will progress to stage III.
Stage III (incipient nephropathy)	Persistence of hyperfiltration and onset of microalbuminuria (20–200 µg/min). GFR eventually decreases, and hypertension begins.
Stage IV (overt nephropathy)	Fixed proteinuria of greater than 500 mg/24 hours. Hypertension and decreased GFR are present. Progressive renal insufficiency occurs.
Stage V (end stage)	Dialysis or renal transplantation is necessary. The average patient progresses from stage IV to V in 5 to 7 years. Average life expectancy $<$ 2 years afer requiring dialysis.

years after beginning dialysis, due to the extensive vascular disease already present. Renal transplantation may greatly prolong the life span in these persons.

Q: What is urine microalbumin?

A: **Microalbumin** refers to urinary albumin that is present in an insufficient amount to be detected by urine dipstick (lower limit = 300 mg/day [500 mg/day total protein] or 200 μg/min). **Microalbuminuria** therefore refers to albumin excretion of 30–300 mg/day (total protein 50–500 mg/day) or 20–200 μg/min. Its presence in type 2 diabetes is a strong predictor of cardiovascular disease; approximately 80% of type 2 diabetics with microalbuminuria die within 10 years. Its presence in those with type 1 diabetes is a strong predictor of the development of overt albuminuria.

Q: What is the treatment of diabetic nephropathy?

A: For microalbuminuria, the measurements should be repeated to confirm the diagnosis, given day to day variation and possible confounding factors (e.g., urine contaminated with menstrual blood, or urine from a person with a urinary tract infection). Good glycemic control is the most important step, as it slows or prevents the progression to overt albuminuria.

Angiotensin-converting enzyme (ACE) inhibitors decrease intraglomerular pressure and peripheral vascular resistance. They also slow the decline of glomerular filtration rate (GFR). They are typically the drugs of choice in patients with hypertension caused by the renal protective effect, but they should be avoided in those prone to hyperkalemia (e.g., those with type IV renal tubular acidosis). Adverse side effects such as cough (common) and angioedema (rare) may occur. Even normotensive patients with microalbuminuria are felt to benefit from ACE inhibitor administration. ACE inhibitors appear to improve insulin sensitivity and are lipid-neutral.

Calcium channel blockers are another class of antihypertensive agents that appear to be beneficial in patients with microalbuminuria. Like ACE inhibitors, they are lipid neutral. The non–dihydropyridine drugs (verapamil, diltiazem) are preferred over the dihydropyridine drugs (nifedipine, amlodipine).

The angiotensin receptor blocking drugs. (e.g., losartan, irbesartan) act in a similar fashion to the ACE inhibitors. Further clinical studies must be done, but they would appear to be as beneficial as ACE inhibitors in persons intolerant of these medications.

Moderate protein restriction (0.8–1.0 mg/kg/day) is also recommended in many diabetic patients with microalbuminuria. Substitution of vegetable for animal protein is also advised, as this will help prevent decline in renal function.

Patients with overt (stage IV) nephropathy will progress to complete renal failure in time. Good glycemic and blood pressure control will slow the progression, however. A more intensive protein restriction (0.6–0.8 g/kg/day) is recommended in those with renal insufficiency. ACE inhibitors are again the drugs of choice.

Progression to dialysis may be predicted by plotting the reciprocal of the serum creatinine value versus time (Fig. 5-7). The time to a dialysis-requiring creatinine value (e.g., 10 mg/dL) may then be predicted. Although renal failure will eventually occur in those with chronic renal insufficiency, the time course may be altered significantly by the treatments above.

Q: What are standards of care for diabetes?

A: "Standards of care" refer to the routine laboratory tests and examinations that should be done on a yearly basis for persons with diabetes. These tests are to screen for complications of diabetes, such as nephropathy, neuropathy, and retinopathy. The recommendations for the initial visit are shown in Table 5-7. The standards of care for continued management are shown in Table 5-8.

Q: What is diabetic ketoacidosis?

A: **Diabetic ketoacidosis** (DKA) is a common derangement of glucose metabolism that leads to metabolic acidosis, dehydration, and fluid/electrolyte depletion (Fig. 5-8). In the normal individual, basal insulin levels in the fasting state allow gluconeogenesis and glycogenolysis to occur in a balanced fashion. With lack of insulin, glyco-

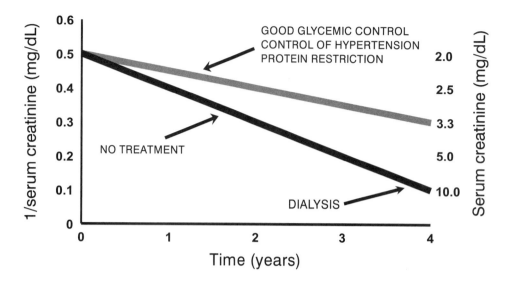

Figure 5-7. Predicting renal failure in diabetics.

genolysis, lipolysis, ketogenesis, and proteolysis occur in an effort to obtain energy from these sources (as many cells depend on insulin for glucose uptake).

So begins a vicious cycle in which glucose levels are elevated by glycogenolysis (due to increased counterregulatory hormones such as glucagon and epinephrine), but glucose is not being taken up peripherally, resulting in even more glycogenolysis—the body thinks it is in a "starved" state. Hyperglycemia raises serum osmolality, causing osmotic diuresis and severe fluid depletion. Free fatty acids and glycerol are produced by lipolysis and help promote the gluconeogenic pathway, but since glucose is not taken up, this cycle continues. Then, ketonuria promotes electrolyte depletion via obligatory loss of cations (K^+). Ultimately, metabolic acidosis occurs from ketonemia, and death results if the condition is not untreated.

Q: What is the most common cause of diabetic ketoacidosis?

A: The most common cause of DKA is infection, followed by inadvertent cessation of insulin and new-onset type 1 diabetes.

Q: What are the laboratory findings in diabetic ketoacidosis?

A: In DKA, serum glucose is typically elevated (usually > 300 mg/dL), but DKA can occur with a normal blood glucose. An elevated anion gap acidosis occurs due to accumulation of the ketoacids β-hydroxybutyrate (BOH) and acetoacetate; acetone is also present (Fig. 5-9). Typically, the BOH to acetoacetate ratio is about 3:1 to 15:1. An important point is that the typical (nitroprusside) laboratory test for quantitative ketones detects acetoacetate but not BOH. With treatment, BOH (which is the predominant ketoacid) is converted to acetoacetate, which is detected by the assay; so it may appear that the patient is getting worse because the measured ketone "level" rises erroneously. Modern laboratories can measure BOH, which eliminates this problem.

An alternative to measuring BOH is simply to monitor the anion gap. This is a measure of the unmeasured anions (sulfate, phosphate, lactate, ketoacids, albumin) and is usually 10–12 mEq/L. It is calculated by subtracting the sum of serum chloride and bicarbonate concentrations from the sodium (Na^+) concentration:

$$\Delta = Na^+ - (Cl^- + HCO_3^-)$$

The actual measured serum sodium should be used to calculate the anion gap. Hyperglycemia lowers serum Na^+ as the high osmotic load in serum draws water from the cells into plasma, resulting in hyponatremia. This is a true hyponatremia, not a pseudohyponatremia caused by an interfering substance. A "correction factor" may

TABLE 5-7.   Initial Visit Recommendations for Patients with Diabetes

HISTORY	PHYSICAL EXAMINATION
Symptoms, results of laboratory tests, and special examination results related to the diagnosis of diabetes	Cardiac examination
Eating patterns, nutritional status, and weight history; growth and development in children and adolescents	Blood pressure determination (with orthostatic measurements when indicated) and comparison to age-related norms
Family history of diabetes and other endocrine disorders	Evaluation of pulses (by palpation and auscultation), and hand/finger examination
Details of previous treatment programs, including nutrition and diabetes self-management training	Ophthalmoscopic examination (preferably with dilation)
Current treatment of diabetes, including medications, meal plan, and results of glucose monitoring and patient's use of monitoring data	Neurological, thyroid, abdominal, oral examination
History and treatment of other conditions, including endocrine and eating disorders	Skin examination (including insulin-injection sites)
Prior or current infections, particularly skin, foot, dental, and genitourinary infections	Foot examination
Lifestyle and cultural, psychosocial, educational, and economic factors that might influence management of diabetes; exercise history	Height and weight measurement (and comparison to norms in children and adolescents)
Symptoms and treatments: chronic eye, kidney, and nerve conditions; genitourinary, bladder, and gastrointestinal function; heart, peripheral vascular, foot, and cerebrovascular complications associated with diabetes	
Risk factors for atherosclerosis: smoking, hypertension, obesity, dyslipidemia, and family history	
Gestational history: hyperglycemia, delivery of an infant weighing >9 lb, toxemia, stillbirth, polyhydramnios, or other complications of pregnancy	

be used to estimate what the Na⁺ concentration would be without the hyperglycemia; this estimates how much water has been removed from the cells. The correction factor is to add 1.6 mEq/L to the serum Na⁺ for each 100 mg/dL above normal (100 mg/dL) that the serum glucose is elevated. For example, if the glucose is 1000 mg/dL and Na⁺ 122 mEq/L, the correction factor would be

$$\frac{1000-100}{100} \times 1.6 = 9 \times 1.6 = 14.4 \text{ mEq/L}$$

The "corrected" Na⁺ is therefore 122 + 14.4 = 136 mEq/L. Remember that this only helps estimate what the Na⁺ will be after the hyperglycemia has been corrected; the true Na⁺ is still 122. The actual measured Na⁺ should be used when calculating the anion gap.

Because of the osmotic diuresis, potassium (K⁺) is also depleted in DKA. K⁺ may initially be high at presentation due to the metabolic acidosis (which causes a transcellular shift from extracellular to intracellular fluid). After the acidosis improves, K⁺ will become low and require treatment. Phosphate also may be initially elevated due to transcellular shifts, but a total body deficit generally exists.

Q: What is the treatment of DKA?

A: Immediate resuscitation may be required, including intubation if the patient is comatose, and treatment of arrhythmia. Fluid administration is essential as the typical fluid deficit is 5 to 10 liters. Initially replace fluid rapidly with 0.9% NaCl (normal saline), usually at least 2 to 3 liters. As

TABLE 5-8. Standards of Care for Patients with Diabetes

EACH VISIT	YEARLY
Height (until maturity), weight, blood pressure	Lipid profile
Glycated hemoglobin	Electrocardiogram (ECG) in adults
Foot examination (assess vascular system, skin, presence of ulcerations)	Creatinine clearance and microalbumin determination; start at 5 years from diagnosis in type 1, initially at diagnosis in type 2
Screening for neuropathy in at-risk patients	Thyroid function studies (when indicated)
Frequency, causes, and severity of hypoglycemia or hyperglycemia	Dilated fundoscopic examination
Results of SMBG	
Review current medications	
Psychosocial issues, and lifestyle changes (e.g., regarding tobacco and alcohol use, exercise)	

serum glucose levels fall, water will shift back into the intracellular space; therefore, it is best to avoid hypotonic solutions initially. After several liters have been administered, maintenance fluids are given. Invasive cardiovascular monitoring may be required in patients with cardiac or renal disease. After the glucose is lowered to 250 mg/dL, it is advisable to add glucose to the intravenous solution to prevent hypoglycemia; for example, the solution would be changed to D_5NS (normal saline with 5% glucose), 5 grams per 100 mL.

Insulin is initiated by giving a "loading" bolus of 0.2 units/kg. An infusion is then started, often at 0.1 units/kg/hour (e.g., 5 units/hour for a 100 kg

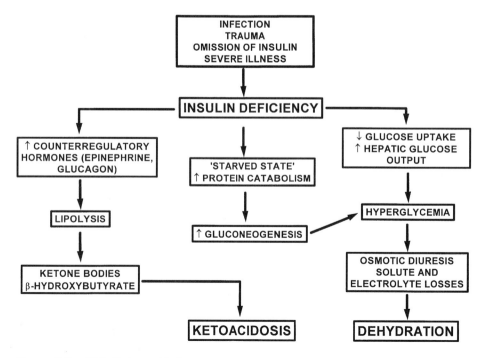

Figure 5-8. Diabetic ketoacidosis.

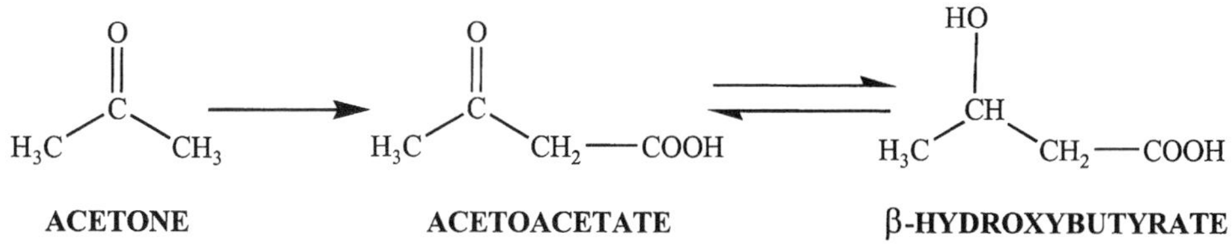

Figure 5-9. Ketones and ketoacids in DKA.

person). Human regular insulin is used; there is no advantage in using lispro, as both the human and synthetic insulins are equally potent and dissociate into monomers instantly at their low concentrations in plasma.

The goal is a decrease of serum glucose by 80–100 mg/dL/hour, so the infusion is continued until the acidosis is resolved. Because most of the hyperglycemia is due to dehydration, the acidosis has not always resolved by the time the glucose normalizes. The infusion must be continued until the anion gap normalizes (12 or less) or the BOH lowers to an acceptable level (less than 2 mmol/L). Occasionally, the glucose will become low even though the acidosis persists; in this case, the insulin infusion is continued and the glucose concentration in the intravenous fluid is increased; for example, the infusion would go from D_5 (5% glucose) to D_{10} (10% glucose).

The K^+ levels must be followed meticulously, as there is typically a total body deficit. If K^+ is initially elevated, do not give supplements until the level falls below 5 mEq/L. After this, intravenous KCl may be given. Phosphate levels also may be low; cautious replacement is recommended. Overly aggressive phosphate repletion can cause hypocalcemia.

Therapy with bicarbonate (HCO_3^-) is controversial. It is usually not necessary, as HCO_3^- is produced during insulin treatment. It also can be hazardous, as it may cause rapid falls in K^+ levels (due to transcellular shifts) and cardiac arrhythmias. Bicarbonate may actually exacerbate acidosis in the cerebrospinal fluid and increase hepatic ketogenesis, so it is not recommended unless the patient has severe acidosis (pH 7.0), is in shock and not responding to fluid therapy, or has life-threatening hyperkalemia.

Most patients with DKA have an ileus from the acidosis and thus should not eat. Very ill patients will require a nasogastric tube to prevent aspiration of gastric contents. After the acidosis clears and bowel function returns, food may be slowly re-instituted. Any secondary problems such as urinary tract infection, pneumonia, or myocardial infarction should be treated appropriately.

Subcutaneous insulin is restarted after the acidosis clears. It must be started at least 1 hour before stopping the infusion. If the patient was on insulin previously, this dose can be restarted; if not, a starting dose is given. An approximation using 0.4–0.7 U/kg/day of insulin can be made using the "2/3 to 1/3" rule (see "How much insulin do I start?" below).

Q: What is the hyperosmolar nonketotic syndrome?

A: **Hyperosmolar nonketotic syndrome** (HNKS) is a syndrome of severe hyperglycemia (600–1000 mg/dL), severe dehydration, and lack of significant ketoacidosis. The anion gap is often normal to slightly elevated, and BOH is only slightly elevated. Glucose is often higher than that seen in DKA. HNKS differs from DKA in that patients with the former have sufficient insulin to prevent lipolysis and metabolic acidosis. However, there is enough relative insulin deficiency to cause hyperglycemia and protein/carbohydrate catabolism, leading to osmotic diuresis with fluid and electrolyte depletion.

HNKS is commonly the presenting manifestation of diabetes in elderly patients and is typically associated with a concurrent illness (such as infection, myocardial infarction, or stroke). The treatment of HNKS centers on fluid and electrolyte repletion. This must be done with caution in patients with cardiovascular or renal disease, who may require invasive monitoring. Insulin is also given after rehydration has been started, in a similar fashion to patients with DKA. Serum glucose is the main parameter followed, as acidosis is not present. K$^+$ and PO$_4^-$ are also given as needed.

Patients are switched to subcutaneous insulin after the hyperglycemia resolves. Underlying conditions (e.g., urosepsis) are treated, and insulin sensitivity usually improves. Because HNKS patients lack acidosis and by definition have type 2 diabetes, many will be able to take oral agents and discontinue insulin.

Q: What is the therapy of type 1 diabetes?

A: Insulin is the only therapy for type 1 diabetes, and it should be started as soon as possible. Admission to the hospital may be advisable so that the patient may learn "survival skills" such as insulin administration, use of the meter, and treatment of hypoglycemia under expert supervision. Aggressive therapy may preserve residual β-cell function.

Q: How is insulin given?

A: Insulin is a polypeptide that is not absorbed well orally, as it is degraded in the gastrointestinal tract. Currently it must be given by injection, either subcutaneously or intravenously. It is also well absorbed intraperitoneally and may be given this way in certain patients, such as those on peritoneal dialysis. Other routes of insulin administration (e.g., nasal, inhaled aerosol) are being studied experimentally.

Q: What are the pharmacokinetics of insulin?

A: Insulin pharmacokinetics are outlined in Table 5-9. The most commonly used insulins are the NPH, lente, regular, and ultralente series. Human lispro, a modified human insulin analog, is used because of its rapid onset of action. Note that human insulin is significantly shorter acting than is animal insulin, which must be remembered when switching patients from animal to human insulin. Although animal insulins have been discontinued, they may still be available and some patients still use them.

Q: How is insulin absorbed after injection?

A: Insulin is traditionally given as a subcutaneous injection. Regular or soluble insulin normally associates into a hexameric form (around a zinc atom) at the concentrations present in the vial (Fig. 5-10). After injection, it gradually becomes diluted by body fluids and dissociates into dimeric and monomeric forms when the concentration becomes low enough. Very little insulin is absorbed into the bloodstream as the hexameric form; some is absorbed as dimers, but monomers are most rapidly absorbed (Table 5-10). The intermediate- or long-acting insulins (e.g., NPH, lente, ultralente) use retarding agents that cause the insulin molecules to form larger particles and dissociate more slowly, increasing the duration of action. These larger particles convey a cloudy appearance to these insulins, and some patients may refer to these preparations as "cloudy" and to

TABLE 5-9.   Insulin Pharmacokinetics

INSULIN	ONSET (HOUR)	PEAK (HOUR)	DURATION (HOUR)
Animal origin			
Regular	0.5–2.0	3–4	6–8
NPH/Lente	4–6	8–14	20–24
Ultralente	8–14	Minimal	24–36
Human (recombinant DNA origin)			
Regular	0.5–1.0	2–3	4–6
NPH/Lente	2–4	4–10	14–18
Ultralente	6–10	12–16	20–30
Human insulin analog			
Lispro	0.25	0.5–1.5	< 5

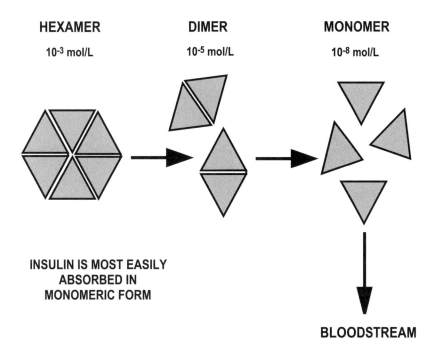

HEXAMER	DIMER	MONOMER
10^{-3} mol/L	10^{-5} mol/L	10^{-8} mol/L

INSULIN IS MOST EASILY ABSORBED IN MONOMERIC FORM

BLOODSTREAM

Figure 5-10. Absorption of subcutaneous insulin.

regular as "clear." Lente and ultralente use zinc as the retarding agent; NPH (short for neutral protamine Hagedorn) uses the protein protamine.

Q: What is lispro insulin?

A: **Lispro** is a synthetically modified human insulin (reversing lysine and proline at amino acids 28 and 29, hence the name "lyspro" or lispro) that dissociates into monomeric form at a higher concentration than regular insulin. It is much more rapidly absorbed from subcutaneous tissue than regular insulin and is taken right before a meal. In contrast, regular insulin is taken 30 to 45 minutes

before eating. Lispro's rapid onset of action much more closely approximates normal insulin secretion than does regular insulin (Fig. 5-11). Many patients treated with regular insulin also experience hypoglycemia several hours after eating, due to its relatively long duration of action. Lispro insulin is eliminated much more rapidly, helping to avoid this problem.

Q: Who are good candidates for lispro?

A: Type 1 patients, especially those who experience hypoglycemia several hours after meals (due to the long action of regular insulin), are good candi-

TABLE 5-10.   Factors Affecting Insulin Absorption

DECREASED (SLOWER) ABSORPTION TIME	INCREASED (FASTER) ABSORPTION TIME
Cold	Heat
Smoking	Exercise
Increased volume	Decreased volume
Increased concentration (U-500 insulin)	Decreased concentration
Edema	Massage
Lipohypertrophy	Use of monomeric insulin analogs (lispro)

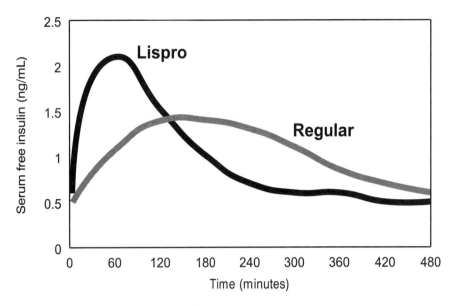

Figure 5-11. Lispro versus regular insulin.

dates for lispro. Lispro may be given before each meal along with long-acting or intermediate insulin. One advantage of lispro is that it can be taken right before a meal (as opposed to 30 to 45 minutes before a meal for regular insulin). This schedule may be more convenient for the patient and allow a more flexible lifestyle. Type 2 patients may also benefit for the same reasons. Lispro is not approved for use in pregnancy.

Q: I want to convert my patient on regular insulin to lispro. How do I do that?

A: Unit for unit, the lispro and regular insulin are equipotent. The only difference is that lispro dissociates into a monomer at a much higher concentration, speeding absorption. Thus, it is reasonable to substitute unit for unit. In practice, one usually ends up increasing the basal (long-acting or intermediate insulin) by about 20% and giving less lispro than regular insulin. This is because regular has a significant "tail" effect, which essentially adds to the effect of the longer-acting insulin.

Q: How much insulin do I start?

A: There is no 'magic formula' to determine how much insulin a person needs. A normal person secretes approximately 0.5–0.7 units of insulin/kg/day, so this is a reasonable dosage for a type 1 diabetic. Given that most type 1 patients go through a honeymoon period after beginning treatment in which some residual insulin secretion returns, it is often wise to start newly diagnosed patients at a lower dose (0.4–0.5 U/kg/day) to prevent hypoglycemia.

Type 1 patients should take intermediate or long-acting insulin along with a fast-acting (soluble) insulin (regular or lispro). A good starting point is to give 2/3 as long-acting or intermediate-acting insulin and 1/3 as soluble insulin. If lente or NPH insulin is given, a good starting point is to give 2/3 of the total dose in the morning, and 1/3 in the evening. If a long-acting insulin is used (ultralente), it is often desirable to divide the doses evenly morning and evening. The remaining 1/3 of the insulin is given as fast-acting or soluble insulin. Regular insulin is typically given before breakfast and supper, and lispro is typically given before each meal. Insulin is adjusted after review of self-blood glucose readings.

It is very difficult to predict how much insulin will be required in a type 2 patient, since insulin resistance varies. One approach is to begin an intermediate or long-acting insulin only at supper time in an effort to control the morning blood glucose. If adequate control cannot be obtained on once-daily insulin, then twice-daily insulin must be instituted. A small dose (10–20 units of NPH, lente, or ultralente) may be started and adjusted from there.

Q: What are some common insulin dosing regimens?

A: For good control, all type 1 patients require some combination of intermediate- or long-acting insulin plus fast-acting insulin (regular or lispro), or a continuous subcutaneous infusion of insulin (insulin pump). Many type 2 patients will achieve good control on a single insulin alone, or with premixed insulin combinations. Some common insulin regimens are shown in Figures 5-12, 5-13, and 5-14. Other regimens are possible. What may work for one patient may not work well for another.

Q: How do I adjust insulin doses?

A: Insulin is adjusted based on the glucose level that it affects (Table 5-11). The best possible control is achieved when the patient monitors frequently (four or more times daily). The fewer times the patient monitors, the fewer data points are available. How much to increase or decrease the doses depends on the patient and personal experience.

A good rule of thumb is 10% for a minor change, 20% for a large change. More or less may be needed, depending on the individual patient.

Q: How is ideal body weight calculated?

A: In calculating ideal body weight (IBW) for men, allow 106 pounds for the first 5 feet of height, and add 6 pounds for each additional inch (medium frame). For men with a small frame, subtract 10%; for a large frame, add 10%. To determine the patient's frame size, ask him to grasp his wrist with the opposite hand: if the thumb and 3rd finger overlap, he has a small frame; if they just touch, he has a medium frame, and if a gap exists, his has a large frame. For example, a man who is 6 feet tall with a medium frame has an IBW of 106 + (12)(6) = 106 + 72 = 178 lb. If he had a large frame, IBW = 178 + (178)(0.10) = 196 lb.

For women, allow 100 lb for the first 5 feet, and add 5 lb for each additional inch of height. Add

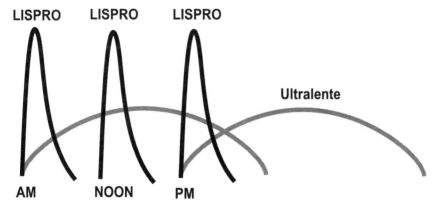

Figure 5-12. Ultralente and pre-meal lispro insulin.

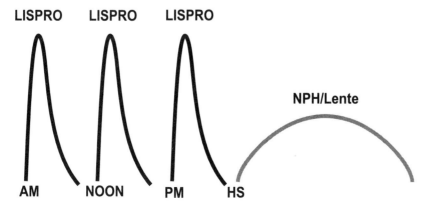

Figure 5-13. Bedtime NPH and pre-meal lispro insulin.

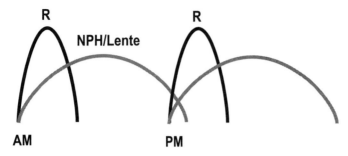

Figure 5-14. Twice-daily NPH/lente and regular insulin.

and subtract based on frame size as with males. For example, a woman 5 feet 5 inches tall with a medium frame should weigh 100 + (5)(5) = 100 + 25 = 125 pounds.

Q: How is caloric expenditure calculated?

A: There are many methods, of varying complexity, for calculating caloric expenditure. A common method is the Harris-Benedict equation, which uses height, weight, age, and sex to arrive at basal energy expenditure (BEE). The Harris-Benedict equation is as follows:

$$\text{Males: BEE (kcal)} = 66 + 13.7 \times \text{Weight (kg)} + 12.7 \times \text{Height (in)} - 6.8 \times \text{Age (years)}$$

$$\text{Females: BEE (kcal)} = 655 + 9.6 \times \text{Weight (kg)} + 4.3 \times \text{Height (in)} - 4.7 \times \text{Age (years)}$$

Stress or activity factors may be added to compensate for severe illness or increased activity. For example, a patient with sepsis or severe trauma might require twice as many calories as a normal person at rest.

Q: What is the diet therapy of diabetes?

A: Nutrition therapy is as important as medication for good control of diabetes. Unfortunately, many patients who are perfectly willing to take insulin or oral agents are unable to follow a diet. The goals should be tailored to the patient; for example, some patients may be unable to follow an excessively complex diet plan.

In the past, diet prescriptions were complex regimens that involved weighing of food and rigid adherence. Today, diet therapy is much more flexible. In 1994, the American Diabetes Association (ADA) replaced the "diabetic," and "ADA diet" guidelines with new guidelines for therapy:

- Limit cholesterol to 300 mg daily.

- Decrease total dietary fat to 30% or less of total calories with emphasis on decreasing saturated and polyunsaturated fat to less than 8% to 9% of total calories. Remainder of fat to be monounsaturated.

- Daily protein intake of 10% to 20% total calories.

TABLE 5-11.   Adjustments in Insulin Dose

INSULIN	DECREASE IF:	INCREASE IF:
AM NPH/lente/ultralente	supper BG too low	supper BG too high
AM regular/lispro	noon BG too low	noon BG too high
Noon regular/lispro	supper BG too low	supper BG too high
PM or bedtime NPH/lente/ultralente	fasting BG too low	fasting BG too high
PM regular/lispro	bedtime BG too low	bedtime BG too high

BG = blood glucose.

- Moderate caloric restriction (250–500 kcal/day less than average daily intake) in overweight individuals.

- Moderate increase in protein intake for children, adolescents, and pregnant women.

- No set amount of carbohydrate; amount tailored to individual, considering factors such as age and activity level.

The simplest method of attaining a sensible diet is to follow the **food pyramid** (Fig. 5-15). Foods at the top of the pyramid should be eaten sparingly or not at all (high fat foods, desserts, and alcoholic beverages). Those at the bottom (e.g., cereals) can be eaten in much larger portions. This is a relatively simple plan that most persons can follow.

A more advanced method of meal planning is the **exchange list.** Exchange lists are a simple way of making food choices. Each person has a certain number of each exchanges for each meal. If, for example, another carbohydrate is desired, the person simply makes a substitution for the equivalent amount of another exchange. In the exchange list, foods are grouped into carbohydrate, meat/meat substitute, and fat groups. The carbohydrate group is subdivided into starches (e.g., bread), fruit, milk, and vegetables. Each carbohydrate exchange contains approximately 15 grams of carbohydrate

(60 kcal), except for vegetable exchanges, which contain 5 grams of carbohydrate. One meat/meat substitute exchange contains approximately 7 grams of protein. The number of calories depends on the type of meat; high-fat meat has more calories than lean meat. A fat exchange equals 5 grams of fat (45 kcal); the fats are divided into monounsaturated, polyunsaturated, and saturated, of which the monounsaturated fats are preferable.

Carbohydrate counting is a sophisticated method of determining how much carbohydrate is eaten with each meal. It has been shown that carbohydrate is the major substance affecting postprandial glucose levels. Through trial and error, the amount of insulin for the carbohydrate eaten is determined. For example, a person might use 1 unit of lispro for 15 grams of carbohydrate; if the person consumes 75 grams (300 kcal), then he or she would use 5 units lispro to cover. This system provides more eating flexibility for those that can master it, particular those diabetics who have erratic schedules.

Q: How do the diet recommendations for type 1 and type 2 diabetes differ?

A: Type 2 diabetics are often overweight, so the goal is a modest weight loss. Radical, reduced-calorie diets are not recommended. A deficit of 250–500 kcal per day is desirable, resulting in a weight loss of up to 1 pound (3500 kcal) per week. Those with type 2 often have hyperlipidemia, and low-fat diets are advocated.

Q: May insulin be combined with oral agents?

A: Insulin can be combined with oral agents, but some combinations may not be practical or useful. There are dozens of possible combinations of available therapies, and it may require trial and error to determine what will be effective in the individual patient. For example, if the patient is already on twice daily insulin, the addition of a sulfonylurea or metformin may not add much benefit. Bedtime insulin and daytime sulfonylurea (BIDS) is a commonly used regimen in which long- or intermediate-acting insulin is given at supper or bedtime with sulfonylurea in the morning. This may be of use in patients who predominantly have elevated fasting glucose levels, which

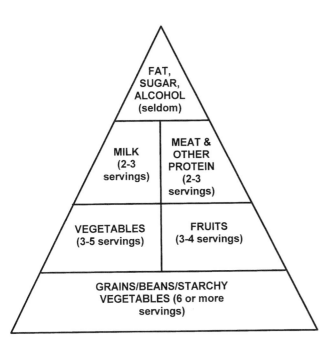

Figure 5-15. The food pyramid.

improve during the day. This approach may obviate the need for twice daily insulin. Troglitazone is an insulin-sensitizing agent that may lower the patient's insulin requirements and be useful as combination therapy.

Q: What is U-500 insulin?

A: U-500 is a special kind of regular insulin with 500 units per mL (instead of the 100 units per mL of U-100 insulin). It is currently available in synthetic human form. Although it is regular insulin, it acts as a long-acting insulin because of its high concentration—it is released (i.e., dissociates into monomers) very slowly. For this reason it is used by itself and not with any other long-acting insulins. U-500 is used when the patient is on so much conventional insulin that it becomes difficult to give.

Q: What is continuous subcutaneous insulin infusion?

A: **Continuous subcutaneous insulin infusion** (CSII) is a method by which short-acting insulin is continuously infused by use of an **insulin pump.** External pumps are small devices (about the size of a pocket pager) that contain insulin (Fig. 5-16). Insulin in the pump may be either buffered regular or lispro. The pump is connected to the patient by a thin plastic tube that is inserted into subcutaneous fat and is changed every 48 hours. The patient programs the pump to give a set amount of *basal* insulin continuously (Fig. 5-17). For meals, the patient has the pump give additional insulin (the **meal bolus**). The pump cannot sense the patient's

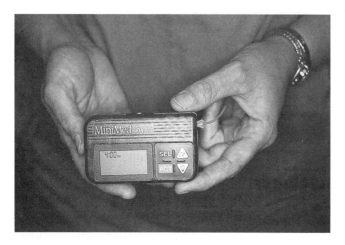

Figure 5-16. External insulin pump.

blood sugar, so he or she must still monitor capillary glucose several times daily.

Internal insulin pumps are implanted into the abdomen and infuse insulin into the peritoneal cavity. These are still experimental and not available for mainstream use.

Q: What are the advantages of insulin pump therapy?

A: Conventional insulin therapy relies on intermediate- or long-acting insulin to provide basal coverage. Absorption of these depot insulins may be erratic, leading to early peaking at times (hypoglycemia) and late peaking at others (hyperglycemia). Continuous infusion of short-acting insulin avoids this problem and most closely approximates secretion of insulin by a normal pancreas.

It is also difficult to give subcutaneous insulin in increments of less than one unit; pumps can accurately deliver insulin in increments of 0.1 unit. This is advantageous for the patient on small doses of insulin in whom small increments are very significant. More accurate insulin delivery helps decrease hypoglycemia and improve overall control.

CSII also allows for a more flexible lifestyle. Patients control their own insulin at all times; they do not have to worry about a long-acting insulin peaking at a certain time. This is useful for persons with active lifestyles whose mealtimes vary, and those involved in strenuous physical activity (which can cause hypoglycemia).

Q: What are the disadvantages of pump therapy?

A: *CSII is not for everyone.* The relative complexity of the device demands a higher degree of compliance than injections. The patient obviously must physically and intellectually be able to master it. It is much more expensive, and patients must have adequate insurance or financial resources.

Because CSII only uses short-acting insulin, the patient will develop problems rapidly if the pump or plastic tubing is damaged. Damaged tubing is usually the culprit, either developing a tear or becoming clogged. If the problem is not corrected immediately, ketoacidosis may result in hours. A clue that a "pump emergency" has developed is the presence of unexplained hyperglycemia. If the

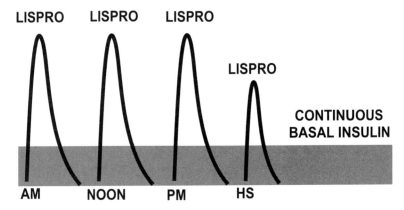

Figure 5-17. Insulin profile: continuous subcutaneous insulin infusion (CSII).

patient does not check faithfully, there is little warning, and hospitalization may result for DKA. If patients do develop unexplained hyperglycemia, they should immediately draw up insulin in a syringe (according to coverage scale) and inject immediately; the pump problem should then be corrected. Prompt attention to this avoids DKA in the majority of cases.

Q: Can the pump sense blood glucose levels?

A: The pump cannot sense blood glucose levels, so the wearer must tell it how much insulin to give. An implantable glucose sensor would allow continuous monitoring of glucose levels and adjustment accordingly. Unfortunately, a sensor that would be reliable for long periods of time is not yet available. Development of such a device would truly permit a closed-loop system of diabetes control, with less intervention required by the patient.

Q: What is a glucagon emergency kit?

A: **Glucagon** is a hormone that promotes glycogenolysis and is used in diabetics who suffer a severe hypoglycemic reaction that cannot be treated orally. It is generally not safe to give an unconscious person something by mouth (other than glucose gel, which is absorbed in the buccal mucosa). Glucagon is available in 1-mg vials and must be reconstituted with sterile water before being given intramuscularly. Those who live or work with the patient should be trained in its administration, as it may be life saving.

Q: What are "sick day" rules?

A: These are instructions for patients with type 1 diabetes who have nausea, vomiting, and are not eating well. One of the most common reasons for DKA is omission of insulin on sick days. Patients need more insulin, not less, when ill. Patients who are sick should always take the long-acting insulin; short-acting insulin (regular or lispro) should be given every 4 hours according to a coverage scale. They should check urine for ketones if glucose is over 240; if ketones are moderate to large, a physician should be called (trace ketones may be present simply from fasting). If the patient cannot be managed at home, he or she should come into the hospital for intravenous hydration and insulin.

Q: What is a "sliding scale"?

A: A **sliding** or **coverage scale** is designed to supplement existing insulin when the glucose level is high, as when a patient is sick. The amount of supplemental insulin given depends on the amount of total daily insulin taken; a person taking 100 units daily needs to take more than a person on 10 units daily.

Supplemental insulin doses can be calculated using the "1500 rule": divide 1500 by the total daily amount of insulin to get the amount that one unit of insulin will theoretically lower the glucose level. For example, if the patient is on 75 units of insulin daily, dividing 1500 by 75 = 20, which is the amount that a unit of insulin will lower the glucose. So, if we want to lower the glucose by 40,

2 units would be administered. A sample coverage scale would be as follows:

> 140   2 units

> 180   4 units

> 220   6 units

> 260   8 units

> 300   10 units

> 340   12 units

> 380   14 units

If the person were on, say, 40 units, 1500/40 = 37.5 ~ 40; so a unit of insulin lowers the glucose by 40, instead of by 20 as in the last example. It stands to reason that for a person on less insulin, less coverage would be needed. So, for this patient, we might use increments of 1 unit instead of 2.

A sliding scale is meant to supplement insulin, not replace it. The patient's scheduled insulin should not be stopped. All too often a patient's scheduled insulin is stopped when he or she comes into the hospital, and only a coverage scale is given. There is no reason not to give the person's insulin in the hospital; omission of insulin may lead to unwanted hyperglycemia and even ketoacidosis, especially in type 1 patients.

Q: How should insulin be administered in hospitalized patients?

A: Insulin should never be stopped in type 1 patients, as it is required for life. Insulin in some form must be given to meet basal needs; a sliding scale alone is inadequate.

For the patient who is eating normally, the best thing to do is simply continue the usual insulin plus a coverage scale as per the 1500 rule above. An ill patient who is not eating can be managed using sick day rules (giving the intermediate- or long-acting insulin plus coverage every 4 hours). The scheduled insulin may need to be decreased, but it should never be stopped in a type 1 patient. Very ill patients require the use of an insulin infusion.

Type 2 patients, while resistant to ketoacidosis, may still experience adverse metabolic problems from uncontrolled hyperglycemia during hospitalization. In most cases, insulin should be continued according to the rules above.

Q: What instructions should I give my patient who is going to surgery?

A: Patients undergoing a minor procedure for which they will be NPO (unable to eat) should be instructed to take approximately 1/2 of the morning intermediate- or long-acting insulin and no soluble (regular or lispro) insulin. Those on oral agents should not take them on the morning of surgery, with the exception of troglitazone, which is safe. Metformin especially should not be taken on the day of surgery.

Patients on insulin who are undergoing a major surgical procedure may require insulin infusions to regulate glucose levels prior to surgery and after the procedure. Because of the rapid onset and short (8-minute) half-life of intravenous insulin, it is easier to titrate than subcutaneous insulin.

Q: How is hypoglycemia treated?

A: If the patient is awake, the treatment for hypoglycemia should consist of 15 grams of carbohydrate (6 oz regular soft drink, 4 oz juice); the level should be rechecked in 15 minutes. If the patient's level is still low, he or she should be treated again. An injection of glucagon should be given to those who are unconscious or who are otherwise unable to take oral glucose.

Q: What is the team approach to diabetes?

A: Good diabetes care requires more than the physician can provide in a single office visit. Other health care providers, who provide specialized care, are necessary. Successful management of diabetes requires intensive education so that patients may take care of themselves. The diabetes team consists of the physician, diabetes nurse educator, registered dietitian, podiatrist, ophthalmologist/optometrist, and other specialists as needed (vascular surgeon, nephrologist, social worker, mental health professionals, clergy).

Q: What is a certified diabetes educator?

A: A Certified Diabetes Educator (CDE) is a health care professional (physician, registered nurse, registered dietitian, or registered pharmacist) who has an interest in and has received advanced training in the care and education of patients with diabetes. These individuals must take a rigorous qualifying examination and be periodically recertified. CDEs should be the major resource in teaching patients about diabetes care.

A diabetes clinical nurse specialist (CNS) is a registered nurse with a master's or doctoral degree with a specialization in clinical diabetes. He or she may also be a CDE and is an advanced practitioner who can function more autonomously.

Q: What are oral hypoglycemic agents?

A: True oral hypoglycemic agents include the sulfonylureas and repaglinide, both of which enhance insulin secretion from β-cells. They may cause hypoglycemia in normal individuals, hence their name. Metformin, thiazolidinediones, and α-glucosidase inhibitors are not properly called oral hypoglycemic agents as they do not produce hypoglycemia, although hypoglycemia may of course occur if they are combined with hypoglycemic agents.

Sulfonylureas include the first-generation agents (chlorpropamide, acetohexamide, tolbutamide, tolazamide), and the second-generation agents (glipizide, glyburide, glimepiride). The second-generation agents are generally superior and are preferred.

Q: What are sulfonylureas?

A: **Sulfonylureas** are modified sulfonamide antibiotics that possess hypoglycemic properties (Table 5-12). They were first discovered during World War II when new antibiotics were being developed; researchers found that several patients died

TABLE 5-12.   Sulfonylureas

FIRST GENERATION	SECOND GENERATION
Chlorpropamide	Glyburide
Tolbutamide	Glipizide
Tolazamide	Glimepiride
Acetohexamide	

of hypoglycemia. Carbutamide was the first sulfonylurea used but it had adverse clinical effects.

The so-called first-generation agents, introduced in the late 1950s, included tolbutamide and chlorpropamide. Acetohexamide and tolazamide were introduced later. Later, the second-generation sulfonylureas were introduced; these include glyburide and glipizide. The newest second-generation agent is glimepiride.

Sulfonylureas act by sensitizing the pancreatic β-cells to glucose, and this results in increased insulin secretion. As intact β-cells are required, these agents are not useful in type 1 diabetics. They also appear to decrease hepatic glucose production, decrease glucagon levels, and increase peripheral sensitivity to insulin. The second-generation agents are generally preferred over the first-generation agents because of their increased efficacy.

Q: What adverse effects may occur with sulfonylureas?

A: Because sulfonylureas enhance endogenous insulin secretion, hypoglycemia may occur. Patients with prolonged hypoglycemia require admission to the hospital, as sulfonylureas have a relatively long duration of action.

Chlorpropamide has a very long half-life and should be used cautiously. Chlorpropamide can have several adverse effects. It simulates the hypothalamic release of antidiuretic hormone and potentiates its action, and may result in SIADH, with resultant hyponatremia. It also may produce a disulfiram-like reaction when alcohol is consumed, with resultant flushing, headache, nausea, and vomiting. For these reasons, chlorpropamide therapy cannot be routinely recommended.

The rare side effects of sulfonylureas include hepatic disease, leukopenia, agranulocytosis, photosensitivity, and aplastic anemia. Rash, anorexia, nausea, and heartburn are more common. Most patients experience no adverse effects. A study done in 1970 (University Group Diabetes Program) showed increased cardiovascular mortality in persons taking tolbutamide, but this was felt by most experts to be a poor study; sulfonylureas are not generally thought today to cause cardiovascular disease. In the UKPDS study, sulfonylureas used alone or with insulin were not associated with adverse cardiovascular outcomes. Cardiovascular mortality increased with patients taking sulfonylurea and metformin; the significance of this is unknown, as these data have not been confirmed by epidemiological or meta-analysis.

Q: What is the initial therapy of type 2 diabetes?

A: The therapy for type 2 diabetes is progressive management (Fig. 5-18). Asymptomatic individuals require diabetes education, meter instruction, and dietary counseling. Those with moderate to severe symptoms (polyuria, weight loss) may require oral-agent or insulin therapy initially. Those who do not respond to diet alone begin therapy with a single oral agent (e.g., sulfonylurea, metformin, or troglitazone). Other oral agents (repaglinide, acarbose) might then be tried if the initial agents yield suboptimal control.

Insulin therapy should be considered if all else fails; the natural course of type 2 diabetes is eventual progression to insulin therapy after many years. Thus, the need for insulin should not be looked upon as a failure by the patient or physician, but instead as a way to "take control" of the disease.

Q: Is insulin bad for the patient with type 2 diabetes?

A: We know that hyperinsulinemia itself may cause deleterious effects such as hypertension, hyperlipidemia, and hyperandrogenism. Therefore, it can be postulated that addition of insulin to an already insulin-resistant individual might be harmful. However, hyperglycemia is also harmful, so the glucose level must be controlled, even if high insulin doses are needed. Insulin-sensitizing drugs (e.g., troglitazone) are theoretically useful, as they may reduce the requirement for exogenous insulin.

Q: What is metformin?

A: **Metformin** is in a class of drugs known as **biguanides** and is the biguanide of choice in most countries. It is preferred over an older drug, phenformin, which has a much higher incidence of lactic acidosis. Although it was first approved for U.S. use in 1995, metformin had already been used for over 20 years in other countries. Its main mechanism of action is to decrease hepatic glu-

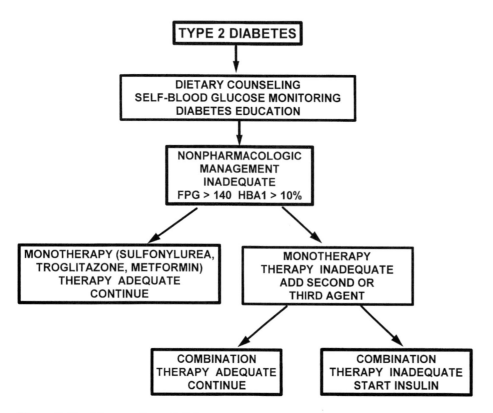

Figure 5-18. Therapy of type 2 diabetes.

cose output. It also appears to enhance insulin receptor binding. It may be used as monotherapy or in conjunction with other oral agents or insulin. It is best given with meals, because the most common side effects are gastrointestinal (nausea, vomiting, diarrhea).

Although metformin itself does not cause hypoglycemia, it can cause hypoglycemia when combined with hypoglycemic agents. Thus, doses of other agents should be reduced, as they can add to the effect of metformin.

Metformin very rarely causes lactic acidosis (incidence 3 per 100,000), which can be fatal. This condition typically occurs in persons with renal or hepatic disease, so the agent should not be used in these patients. Fortunately, this side effect is much less common with metformin than it was with phenformin, which was long ago taken off the market in the United States. The contraindications for metformin therapy are shown in Table 5-13.

For hospitalized patients, a good rule of thumb is that if the person is sick enough to be in hospital, metformin should be discontinued. The reasoning is that acute illness (such as myocardial infarction, sepsis, or surgery) may predispose the patient to a fatal acidosis. Exceptions to this rule might include patients undergoing chemotherapy, thyroid cancer patients receiving radioiodine, patients with deep venous thrombosis, or patients in psychiatric or chemical dependency services. Metformin also should be stopped for 48 hours prior to a contrast-requiring x-ray procedure (e.g., cardiac catheterization). The contrast might potentially induce renal failure and predispose the

patient to lactic acidosis. Metformin may be safely restarted after the procedure is completed.

Q: What is troglitazone?

A: **Troglitazone** is a unique drug of the thiazolidinedione class that acts to decrease insulin resistance by increasing peripheral glucose uptake. It also decreases hepatic glucose output. Thus, it is useful for monotherapy or for those poorly controlled on insulin and/or other oral agents.

Although troglitazone itself does not cause hypoglycemia, it may potentiate the effect of hypoglycemic agents (e.g., insulin); the dosage of insulin and/or sulfonylurea may need to be reduced after starting the patient on troglitazone. Another such agent is rosiglitazone, which has just been approved for use.

Q: Are there any contraindications for troglitazone use?

A: Because troglitazone rarely can cause hepatotoxicity, it should be used with caution in patients with hepatic disease. Serum transaminases should be obtained initially, once monthly for 8 months, then every 2 months for next 4 months and as needed thereafter (every 3 to 6 months). Those with transaminase elevation should not be placed on troglitazone. The drug should be discontinued when transaminase elevations occur while on the medication. At this time the effects of the other thiazolidinedione drugs on the liver are unknown.

Like any oral agent, troglitazone is not recommended for use during pregnancy. It may improve hyperandrogenism in women with anovulation and polycystic ovary syndrome (PCOS), and such users should not become pregnant and start ovu-

TABLE 5-13.   Contraindications to Metformin Therapy

Renal insufficiency: serum creatinine ≥ 1.5 mg/dL in men, or ≥ 1.4 mg/dL in women

Hepatic failure

Severe cardiovascular disease

Severe pulmonary disease

Severe illness (sepsis, shock, trauma requiring hospitalization)

Pregnancy

lating. It also appears to decrease the effectiveness of estrogens used for contraception.

Q: What are α-glucosidase inhibitors?

A: **Acarbose** and **miglitol** are α-glucosidase inhibitors that inhibit postprandial absorption of glucose. Glucose is instead broken down in the large intestine by bacteria, leading to flatulence, the major side effect of these drugs. This agent is useful for mild hyperglycemia, but studies with acarbose show only a minimal improvement in glycated hemoglobin (1%). If a patient on these drugs is also on other agents that can cause hypoglycemia, such as insulin or sulfonylureas, the hypoglycemia cannot be treated with *glucose*; rather, the patient may consume more complex sugars (e.g., in milk) or use oral glucose gel, which is absorbed through the buccal mucosa.

Q: What is repaglinide?

A: Repaglinide is a drug of the meglitinide class that stimulates insulin release from the β cell. It therefore acts in a similar fashion to the sulfonylureas, although their structures differ. Unlike the sulfonylureas, repaglinide has a very short half-life and is therefore suitable for preprandial administration. It is not taken unless a meal is eaten. Repaglinide is cleared hepatically and needs no adjustment for patients with renal insufficiency. As with sulfonylureas, hypoglycemia may occur.

Q: What is amylin?

A: Amylin is a 37-amino acid peptide hormone that (like insulin) is secreted by pancreatic β cells in response to food. It appears to enhance gastric emptying and glucose utilization. Patients with type 1 (and some with type 2) diabetes are deficient in amylin, and synthetic analogs are being studied experimentally. One such amylin analog, pramlinitide, has been shown in clinical trials to decrease postprandial hyperglycemia and improve 24-hour glucose control without increasing the risk of hypoglycemia.

Q: Can type 1 diabetes be cured?

A: There is no cure for type 1 diabetes. The closest option is restoration of the patient's β-cell mass by transplantation of the whole pancreas (pancreas transplantation) or of the islets themselves (islet cell transplantation). Typically, a cadaveric organ is used. Autotransplantation of the patient's own islets can be done for those undergoing pancreatectomy for benign disease (e.g., pancreatitis). The advantage of these procedures is that normal or near-normal glycemic control can be achieved with freedom from insulin, thus reducing the likelihood of long-term complications and improving the patient's quality of life.

Because of the risks of long-term immunosuppressive drugs, pancreas transplants are usually reserved for patients with renal failure who are also candidates for a renal transplant. In such cases, immunosuppressive drugs would be required anyway, so pancreas transplantation carries little additional risk. However, several centers are now performing pancreas-only transplantation for diabetics with severe complications.

In a pancreas transplantation, the whole pancreas is transplanted into the pelvis, and exocrine secretions are usually drained into the bladder. Urinary amylase concentration is therefore a convenient indicator of pancreatic function. The mortality rate of pancreas transplantation is similar to that of renal transplants. The 1-year pancreas survival is approximately 75%, and 5-year survival is about 60%.

Pancreatic islets themselves may be transplanted, although islet cell purification is technically quite difficult. These cells can be injected into the portal vein, and they will lodge inside the liver where they secrete insulin in response to hyperglycemia. Insulin secretion is not entirely normal in these patients, and some may still require additional insulin. Other patients are able to come off insulin entirely. Glucagon secretion is not normal. In any case, patients with a functional graft have a significantly better quality of life than before.

Q: Can type 1 diabetes be prevented?

A: Clinical trials in the United States have examined persons at high risk for development of IDDM (e.g., those with affected first-degree relatives). These persons were monitored for the development of autoantibodies and/or hyperglycemia. Persons who develop autoantibodies received immunosuppressive drugs (azathioprine, cyclosporine), which reduced antibody levels and delayed the onset of type 1 diabetes. Relapses occurred in some individuals taking the drugs, and insulin was required a few weeks after the drug was discontinued. The benefits of this sort of therapy must be weighed carefully against the side effects of these potentially toxic drugs.

A derivative of nicotinic acid, nicotinamide, appears to preserve β-cell mass in animals, via several immunologic actions. Clinical trials in humans have yielded conflicting results. Vaccination with BCG (bacille Calmette-Guérin) appears to prevent diabetes in the mouse; further studies are required in humans.

First-degree relatives of persons with IDDM have been given oral insulin or GAD-65 (glutamic acid decarboxylase antibodies) in an attempt to induce "tolerance" to the antibodies. This potentially may delay the onset of type 1 diabetes in these persons.

In persons with new onset IDDM, intensive insulin therapy has been shown to preserve existing β-cell mass and enhance long-term glycemic control.

Q: What is hypoglycemia?

A: **Hypoglycemia** is the condition of low serum glucose levels. The low glucose itself is not enough to make a diagnosis, but rather the criteria of **Whipple's triad** must be met:

1. The person must have unequivocal hypoglycemia (< 60 mg/dL).

2. The person must have symptoms at the time the glucose is low.

3. Symptoms must improve after treatment of the low serum glucose.

All three must occur simultaneously. For example, low serum glucose without symptoms, plus symptoms at another time with normoglycemia cannot satisfy Whipple's triad, and a diagnosis cannot be made. Although it is often cited in the popular media as a cause of multiple ailments, true hypoglycemia is very rare except in diabetics treated with insulin or oral hypoglycemic agents.

Q: What is the body's normal response to hypoglycemia?

A: In hypoglycemia, insulin levels decline, and glucagon levels increase. Glucagon stimulates gluconeogenesis and glycogenolysis. Epinephrine also plays a key role in facilitating these two processes. Type 1 diabetics lose glucagon secretion along with insulin secretion, diminishing their response (hypoglycemia unawareness). Those with long-standing diabetes may develop autonomic neuropathy and deficiency in the epinephrine response.

Cortisol and growth hormone are also important in the delayed response to hypoglycemia. Persons with adrenal insufficiency may develop hypoglycemia as a presenting complaint.

Q: What is reactive hypoglycemia?

A: The normal response to an oral glucose load is secretion of an appropriate amount of insulin by the pancreas, resulting in euglycemia. In those with **reactive hypoglycemia,** the insulin response is exaggerated, leading to postprandial hypoglycemia with resultant symptoms. True reactive hypoglycemia is actually quite rare in the absence of gastrointestinal tract abnormalities, contrary to many people's beliefs. It is an over-diagnosed illness, usually by inappropriate use of the 100-gram OGTT. If true reactive hypoglycemia is present, it is not a life-threatening disorder, and may be managed with smaller, more frequent meals and avoidance of concentrated sweets.

Patients with abnormal gastric emptying (e.g., post-gastrectomy) have rapid "dumping" of food into the intestinal tract, which may result in hyperinsulinism and postprandial hypoglycemia. Treatment involves smaller, more frequent meals.

Patients with impaired glucose tolerance occasionally have delayed insulin release 1 to 2 hours after a meal, which may result in mild postprandial hypoglycemia. Treatment is weight loss and dietary management. It is common for a patient with type 2 diabetes to mention that he or she had "hypoglycemia" when younger or to have brothers and sisters with "hypoglycemia."

Q: Should an oral glucose tolerance test be used to make the diagnosis of hypoglycemia?

A: No. Although the 100-gram OGTT has been widely employed to test for reactive hypoglycemia, it is a non-physiologic test, as 400 kcal of glucose are consumed at once. Many normal persons will have at least one hypoglycemic reading during the OGTT, without symptoms; others will have symptoms without hypoglycemia. Because of this poor specificity, it is no longer indicated for the evaluation of reactive hypoglycemia. The 100-gram OGTT has only two appropriate uses: evaluation of gestational diabetes mellitus and evaluation of growth hormone hypersecretion (acromegaly).

If desired, a more physiologic test is the **mixed meal challenge,** which is done by giving the patient approximately 25% of the daily calories as a liquid food supplement, then measuring glucose levels at 1, 2, and 3 hours afterward. The vast majority of persons who have an abnormal OGTT will have a normal mixed meal challenge and hence do *not* have reactive hypoglycemia.

Q: What is fasting hypoglycemia?

A: Unlike reactive hypoglycemia, which occurs after a glucose load, **fasting hypoglycemia** occurs after an individual has been without food for several hours (Table 5-14). Typically the patient feels worse in the morning, but feels better after eating. This type of hypoglycemia is ominous, and is associated with either insulin hypersecretion or glucose underproduction.

Q: How is insulinoma diagnosed?

A: For **insulinoma,** fasting hypoglycemia must occur along with elevated insulin and C-peptide levels. It is most helpful if the patient presents spontaneously in this fashion. If not, a prolonged fast may be required to provoke hypoglycemia; typically, the patient is subjected to a 72-hour fast in the hospital. Almost every patient with insulinoma will develop a hypoglycemic episode during this time, and the hospital setting is necessary owing to the potential hazards of this procedure.

Both serum insulin and C-peptide levels should be obtained at the time of hypoglycemia, and both should be elevated with true endogenous insulin hypersecretion. Proinsulin levels may be more specific than insulin levels alone in some patients and are elevated in persons with insulinoma. With factitious use of insulin, the insulin level will be high but C-peptide (the fragment cleaved from proinsulin) will be suppressed, indicating an exogenous source of insulin. Patients with hypoglycemia due to underproduction of glucose (e.g., adrenal insufficiency) will have suppressed insulin and C-peptide levels. The euglycemic clamp study (an experimental test) demonstrates that very high glucose infusion rates are necessary to maintain euglycemia.

Once endogenous hyperinsulinemia has been confirmed, localization procedures are in order. Abdominal CT scan may be able to localize the tumor. Portal venous sampling may be done for a

TABLE 5-14.   Causes of Fasting Hypoglycemia

INSULIN EXCESS	GLUCOSE UNDERPRODUCTION	PARANEOPLASTIC (? HUMORAL FACTOR, INCREASED UTILIZATION)
Insulinoma	Adrenocortical insufficiency	Large mesenchymal sarcomas (fibrosarcomas, rhabdomyosarcomas)
Sulfonylurea or meglitinide ingestion	Alcohol intoxication	Adenocarcinomas (hepatomas)
Factitious use of insulin	Severe hepatic disease	Carcinoid tumors
Insulin-treated diabetes	Drugs (e.g., propranolol, pentamidine)	
Autoimmune (insulin release; insulin receptor antibodies)	Renal insufficiency	
β-cell hyperplasia (nesidioblastosis)	Inborn errors of glucose metabolism	

tumor that cannot be seen, as a means of measuring a "step-up" in insulin level. Intraoperative ultrasound may demonstrate a tumor not seen by other means. Radiolabeled octreotide scans are also useful in isolating an isulinoma.

Treatment of insulinoma is surgical resection. Diazoxide, which is administered preoperatively to restore euglycemia, is the definitive treatment for patients with inoperable tumors. The long-acting somatostatin analog octreotide suppresses insulin secretion and has been used with some success.

Q: How does alcohol cause hypoglycemia?

A: Ethanol is metabolized by alcohol dehydrogenase, which requires the cofactor nicotinamide adenine dinucleotide (NAD$^+$). Alcohol intoxication may deplete NAD$^+$, which is also required in gluconeogenesis. Glycogenolysis is not affected, so hypoglycemia does not occur until after approximately 12 hours after the patient has eaten.

Q: How does adrenocortical insufficiency cause hypoglycemia?

A: Cortisol, a "stress" hormone, enhances gluconeogenesis and glycogen mobilization. Cortisol deficiency therefore impairs these processes, and hypoglycemia may occur in susceptible individuals.

Q: What are some other causes of glucose underproduction?

A: Most gluconeogenesis occurs in the liver, so patients with severe hepatic disease often develop hypoglycemia. As the kidney also contributes to gluconeogenesis (10%), persons with renal failure on dialysis also may develop hypoglycemia. Those with septic shock may develop hypoglycemia from excessive glucose consumption. Persons with inborn errors of glucose metabolism (e.g., glycogen storage diseases) often have hypoglycemia.

Q: What is autoimmune hypoglycemia?

A: In rare patients, circulating anti-insulin antibodies bind insulin and circulate in plasma. This generally results in postprandial hypoglycemia when the excess insulin is released from the antibodies. Another rare syndrome is that of insulin receptor autoantibodies, which have a stimulatory effect on the insulin receptor. Interestingly, these patients also have insulin resistance and acanthosis nigricans (type B insulin resistance); they may also develop type 2 diabetes.

Q: What is nesidioblastosis?

A: **Nesidioblastosis** is β-cell hyperplasia that involves most or all of the pancreas. This is in contrast to insulinoma, which is a focal pancreatic tumor. Nesidioblastosis occurs most commonly in infants and children.

BIBLIOGRAPHY

Alpers DH, Clouse RE, Stenson WF. Protein and calorie requirements. In: Alpers DH, Clouse RE, Stenson WF. Manual of nutritional therapeutics. 2nd ed. Boston: Little, Brown, 1988:129–130.

American Diabetes Association. Implications of the United Kingdom prospective diabetes study. Diabetes Care 1998;21:2180–2184.

American Diabetes Association. Nutrition recommendations and principles for people with diabetes mellitus (position statement). Diabetes Care 1998; 11(suppl 1):S32–S35.

Bretzel RG, Hering BJ, Federlin KF. Transplantation of the pancreas and pancreatic islets. In: Pickup JC, Williams G, eds. Textbook of diabetes. 2nd ed. Cambridge, MA: Blackwell Scientific, 1997:86.1–86.6.

Davidson MH. "Diabetic ketoacidosis and hyperosmolar nonketotic syndrome." In: Davidson MB. Diabetes mellitus: diagnosis and treatment. 4th ed. Philadelphia: W.B. Saunders, 1998:159–190.

Davidson MB. Oral antidiabetes agents. In: Davidson MB. Diabetes mellitus: diagnosis and treatment. 4th ed. Philadelphia: W.B. Saunders, 1998:127–141.

Dupré J, Mahon JL, Stiller CR. Prevention of development or progression of β-cell damage in insulin-dependent diabetes mellitus. In: Pickup JC, Williams G, eds. Textbook of diabetes. 2nd ed. Cambridge, MA: Blackwell Scientific, 1997:82.1–82.10.

Franz MJ, Horton ES, Bantle JP, Beebe CA, et al. Nutrition principles for the management of diabetes and related complications. Diabetes Care 1994;17: 490–518.

Karam JH. Hypoglycemic disorders. In: Greenspan FS, Strewler GJ, eds. Basic and clinical endocrinology. 5th ed. Norwalk, CT: Appleton & Lange, 1997: 664–677.

Olson DR, Stevenson JM. Diabetes surveillance at the centers for disease control. In: Davidson JK, ed. Clinical diabetes mellitus: a problem-oriented approach. New York: Thieme Medical, 1991:808–811.

Tattersall RB. Maturity-onset diabetes of the young (MODY). In: Pickup JC, Williams G, eds. Textbook of diabetes. Cambridge, MA: Blackwell Scientific, 1991:243–246.

Weir GC, Nathan DM, Singer DE. Standards of care for diabetes. Diabetes Care 1994;17:1514–1522.

REVIEW QUESTIONS

I. SHORT ANSWER

1. A disorder of glucose metabolism resulting in hyperglycemia is called _____. Type ____ occurs in individuals who do not make insulin and depend on exogenous insulin for life. Type ____ is more common and is a disorder of impaired insulin action rather than absent insulin secretion.

2. The classic signs and symptoms of diabetes include the triad of _____, _____, and _____.

3. Diabetes may be diagnosed when two fasting serum glucose values equal or exceed _____. It can also be diagnosed when the patient presents with _____ and a random glucose equal to or over _____. Finally, diabetes is present if a 2-hour glucose value and any intermediate value after a 75-gram oral glucose load equals or exceeds _____.

4. Patients with elevated glucose levels that do not fulfill the criteria for diagnosis of diabetes are said to have _____.

5. _____ is a peptide produced by the β cells of the pancreas. It is produced by cleavage of the prohormone _____ into it and another, biologically inactive, peptide, _____. The latter can be used as a marker of _____.

6. Insulin levels increase in response to _____, and decrease in response to _____. Insulin is an anabolic hormone that promotes energy _____.

7. A peptide hormone made in the α cells of the pancreas is _____. In contrast to insulin, it is a _____ hormone that helps provide increased energy for cells.

8. Type ____ diabetes results when the pancreas no longer makes insulin in sufficient amounts. The cause is usually _____. Without treatment, _____ and _____ result.

9. Early in the course of type 1 diabetes, a brief period of insulin secretion returns, called the _____.

10. Patients predisposed for developing type 1 diabetes carry the HLA haplotypes _____ and _____ on chromosome 6. _____, seen in 70% of patients at the time of diagnosis, result in _____.

11. Type ____ diabetes is caused by impaired insulin utilization or insulin _____. In contrast to type 1 diabetes, insulin levels are often _____ at the time of diagnosis. Most with this disorder are _____, although some are normal weight.

12. Hyperglycemia may actually impair insulin secretion in type 2 diabetics, resulting in _____.

13. In addition to hyperglycemia, impaired insulin utilization may also result in _____, _____, and _____. These disorders are often referred to collectively as _____.

14. An unusual form of type 2 diabetes occurring in teenagers or young adults is _____. Unlike typical type 2 diabetes, which is multi-factorial in inheritance, this disorder is inherited as _____.

15. Diabetes developing during pregnancy is called _____. It is usually caused by the diabetogenic effects of the _____ in the late second and third trimester. This disorder typically _____ after the pregnancy ends. These women are at higher risk for developing _____ later in life.

16. Women with poorly controlled diabetes in the first trimester place the fetus at risk for _____. Poor control late in pregnancy may result in _____ and _____.

17. Patients may monitor glucose levels at home with a _____. _____ glucose does not accurately reflect serum levels, so it is not a routinely recommended test.

18. Glucose irreversibly attaches to hemoglobin A, resulting in _____. Of these molecules, the most specific is _____. This reflects average serum glucose levels for the previous _____. This test is not accurate in persons with abnormal _____ molecules. A similar test for _____ is an estimate of glycated albumin.

19. Coronary artery and cerebrovascular disease are called _____ complications of diabetes. Retinopathy and nephropathy are _____ complications.

20. Neuropathies may be _____ or _____. The most common form of neuropathy is _____. A form in which the patient does not recognize hypoglycemia is _____. _____ causes nausea and early satiety as a result of gastrointestinal denervation.

21. Most patients with long-standing diabetes develop _____ retinopathy, which is of minimal clinical significance. Exudates occurring in the macula may result in _____ and visual loss. Neovascularization of blood vessels causes _____ retinopathy, which can result in _____, _____, and _____.

22. The first indicator of diabetic nephropathy is an increase in _____. _____ occurs next, defined as protein excretion of between _____ μg/min. At this point, nephropathy is potentially _____. _____ is said to occur when the protein excretion exceeds _____ mg/day. In time, persons at this stage will invariably progress to _____, although the progression can be slowed.

23. The most important factor in slowing the progression of diabetic nephropathy is _____. Control of _____ and administration of _____ drugs are also beneficial. Restriction of dietary _____ is also advocated.

24. _____ is a disorder of glucose metabolism resulting in metabolic acidosis and dehydration. It is due to a deficiency of _____. An increase in _____ hormones results in lipolysis, leading to _____ formation. _____ catabolism also occurs, resulting in increased _____. Hyperglycemia results in _____ and _____.

25. Ketone bodies and ketoacids in DKA include _____, _____, and _____. The primary molecule is _____, which can be measured and is a useful parameter to follow in treatment. Another useful laboratory parameter is the _____.

26. _____ is depleted in DKA and should be replenished, unless renal failure is present. Levels may be elevated at presentation due to _____ and _____, even though total body stores are low.

27. Immediate treatment of DKA includes administration of _____. _____ is then started, first with a "loading dose" which is then followed by a continuous infusion. The infusion is continued until the _____ has resolved. At that point, _____ can be started, and the infusion may be safely stopped.

28. _____ is different from DKA in that significant _____ is not present. Glucose levels are often _____ than those in DKA. The cornerstone of therapy is _____ administration. _____ plays a lesser role than in DKA.

29. Regular or soluble insulin is arranged as a _____ at high concentrations. After injection, it dissociates into _____ and then is absorbed. _____ is a synthetically modified insulin that dissociates into _____ at a _____ concentration than regular insulin and is thus absorbed faster.

30. Long-acting insulins use retarding agents such as _____ or _____ to slow dissociation and prolong action.

31. _____ is the administration of short-acting insulin by an infusion device. The patient receives a set amount of _____ insulin continuously, and administers an insulin _____ at meal time. _____ results rapidly if something happens to the infusion pump or tubing.

32. Patients should supplement their insulin dose with a _____ when glucose levels are high.

33. _____ are agents that enhance insulin secretion and thus may produce _____. They include the older _____ agents and the newer drug _____.

34. _____ is an antihyperglycemic agent of the biguanide class. It should be avoided in persons with _____ or _____ disease. A common side effect is _____. A rare and potentially lethal side effect is _____.

35. A novel antihyperglycemic agent that improves insulin sensitivity is _____. It must be avoided in persons with _____ disease. _____ must be monitored often.

36. _____ and _____ are inhibitors of α-glucosidase and thus inhibit glucose absorption from the intestine. A frequent side effect is _____.

37. The diagnosis of hypoglycemia requires the presence of the signs and symptoms called _____.

38. The most important counterregulatory hormones in the body's response to hypoglycemia are _____ and _____.

39. An exaggerated insulin response to food resulting in hypoglycemia is known as _____. A poor method of testing for this disorder is the _____. Mild postprandial hypoglycemia is common in persons who are destined to develop _____.

40. Hypoglycemia occurring many hours after food ingestion is termed _____ hypoglycemia. Unlike _____ hypoglycemia, it may be lethal.

41. A tumor resulting in insulin excess and hypoglycemia is an _____. It is suggested by spontaneous hypoglycemia associated with ele-

vated _____ and _____ levels. In contrast, persons who factitiously use insulin to produce hypoglycemia have elevated _____ and low _____ levels.

II. MULTIPLE CHOICE

Select the one best answer.

42. Which is true of gestational diabetes mellitus?
    a. It always requires insulin for control.
    b. It may be treated with oral antidiabetic agents.
    c. It typically is diagnosed in the first trimester of pregnancy.
    d. It usually goes away after giving birth.
    e. It places the patient at no greater risk for developing overt diabetes mellitus later in life than a woman without gestational diabetes.

43. A patient is on 70/30 insulin, 28 units twice daily (b.i.d.). You want to switch her over to mixed N and R insulin. The correct dosage would be:
    a. N 24, R 4 b.i.d.
    b. N 16, R 12 b.i.d.
    c. N 20, R 8 b.i.d.
    d. N 8, R 20 b.i.d.
    e. N 22, R 6 b.i.d.

44. A 22-year-old Caucasian man is admitted to the hospital for treatment of newly diagnosed diabetes. He presented with nonketotic hyperglycemia and classic symptoms of diabetes. He is thin and without family history of diabetes. After starting insulin, his glucose levels returned to normal and he goes home. Several weeks later he noticed that his glucose levels remained normal even though he forgot to take his insulin several times. The most likely explanation for his glucose levels remaining normal despite not taking insulin is:
    a. he has MODY (maturity-onset diabetes of the young).
    b. he had "glucose toxicity" initially when he was diagnosed, and now his β-cell function has returned.
    c. he is going through the honeymoon period of type 1 diabetes, and his insulin requirements will increase in time.
    d. he probably does not have diabetes, and the diagnosis was a mistake.
    e. his glucometer is probably broken.

45. Which one of the following features is not characteristic of type 2 diabetes?
    a. absent insulin secretion
    b. insulin resistance
    c. accelerated rate of hepatic glucose output
    d. increased insulin secretion early and decreased insulin secretion late in the disease process
    e. predisposition to hypertension and hypertriglyceridemia

46. The half-life of regular insulin in serum is:
    a. < 10 minutes
    b. 30 minutes
    c. 1 hour
    d. 3 hours
    e. 6 hours

47. A 16-year-old girl with known type 1 diabetes is brought to the emergency room, unresponsive. She is breathing rapidly, and her breath has a fruity odor. Her blood pressure is 60/40, and pulse is 140. The first thing you should do is:
    a. give an ampule of D_{50} intravenously, as she is probably hypoglycemic.
    b. obtain a serum glucose level and wait for it to return before recommending further treatment.
    c. give 10 units human insulin, intravenously.
    d. begin vigorous intravenous fluid administration.
    e. start dopamine, 3 μg/kg/hour.

48. A woman 5 feet 9 inches tall, and weighs 200 pounds. You ask her to grasp her wrist with the

other hand, and the fingers do not touch. Her ideal body weight is approximately:

   a. 135 lb

   b. 145 lb

   c. 160 lb

   d. 172 lb

   e. 180 lb

49. The rapid absorption of lispro insulin (as compared to regular insulin) is due to:

   a. its shorter half-life in serum.

   b. its greater potency on a unit for unit basis.

   c. its ability to dissociate into monomers at a higher concentration.

   d. its decreased protein binding.

   e. its ability to resist degradation by proteolytic enzymes in the skin.

50. A 23-year-old woman with type 1 diabetes monitors blood glucose five times daily. She is on twice-daily human ultralente insulin and pre-meal regular. She has no complications from diabetes, recognizes hypoglycemia well, and lives with her husband. Her glucose values are as follows:

3 AM	PRE-BREAKFAST	PRE-LUNCH	PRE-SUPPER	BEDTIME
76	165	43	122	104
123	175	37	89	98
—	182	62	134	123
107	155	—	101	118
—	142	67	—	—

Of the following, the most logical insulin change would be:

   a. decrease both doses of ultralente, leave regular the same.

   b. decrease PM ultralente and increase AM regular.

   c. increase PM ultralente and AM regular.

   d. add regular at bedtime.

   e. increase PM ultralente and decrease AM regular.

51. A 32-year-old man with type 1 diabetes is admitted to the intensive care unit for treatment of ketoacidosis. Two days later, he is stabilized and transferred out to the medical floor on twice-daily NPH and regular insulin. His most recent glucose is 137 mg/dL; β-hydroxybutyrate and anion gap are normal. You are called because he still has ketones in his urine. You examine him and note no abnormalities. You should:

   a. transfer him back to the ICU and start an insulin infusion.

   b. continue the current treatment.

   c. switch him over to lispro (Humalog) insulin.

   d. order an arterial blood gas.

   e. increase the calories in his diet.

52. A 45-year-old man complains of frequent weakness and diaphoresis 2 hours after his daily breakfast of sugary cereal and a doughnut. A glucometer in the factory nurse's office, 2 hours after breakfast, was 67 mg/dL. Examination demonstrates an overweight male with acanthosis nigricans and multiple skin tags. Fasting insulin and C-peptide levels are approximately twice normal; fasting glucose is normal.

A. Which of the following is true about this patient?

   a. He likely has an insulinoma.

   b. He is probably injecting insulin surreptitiously.

   c. He likely has adrenocortical insufficiency.

   d. He likely has impaired glucose intolerance and is at high risk for developing type 2 diabetes in the future.

   e. He has reactive hypoglycemia.

B. The most appropriate next step in management should be:

   a. hydrocortisone, 30 mg daily

   b. exercise regimen and consultation with a dietitian for weight loss

   c. CT scan of the abdomen

   d. 72-hour supervised fast

   e. administration of "hypoglycemic" diet

53. A 25-year-old male with type 1 diabetes uses an external insulin pump. He has been playing basketball all day and has not checked his blood glucose. At 2 PM he checks it and it is 346 mg/dL, and he gives additional sliding scale insulin through his pump. He plays some more basketball, thinking that it will lower his glucose level. Two hours later, his level is 452 mg/dL, and he feels very thirsty and has to urinate frequently. The *first* thing that this man should do is:
    a. program his pump to give additional insulin now.
    b. wait, as the insulin he gave 2 hours ago probably has not kicked in yet.
    c. play more basketball to try and decrease the glucose level.
    d. draw up insulin in a syringe and inject it now.
    e. go home and take a nap, as this will likely help his glucose level.

54. The most common form of diabetic neuropathy is:
    a. cranial nerve palsy
    b. chronic sensory neuropathy ("stocking feet" distribution)
    c. proximal motor neuropathy (amyotrophy)
    d. diabetic gastroparesis
    e. diabetic sudomotor neuropathy (gustatory sweating)

55. The first step in treatment of diabetic neuropathy should be:
    a. narcotic analgesics
    b. tricyclic antidepressants
    c. improvement of glycemic control
    d. gabapentin
    e. topical capsaicin cream

56. A 32-year-old woman is hospitalized with diabetic ketoacidosis. She currently is on an insulin infusion at 2 units/hour, and her last serum glucose was 70 mg/dL. She is receiving D_5 (5% glucose in water) with 0.9% NaCl at 200 mL/hour. Anion gap and β-hydroxybutyrate lev-

els are still significantly elevated. The best action to take at this time is:
    a. stop the insulin infusion and switch to sliding scale insulin only.
    b. decrease the insulin infusion to 1 unit/hour.
    c. stop the insulin infusion and start subcutaneous insulin.
    d. increase the glucose concentration in the intravenous fluid (e.g., D_{10}) and increase the insulin infusion rate.
    e. decrease the insulin infusion rate and glucose concentration in the IV fluid.

57. A 50-year-old sedentary male has type 2 diabetes. He weighs 178 pounds (80 kg) and is 69 inches tall. His daily basal energy expenditure by the Harris-Benedict equation is approximately:
    a. 1200 kcal
    b. 1400 kcal
    c. 1500 kcal
    d. 1700 kcal
    e. 2000 kcal

58. Glucagon would be expected to work *least* well in which one of the following patients with hypoglycemia?
    a. type 2 patient on glyburide
    b. type 1 patient who is intoxicated with ethanol and has not eaten for 10 hours
    c. type 2 patient who is on insulin and metformin
    d. type 1 patient who also has hypothyroidism and is twelve weeks pregnant
    e. patient with severe postprandial hypoglycemia due to gastrectomy and "dumping syndrome"

59. A 25-year-old black male with known thalassemia minor is found to have a slightly elevated glycated hemoglobin level drawn during a routine insurance physical. He has no complaints, and appears in good health. Which is the most appropriate action at this time?
    a. Begin a sulfonylurea.
    b. Test his urine for glucose.

c. Obtain two fasting serum glucose levels.
d. Begin insulin.
e. Begin troglitazone.

III. TRUE OR FALSE

60. A 35-year-old overweight woman with type 2 diabetes wants to become pregnant. She currently takes glipizide and metformin. Correct advice at this time would include the following:
___ a. encourage weight loss
___ b. stop metformin but continue glipizide
___ c. stop glipizide but continue metformin
___ d. stop both oral agents and start insulin
___ e. stop both oral agents and start troglitazone

61. Patients correctly diagnosed as having diabetes mellitus include which of the following?
___ a. patient with a single fasting (serum) glucose of 130 mg/dL and glucometer reading (fasting) of 145 mg/dL in office
___ b. patient with hemoglobin A_{1c} of 8.2% (normal: 4.2–6.5%)
___ c. patient with 2-week history of polyuria, polydipsia, 30-lb weight loss, blood glucose of 897 mg/dL, and anion gap of 23
___ d. patient with 2-hour serum glucose value of 175 mg/dL and 1 hour value of 207 mg/dL after 75-gram glucose load
___ e. patient with 4+ glycosuria on a routine urinalysis for insurance examination

62. Which of the following statements are true concerning insulin?
___ a. Levels are increased during hypoglycemia not due to insulin hypersecretion.
___ b. Facilitates glucose transport across cell membranes by means of GLUT proteins.
___ c. It is structurally identical among animal species.
___ d. It is formed by cleavage of C-peptide into proinsulin and insulin.
___ e. It is absorbed poorly from the gastrointestinal tract.

63. A patient is found comatose with a blood glucose of 39 mg/dL. Serum insulin and C-peptide levels from the same specimen are elevated. Possible reasons for the hypoglycemia include:
___ a. Addison's disease
___ b. MEN I
___ c. surreptitious insulin use
___ d. surreptitious oral hypoglycemic agent use
___ e. alcohol intoxication

64. Which of the following statements are true concerning diabetic ketoacidosis?
___ a. It only occurs with blood glucose > 250.
___ b. It should be treated with IV insulin infusion in very large doses (e.g., 30 units/hour).
___ c. It cannot occur in a type 2 diabetic.
___ d. It commonly results from omission of insulin on "sick days."
___ e. It is expected to occur at least once a year in type 1 diabetics.

65. The Diabetes Control and Complications Trial (DCCT):
___ a. showed that 'tight control' slowed or halted progression of neuropathy, retinopathy, and nephropathy in type 1 and type 2 diabetics.
___ b. showed that "tight control" had no adverse consequences.
___ c. showed that "tight control" halted progression of heart disease and peripheral vascular disease.
___ d. showed that "tight control" is more expensive than conventional control.

66. Poorly controlled gestational diabetes mellitus diagnosed in the late second trimester may result in:
    —— a. congenital organ malformations
    —— b. macrosomia
    —— c. neonatal hypoglycemia
    —— d. neonatal hyperglycemia
    —— e. congenital hypothyroidism

67. Oral medications used to treat diabetes that alone can cause hypoglycemia include:
    —— a. metformin
    —— b. glipizide
    —— c. repaglinide
    —— d. acarbose
    —— e. troglitazone

68. Acceptable treatments for gestational diabetes may include:
    —— a. diet
    —— b. regular insulin
    —— c. glyburide
    —— d. NPH insulin
    —— e. metformin
    —— f. ultralente insulin

69. Which of the following statements are true concerning gestational diabetes?
    —— a. It usually resolves after delivery.
    —— b. 30% to 40% develop type 1 diabetes later in life.
    —— c. Poor control leads to defects in organ development.
    —— d. Poor control may cause neonatal hyperglycemia.
    —— e. All patients require insulin.

70. Conditions that increase the risk for gestational diabetes include:
    —— a. obesity
    —— b. Hashimoto's thyroiditis
    —— c. polycystic ovary syndrome
    —— d. advanced maternal age
    —— e. ovarian hyperthecosis

71. Appropriate treatment for a type 2 diabetic patient with persistent microalbuminuria and elevated creatinine clearance may include:
    —— a. angiotensin-converting enzyme inhibitors
    —— b. good glycemic control
    —— c. moderate dietary protein restriction
    —— d. drinking lots of fluids
    —— e. assessment and modification of cardiac risk factors

72. A 33-year-old woman is seen in your office with chief complaint of polyuria and polydipsia for the last month. Examination reveals a thin female with a small goiter. Serum glucose is 327 mg/dL. Acceptable options at this time include:
    —— a. admission to the hospital to start insulin therapy
    —— b. troglitazone
    —— c. measurement of serum TSH
    —— d. glyburide
    —— e. meeting with a registered dietitian and certified diabetes educator

73. A 40-year-old woman of normal body weight presents with polyuria and serum glucose of 210 mg/dL. Factors that would favor the diagnosis of type 2 diabetes in this individual include:
    —— a. elevated insulin and C-peptide levels
    —— b. non-Caucasian race
    —— c. presence of human leukocyte antigen (HLA) types DR3/DR4
    —— d. necessity of large insulin doses (> 1 U/kg/day) for good control
    —— e. presence of gestational diabetes in a previous pregnancy

74. Second-generation sulfonylureas include:
    —— a. glipizide
    —— b. metformin
    —— c. acetohexamide
    —— d. glyburide
    —— e. chlorpropamide

75. Side effects of chlorpropamide may include:
    ___ a. lactic acidosis
    ___ b. hyponatremia
    ___ c. hypoglycemia
    ___ d. nausea and vomiting when used with alcohol
    ___ e. death from cardiovascular disease

76. A 34-year-old woman with type 1 diabetes wants an insulin pump. Good reasons to advise pump therapy include:
    ___ a. she desires fewer episodes of hypoglycemia.
    ___ b. she has good insurance and support from her family.
    ___ c. she doesn't want to have to worry about her diabetes any more.
    ___ d. she wants more flexible meal schedules.
    ___ e. she has been admitted with ketoacidosis six times within the last year.

77. A 37-year-old woman is found unconscious at home. She is on no known medications, but has a daughter with type 1 diabetes. She awakens after administration of intravenous glucose. Blood drawn by the paramedics before administration of glucose demonstrates a serum glucose of 19 mg/dL (normal: 70–115); serum insulin level 42.2 μU/mL (normal: 0.0–20.0); C-peptide is 4.51 ng/mL (normal: 0.50–2.00). Which of the following is/are appropriate at this time?
    ___ a. consultation with a psychiatrist
    ___ b. measurement of blood sulfonylurea levels
    ___ c. computed tomographic scan of the pancreas
    ___ d. measurement of serum cortisol before and after ACTH
    ___ e. measurement of blood alcohol level

78. Correct use of a 100-gram glucose load includes the evaluation of:
    ___ a. hypoglycemia
    ___ b. acromegaly
    ___ c. gestational diabetes
    ___ d. type 2 diabetes
    ___ e. impaired glucose tolerance

79. Acceptable insulin regimens for a type 1 diabetic without complications include:
    ___ a. once-daily human ultralente insulin
    ___ b. continuous subcutaneous insulin infusion (CSII) via insulin pump
    ___ c. bedtime NPH insulin plus pre-meal lispro insulin
    ___ d. twice-daily NPH insulin
    ___ e. twice-daily human ultralente insulin plus pre-meal regular insulin

80. Regarding the euglycemic clamp study:
    ___ a. It is a type of surgical procedure for those with peripheral vascular disease.
    ___ b. It is designed to measure the in vivo sensitivity of humans to intravenous insulin.
    ___ c. A type 2 diabetic would require more glucose for a given insulin infusion rate than a normal person.
    ___ d. It is a type of insulin pump.
    ___ e. Persons with insulinoma have increased glucose requirements compared to normal individuals.

ANSWERS

1. diabetes mellitus; 1; 2

2. polyuria, polydipsia, polyphagia

3. 126 mg/dL (7.0 mmol/L); classic signs and symptoms (polys), 200 mg/dL (11.1 mmol/L); 200 mg/dL (11.1 mmol/L)

4. impaired glucose tolerance

5. insulin; proinsulin, C-peptide; endogenous insulin secretion

6. hyperglycemia, hypoglycemia; storage

7. glucagon; catabolic

8. 1; autoimmune; ketoacidosis, death

9. honeymoon phase

10. DR3, DR4; islet cell autoantibodies, islet cell destruction

11. 2, resistance; elevated; obese

12. glucose toxicity

13. atherosclerotic disease, hypertension, hyperlipidemia; syndrome X

14. maturity-onset diabetes of the young (MODY); autosomal dominant

15. gestational diabetes; fetoplacental unit (placental growth hormone, placental lactogen, progesterone); goes away; type 2 diabetes

16. organ malformations; macrosomia, neonatal hypoglycemia

17. glucose meter; urine

18. glycated hemoglobin (hemoglobin A_1); hemoglobin A_{1C}; 6 to 8 weeks; hemoglobin; fructosamine

19. macrovascular; microvascular

20. peripheral (somatic), autonomic; distal sensory neuropathy; hypoglycemia unawareness; diabetic gastroparesis

21. nonproliferative (background); macular edema; proliferative, vitreous hemorrhage, retinal detachment, blindness

22. glomerular filtration rate (GFR); microalbuminuria, 20–200; reversible; overt nephropathy, 500 mg/day; renal failure

23. glycemic control; hypertension, angiotensin-converting enzyme inhibitor; protein

24. diabetic ketoacidosis (DKA); insulin; counter-regulatory, ketone; protein, gluconeogenesis; osmotic diuresis, dehydration

25. acetone, acetoacetate, β-hydroxybutyrate (BOH); BOH; anion gap

26. potassium; acidosis, transcellular shifts

27. fluids; insulin; acidosis; subcutaneous insulin

28. hyperosmolar nonketotic syndrome (HNKS), acidosis; higher; fluid replacement; insulin

29. hexamer; monomers; lispro, monomers, higher

30. zinc, protamine

31. continuous subcutaneous insulin infusion (CSII); basal, bolus; ketoacidosis

32. sliding or coverage scale

33. oral hypoglycemic agents, hypoglycemia; sulfonylurea; repaglinide

34. metformin; renal, hepatic; gastrointestinal upset; lactic acidosis

35. troglitazone; hepatic; transaminase levels

36. acarbose; miglitol; flatulence

37. Whipple's triad

38. glucagon, epinephrine

39. reactive hypoglycemia; oral glucose tolerance test; type 2 diabetes

40. fasting; reactive

41. insulinoma; insulin, C-peptide; insulin, C-peptide

42. (*d*). GDM is diabetes that develops during pregnancy. It most typically is a condition of the late second trimester, and results in insulin resistance and hyperglycemia in susceptible individuals. This condition should abate after delivery. It is possible to develop type 1 or type 2 diabetes during pregnancy, in which case the diabetes will persist. Insulin (*a*) is required in many but certainly not all patients. Although gestational diabetes can be diagnosed in the first trimester (*c*), it generally is not diagnosed until later. Those with glucose intolerance in early pregnancy often are older women with

preexisting undiagnosed type 2 diabetes. GDM should never be treated with oral agents, as these can cross the placenta. Approximately 25% to 40% of women with GDM develop type 2 diabetes later in life (*e*).

43. (*c*). For the N component, $0.70 \times 28 = 19.6 \approx 20$; for the R component, subtract the N dosage from the total: $28 - 20 = 8$.

44. (*c*). Persons with newly diagnosed type 1 diabetes typically go through a honeymoon phase in which some residual insulin secretion returns; this may be enough for the patient to be normoglycemic on low doses or even when receiving no insulin. However, it is not recommended that patients stop their insulin, as intensive insulin therapy is believed to preserve the residual insulin secretion. MODY (*a*) is transmitted in an autosomal dominant fashion and is not likely to appear in someone without a strong family history. Glucose toxicity (*b*) occurs commonly in type 2 diabetics; high glucose levels actually inhibit β-cell function. Beta cell function improves after restoration of normoglycemia. It is unlikely that his normal readings are due either to an erroneous diagnosis (*d*) or broken meter (*e*).

45. (*a*). Absent insulin secretion is the hallmark of type 1 diabetes. The other features are typical of type 2 diabetes.

46. (*a*). The short half-life of intravenous insulin means that an infusion should never be discontinued unless subcutaneous insulin is started at least an hour beforehand. If this is not done, stopping the insulin infusion may result in return of ketoacidosis in a type 1 diabetic.

47. (*d*). This girl obviously has ketoacidosis and is hypotensive. The first thing to do is begin fluid administration. Administering insulin first may actually exacerbate the problem; insulin will cause the glucose to go into the cells, taking water with it, resulting in further extracellular dehydration and hypotension.

48. (*c*). For a medium frame, IBW $= 100 + (5)(9) = 145$ lb. She has a large frame, so her IBW $= 145 + (145)(0.10) = 145 + 14.5 = 159.5 \sim 160$ lb.

49. (*c*). Insulin is most active in its monomeric form. In solution, the insulin molecules associate to form hexamers. It is not absorbed until it reaches the monomeric form; the ability of lispro to dissociate into a monomer at a higher concentration than regular insulin accounts for its more rapid onset of action.

50. (*e*). She is having hyperglycemia in the morning with frequent lows at lunch. The evening ultralente should be increased and morning regular decreased. Alternatively, lispro might be considered, as it does not last as long as regular and often helps in preventing late-morning or late-evening hypoglycemia.

51. (*b*). Ketones are fat soluble and may be excreted in the urine for days after a bout with ketoacidosis. They are of no concern as long as the person is doing well clinically. Patients eating too few calories (*e*) may be ketogenic, but this is unlikely in this scenario.

52. A (*d*). This man is overweight and has acanthosis nigricans and skin tags, typical of persons with insulin resistance. He likely has a delayed insulin response to his high-carbohydrate breakfast and is becoming low, hours after ingestion. He should modify his diet and try to lose weight. B (*b*). This man should modify his lifestyle by exercising and losing weight, which will improve his insulin response.

53. (*d*). Something has gone wrong with this man's pump, and he likely has not received insulin for hours. The tubing connecting the pump to his skin may have been damaged. If he had checked his glucose earlier he would have been alerted to this. Trying to give more insulin through the pump (*a*) is futile as there is obviously something wrong. The insulin he gave 2 hours ago (*b*) should have resulted in some decrease. Continuing strenuous physical activity (*c*) is unwise as this could cause deterioration. (It is not recommended that patients participate in athletic activity with glucose levels over 300 mg/dL.) This patient should *immediately* draw up insulin in a *syringe* and inject it. This assures that the insulin has been delivered; after this has been done, the pump prob-

lem can be investigated and corrected. Failure to do this will result in ketoacidosis.

54. (b). Distal extremity sensory neuropathy in a "stocking" distribution (chronic sensory neuropathy) is the most common form of neuropathy.

55. (c). Attainment of euglycemia should be the primary goal. Narcotics (a) should be avoided as they are habit-forming and not effective in the long term. Tricyclics (b), gabapentin (d), and capsaicin (e) are acceptable treatments, but only after improvement of glucose control has been attempted.

56. (d). The patient is still acidotic, but the serum glucose is falling too rapidly and the patient is on the verge of hypoglycemia. The insulin infusion rate must be increased to correct the acidosis. The amount of glucose given must also be increased to allow greater insulinization without hypoglycemia. Decreasing or stopping the insulin infusion would only lead to worsening of the acidosis.

57. (d). BEE = 66 + (13.7)(80) + (12.7)(69) − (6.8)(50) = 1698 kcal.

58. (b). Glucagon works by increasing gluconeogenesis and glycogenolysis. A person who has fasted for 10 hours has depleted most of his or her glycogen stores. Ethanol also inhibits gluconeogenesis, and for both these reasons glucagon would not be very effective.

59. (c). Glycated hemoglobin is not currently recommended for the diagnosis of diabetes. Hemoglobinopathies such as thalassemia result in abnormal glycohemoglobin values. Glycosuria (b) does not necessarily indicate diabetes; there are several benign causes of glycosuria. Causes of nondiabetic mellituria include renal glycosuria (familial, pregnancy), essential pentosuria, and essential fructosuria. Diabetes must be diagnosed by conventional criteria. Drug therapy (a, d, e) should not be started until a diagnosis of diabetes has been made.

60. True (a, d); False (b, c, e). Weight loss in any overweight individual with diabetes is encouraged, especially if she desires pregnancy. Because insulin will likely be required during pregnancy, it is preferable to start it beforehand. Oral agents are not generally recommended during pregnancy.

61. True (c); False (a, b, d, e). Classic signs and symptoms with an elevated glucose (c) confirms the diagnosis. A glucometer (a) should not be used to make a diagnosis; a second serum value should be obtained in this case. A glycohemoglobin (b) should never be used to make a diagnosis of diabetes. The patient in (d) has impaired glucose tolerance. Many disorders other than diabetes mellitus can cause glycosuria (e).

62. True (b, e); False (a, c, d). In normal health, insulin secretion is stimulated by hyperglycemia and inhibited by hypoglycemia. The GLUT glucose transporters are necessary for glucose transport across cell membranes. Insulin molecules typically vary by a few amino acids among species; human insulin differs from pork insulin by only one amino acid but by three amino acids from beef insulin. Proinsulin is cleaved to form insulin and C-peptide in equimolar amounts. Insulin is degraded rapidly in the gastrointestinal tract.

63. True (b, d); False (a, c, e). Persons with MEN I and an insulinoma will produce native insulin, with C-peptide levels also elevated. Sulfonylureas (d) stimulate endogenous insulin production and will cause elevation of both insulin and C-peptide. Exogenous insulin use (c) results in a high insulin level but suppressed C-peptide level. Addison's disease (a) and alcohol intoxication (e) may result in impaired gluconeogenesis and/or glycogen release, resulting in hypoglycemia. Insulin and C-peptide levels should be suppressed, since these disorders cause glucose underproduction.

64. True (d); False (a, b, c, e). One of the most common causes of DKA is mismanagement of sick days by omission of insulin. DKA may certainly occur with a serum glucose < 250 (a). Although type 2 diabetics are normally resistant to ketoacidosis, it may develop given sufficient stress (sepsis, myocardial infarction, etc.). Extremely large doses of insulin (b) were once advocated but this is no longer the case, as only

so many insulin receptors can be saturated at one time. A reasonable starting point is 0.1 unit/kg/hour. Well-educated patients with type 1 diabetes should only rarely develop DKA, if at all, and certainly not once a year (*e*). Patients with frequent DKA need education and counseling to confront possible psychosocial issues.

65. True (*d*); False (*a, b, c*). The DCCT showed that tight control prevented development of microvascular disease (neuropathy, retinopathy, and nephropathy) in type 1 diabetics only; those with type 2 were not studied. The United Kingdom Prospective Diabetes Study showed similar findings in type 2 diabetics. Intensive control (*b*) has the adverse consequence of increased frequency of hypoglycemia, which may not be desirable in certain individuals (the elderly or those with severe cardiovascular disease). The DCCT did not study the effect of good glucose control on macrovascular disease (*c*). Intensive control is more expensive than conventional control, primarily due to the increased testing needed.

66. True (*b, c*); False (*a, d, e*). For congenital defects (*a*) to occur, hyperglycemia must be present in the first trimester; GDM usually presents much later. Macrosomia (*b*) and neonatal hypoglycemia (*c*) are common; the latter is due to chronic fetal β-cell hyperplasia from exposure to high maternal glucose levels. Congenital hypothyroidism (*e*) is not associated with maternal diabetes.

67. True (*b, c*); False (*a, d, e*). Only medications that can themselves cause hypoglycemia are properly referred to as *oral hypoglycemic agents*; the others are termed *antidiabetic* or *antihyperglycemic* agents. Sulfonylureas and repaglinide both stimulate the β cell to produce insulin, and thus can cause hypoglycemia in normal persons. Metformin (*a*) primarily acts by decreasing hepatic glucose output and does not cause hypoglycemia. Acarbose (*d*) inhibits the absorption of glucose in the small intestine. Troglitazone (*e*) works by increasing insulin sensitivity. Endogenous insulin levels will fall

in response to these drugs if glucose levels are lowered, thus preventing hypoglycemia.

68. True (*a, b, d, f*); False (*c, e*). Most patients with GDM can be controlled on diet (*a*). There is no single correct insulin regimen, and any combination of insulin may be used successfully. Oral agents (*c, e*) are not recommended during pregnancy. Sulfonylureas especially should be avoided as they are small molecules that cross the placenta and may produce hypoglycemia.

69. True (*a*); False (*b, c, d, e*). GDM usually resolves after delivery. It is a result of the hormonal effects of pregnancy, resulting in insulin resistance and hyperglycemia in susceptible individuals. Many develop type 2 diabetes later in life, not type 1. (Of course, type 1 diabetes may develop in any individual.) Organ malformation (*c*) does not occur in true GDM, which typically is a disorder of later pregnancy when the organs are already formed. Poor control may lead to neonatal hypoglycemia, *not* hyperglycemia (*d*), due to fetal β-cell hyperplasia from chronic exposure to high glucose levels. The majority of patients do not require insulin (*e*).

70. True (*a, c, d, e*); False (*b*). Obesity, PCOS, advanced age, and ovarian hyperthecosis all predispose an individual to insulin resistance and GDM.

71. True (*a, b, c, e*); False (*d*). ACE inhibitors, good glycemic control, and protein restriction are all beneficial. Patients with microalbuminuria are at higher risk of cardiovascular disease (*e*). Increased fluid intake (*d*) will not change the course of microalbuminuria.

72. True (*a, c, e*); False (*b, d*). This patient has typical signs and symptoms with gross elevation of serum glucose, establishing the diagnosis of diabetes. She most likely is type 1, given her body habitus, and should be started on insulin. In a newly diagnosed patient, this may be best accomplished through hospital admission (*a*). She has a goiter and may also have autoimmune thyroid disease; her thyroid function status (*c*) should be assessed. All diabetics should meet with dietitians and diabetes educa-

tors (*e*). Oral agents (*b, d*) should not be used for treatment of type 1 diabetes.

73. True (*a, b, d, e*); False (*c*). Elevation of insulin levels (*a*) and large insulin doses (*d*) indicate insulin resistance, a hallmark of type 2 diabetes. Type 1 diabetes is less common in non-Caucasians (*b*). Prior GDM (*e*) is a risk factor for subsequent type 2 diabetes. HLA-DR3/DR4 (*c*) are markers for patients with the autoimmune polyglandular autoimmune syndromes, including type 1 diabetes (not type 2).

74. True (*a, d*); False (*b, c, e*). Acetohexamide and chlorpropamide are first-generation agents. Metformin is a biguanide, not a sulfonylurea.

75. True (*b, c, d*); False (*a, e*). Hypoglycemia may occur with all sulfonylureas; SIADH and the disulfiram-like reactions are unique to chlorpropamide. Lactic acidosis is a rare complication of metformin therapy. It is not widely believed that sulfonylureas increase cardiovascular mortality. The UKPDS showed no increased mortality from cardiovascular events with sulfonylurea alone or with insulin; the data from use of sulfonylureas with metformin are conflicting.

76. True (*a, b, d*); False (*c, e*). An insulin pump demands a great deal of compliance, and is not a good choice for someone without dedication (*c*). Any patient admitted six times in a year for ketoacidosis (*e*) is doing something horribly wrong and needs much education before a pump could be considered.

77. True (*b, c*); False (*a, d, e*). Elevated C-peptide and insulin levels with hypoglycemia confirm endogenous hyperinsulinism. This could be caused by an insulinoma, and appropriate imaging studies (*c*) may be ordered. Another possibility is factitious use of sulfonylurea drugs, which stimulate insulin secretion. Factitious use of insulin is excluded by the elevated C-peptide level, so psychiatric counseling (*a*) is not indicated. Adrenocortical insufficiency and alcohol intoxication cause hypoglycemia by underproduction of glucose, and therefore insulin and C-peptide levels are decreased; evaluation of these disorders (*d, e*) is not necessary.

78. True (*b, c*); False (*a, d, e*). Proper uses of a 100-gram glucose load include the evaluation of gestational diabetes and growth hormone hypersecretion (acromegaly or gigantism). In the latter, growth hormone levels should fall to less than 2 ng/mL after the glucose load. A glucose tolerance test is not recommended for evaluation of hypoglycemia (*a*), as the test is not physiologic and many normal subjects will have an abnormal test. Evaluation for nongestational diabetes or impaired glucose tolerance should be done with a 75-gram glucose load.

79. True (*b, c, e*); False (*a, d*). Patients with type 1 diabetes on injections require an intermediate- or long-acting insulin plus soluble (short-acting) insulin. Once-daily ultralente (*a*) or twice-daily NPH (*d*) will not allow acceptable control. Insulin pump therapy (*b*) is extremely useful for the motivated patient.

80. True (*b, e*); False (*a, c, d*). The euglycemic clamp is a closed-loop system in which insulin is infused at a constant rate, and the amount of glucose necessary to keep the glucose normal is recorded. Those who are insulin resistant require less glucose for a given insulin infusion rate. Those with insulinoma exhibit excessive glucose requirements.

CHAPTER 6

CALCIUM METABOLISM

Q: What role does calcium play in the body?

A: **Calcium,** a divalent cation, is important in many processes, including muscle contraction, synaptic transmission in the nervous system, platelet aggregation, coagulation, and secretion of hormones (as an intracellular second messenger).

Q: How is calcium transported in plasma?

A: Approximately 46% of calcium travels as the ionized or active form, 46% is bound to serum proteins, and 8% is complexed to ions such as citrate (Fig. 6-1). Like thyroid hormones, total calcium concentration is affected by amounts of serum proteins. If the serum albumin (in mg/dL) is known, the corrected total calcium (in mg/dL) may be estimated as follows:

$$\text{Corrected } Ca^{2+} = \text{Measured } Ca^{2+} + (0.8)(4 - \text{serum albumin})$$

An alternative to correcting the total calcium is to measure the ionized or active portion, which is not affected by changes in serum proteins.

Q: What hormone is the primary regulator of calcium metabolism?

A: The most important hormone in calcium metabolism is **parathyroid hormone** (PTH), an 84-amino acid peptide secreted by the parathyroid glands (Fig. 6-2).

Q: What are the parathyroid glands?

A: Most persons have four **parathyroid glands,** located in the neck behind the thyroid gland. Occasionally, persons will have fewer or greater than four glands. Extra glands may be in an ectopic location, such as the mediastinum.

Q: What is the stimulus for parathyroid hormone secretion?

A: PTH synthesis and secretion rises rapidly after decrease in serum ionized calcium.

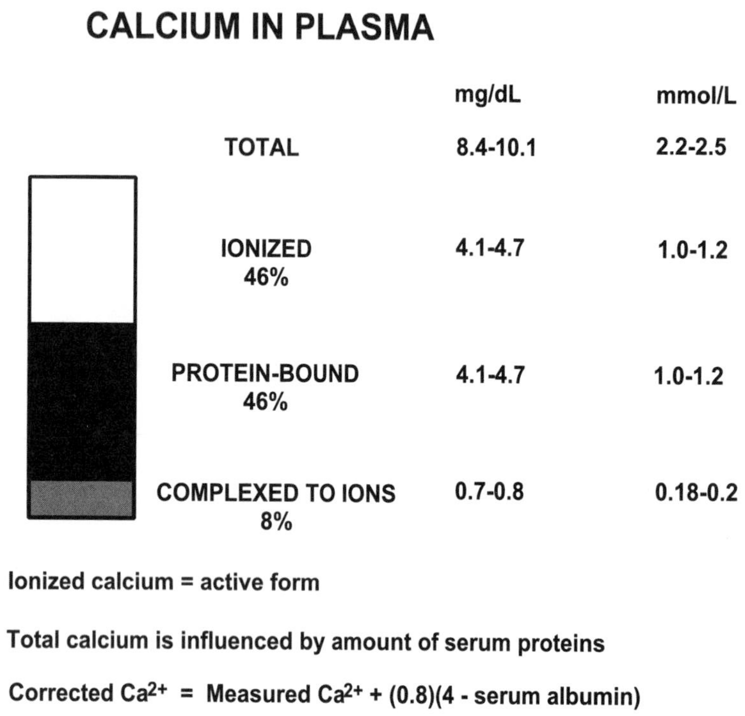

CALCIUM IN PLASMA
mg/dL
mmol/L
TOTAL
8.4-10.1
2.2-2.5
IONIZED
46%
4.1-4.7
1.0-1.2
PROTEIN-BOUND
46%
4.1-4.7
1.0-1.2
COMPLEXED TO IONS
8%
0.7-0.8
0.18-0.2
Ionized calcium = active form
Total calcium is influenced by amount of serum proteins
Corrected Ca2+ = Measured Ca2+ + (0.8)(4 - serum albumin)

Figure 6-1. Calcium in plasma.

LOW IONIZED
Ca2+
CALCITONIN
(weak antagonist)
INCREASED
IONIZED Ca2+
PARATHYROIDS
PTH
VITAMIN D
(Diet, sun)
25OHD3
DIETARY Ca2+
1,25(OH)2D3
Ca2+ reabsorption
PO4- excretion
Ca2+, PO4-
absorption
Ca2+ release

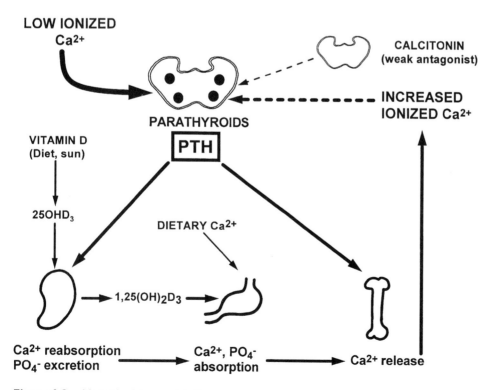

Figure 6-2. Normal calcium metabolism.

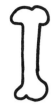

BONE: increased resorption of Ca^{2+}

KIDNEY: increased reabsorption of Ca^{2+}
production of calcitriol
increased secretion of PO$_4^-$

GI TRACT: no direct effect; increased
Ca^{2+} and PO$_4^-$ absorption
via vitamin D

Figure 6-3. Effects of PTH.

Q: What are the actions of parathyroid hormone?

A: PTH acts on the kidney, bone, and indirectly on the small intestine to increase the serum Ca^{2+} concentration (Fig. 6-3).

Q: What is vitamin D?

A: **Vitamin D** is a sterol hormone formed from photogenesis in the skin and absorption from food. It has little activity in itself but is converted to various activated metabolites. A principal one is **calcidiol** (25OHD$_3$) (Fig. 6-4). The most important step in vitamin D metabolism is the conversion of calcidiol to 1,25(OH)$_2$D$_3$ (calcitriol) (Fig. 6-5) in the kidney. **Calcitriol** is the most active metabolite of vitamin D, and its primary effect is to increase calcium and phosphorus absorption in the intes-

tine. Vitamin D receptors are present in other organs but their role is minor.

Q: What is the stimulus for calcitriol formation?

A: Because it facilitates calcium absorption, hypocalcemia increases and hypercalcemia inhibits the synthesis of calcitriol.

Q: What is calcitonin?

A: **Calcitonin** is a 32-amino acid peptide secreted by the parafollicular cells (C-cells) of the thyroid. It is a weak antagonist of PTH and is secreted in response to hypercalcemia. Its importance is negligible in mammals, and no clinical syndrome results from its deficiency. It is very important in salt-water fish, which live in sea water with very

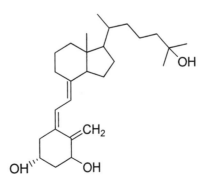

Figure 6-4. 25OHD$_3$ (calcidiol).

Figure 6-5. 1,25(OH)$_2$D$_3$ (calcitriol).

high calcium concentrations. Marine calcitonins (e.g., from the salmon or eel) are often used therapeutically because of their potency. An excess of calcitonin, as can occur with medullary thyroid cancer, may result in symptoms related to calcitonin's vasoactive properties (i.e., diarrhea or flushing), but will not cause hypocalcemia.

Q: What conditions cause hypercalcemia?

A: Table 6-1 lists the causes of hypercalcemia. It is useful to group hypercalcemia into **parathyroid hormone-dependent** and **parathyroid hormone-independent** causes.

Q: What are the symptoms of hypercalcemia?

A: The symptoms of hypercalcemia are listed in Table 6-2.

Q: What is the most common cause of hypercalcemia?

A: In the asymptomatic, otherwise healthy adult, the most common cause is primary hyperparathyroidism. Malignancy is the most common cause in the ill, hospitalized patient. Other causes of hypercalcemia are much less common.

Q: What is primary hyperparathyroidism?

A: Primary hyperparathyroidism (primary HPT) is the most common cause of hypercalcemia in the ambulatory population (incidence 1 in 1000); it appears to be two to three times more common in women than in men. One or more hyperfunctioning glands cause increased PTH secretion, resulting in increased reabsorption of calcium by the kidney, increased release of calcium by bone, and increased calcium absorption from the gut (indirectly via vitamin D). The phosphorus level is usually decreased. *Most patients are asymptomatic and are detected only through routine screening.* Less commonly, symptomatic hypercalcemia and even hypercalcemic crisis can occur. Most cases occur sporadically.

Hyperparathyroidism is also associated with multiple endocrine neoplasia types I and IIa.

Most cases (about 80%) are due to a solitary parathyroid adenoma, and about 18% are due to hyperplasia of all four glands (Fig. 6-6). Parathyroid carcinoma is a very rare and aggressive form of hyperparathyroidism.

TABLE 6-1.   Causes of Hypercalcemia

CAUSE	EXAMPLES

PTH dependent	Hyperparathyroidism
	    Primary (parathyroid adenoma, hyperplasia, carcinoma)
	    Tertiary (long-standing chronic renal disease)

PTH independent	Malignancy
	    Humoral hypercalcemia: PTH-related protein (PTH-rP)
	    Tumor-associated lysis of bone (breast cancer, myeloma)
	    $1,25(OH)_2D_3$ secreting tumors (lymphoma)

Vitamin D dependent	Vitamin D intoxication
	    Granulomatous diseases (tuberculosis, sarcoidosis, berylliosis)
	    $1,25(OH)_2D_3$ secreting tumors

Genetic disorders	FHH (familial hypocalciuric hypercalcemia)
Endocrine disorders	Adrenal insufficiency Hyperthyroidism

Other	Immobilization
	    Milk-alkali syndrome
	    Medications (lithium, estrogens, thiazide diuretics)
	    Vitamin A intoxication

TABLE 6-2.   Symptoms of Hypercalcemia

GENERAL	GASTROINTESTINAL	NEUROMUSCULAR
dehydration	nausea	fatigue
weight loss	vomiting	lethargy
anorexia	constipation	muscle weakness
pruritus		hyporeflexia
polydipsia		confusion
		seizures
		psychosis
		coma

Q: What laboratory findings are seen in primary hyperparathyroidism?

A: In hyperparathyroidism, serum Ca^{2+} is elevated while PO_4^- is decreased. The **intact parathyroid hormone level** is increased: intact PTH is the test of choice as it is the most specific. Other PTH measurements are available (such as C-terminal and N-terminal), but they are less desirable. Calcitriol levels are usually elevated.

Q: What is the treatment of primary hyperparathyroidism?

A: The treatment of choice for primary hyperparathyroidism is surgery. In patients with a solitary adenoma, the adenoma is removed; in hyperplasia, a subtotal parathyroidectomy (3½ glands) is performed. Parathyroid carcinoma is treated by surgery; frequently there is residual disease that is unresectable.

In persons with a solitary adenoma, suppression of the remaining glands occurs. After the adenoma has been removed, the source of excess PTH is gone, and it may take days for the other glands to function sufficiently. **Transient hypocalcemia** is therefore common after parathyroidectomy, but it resolves as the other glands start functioning again.

At this time, there is no effective pharmacologic treatment for hyperparathyroidism. Estrogens may have minimal effect in postmenopausal women and may be tried. Anti-PTH analogs are being studied experimentally.

Q: Should all patients with primary hyperparathyroidism be treated?

A: Not every patient with primary HPT needs to be treated, as some have only a minimal elevation of calcium. Certainly the potential benefits must outweigh the risks. For example, sending an elderly person with severe heart disease to surgery for mild hyperparathyroidism may be too risky with little potential benefit. Doing the same procedure on a healthy 45 year old, however, is less risky with greater benefit. The following are the NIH Consensus Statement indications for surgical treatment of HPT:

Serum Ca^{2+} elevation of 1.0–1.6 mg/dL above the accepted normal range.

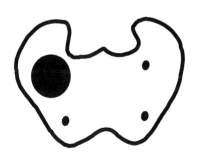

**SOLITARY ADENOMA (80%)
REMAINING GLANDS
SUPPRESSED**

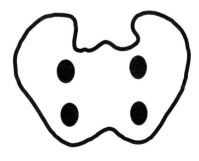

**HYPERPLASIA (~18%)
ALL FOUR GLANDS
ENLARGED**

Figure 6-6. Primary hyperparathyroidism.

Creatinine clearance reduced by 30% compared with those of age-matched normal persons.

Confirmed 24-hour total urine calcium excretion in excess of 400 mg.

Bone mass of less than 2 standard deviations from control persons.

Patient unlikely to return for follow-up.

Patient whose co-existent illness complicates management.

Patients younger than age 50; the outcome of several decades of hyperparathyroidism is unknown.

The following are the recommendations for follow-up of asymptomatic patients who do not meet the surgery criteria:

Semi-annual visits until lack of disease progression has been confirmed; visits every 1 to 3 years thereafter.

Careful history about symptoms relevant to hyperparathyroidism at each visit.

Serum Ca^{2+}, creatinine, and creatinine clearance at each visit.

The 24-hour urinary calcium measurement.

Dual-energy x-ray absorptiometry to detect subtle changes in bone density.

Q: Are any localization studies useful prior to surgery?

A: Ultrasound may help locate an abnormally large gland, but otherwise provides no functional information. Technetium-thallium subtraction may be useful. Technetium is taken up by the thyroid only, whereas thallium is accumulated in both thyroid and parathyroid tissue. By digitally subtracting one from the other, an image of the parathyroid glands is seen. This test can potentially work quite well, but the administration of two different radionuclides makes it technically difficult to perform.

A newer test uses ^{99m}Tc-labeled sestamibi (Cardiolite), a radionuclide frequently used in nuclear cardiology. The test is approximately 85% sensitive in identifying the abnormal area in patients with known hyperparathyroidism. It is *not* a diagnostic test, but only serves to aid the surgeon in working with patients who have known disease based on biochemical data. If a scan is negative, it does not exclude the diagnosis of hyperparathyroidism.

A new technique called **minimally invasive parathyroidectomy** is now being performed in some centers. In this procedure, the abnormal parathyroid tissue is localized intraoperatively by a gamma counter after injection of ^{99m}Tc-labeled sestamibi. The abnormal gland(s) may be removed under local anesthesia, with minimal discomfort to the patient, and with shorter recovery time. A rapid PTH assay (which is completed within 15 minutes) gives confirmation that the abnormal parathyroid tissue has been removed.

Q: What is parathyroid crisis?

A: **Parathyroid crisis** (acute primary hyperparathyroidism or parathyroid storm) is a rare disorder associated with high morbidity and mortality. PTH levels are greatly elevated in this disorder, often 20 times normal or more; the elevated levels are similar with parathyroid carcinoma, which is often in the differential diagnosis. Most patients have a single adenoma, as opposed to hyperplasia. It is not known what causes an uncomplicated case of primary HPT to progress to parathyroid crisis.

The initial treatment for parathyroid crisis is the same as for acute hypercalcemia: rehydration and

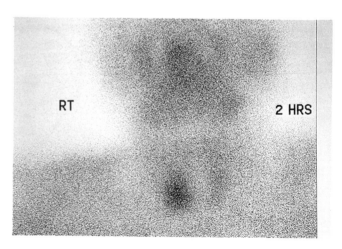

Figure 6-7. Parathyroid scan showing increased right neck activity in man with hyperparathyroidism.

loop diuretics. Parathyroidectomy is done after the patient has been stabilized.

Q: What is the "hungry bone" syndrome?

A: PTH stimulates bone formation and resorption, with the latter predominating in hyperparathyroidism. After hyperparathyroidism has been surgically corrected, the resorptive response decreases, but bone formation may persist for many weeks. The bones therefore are "hungry" for calcium, and their avidity for it may be strong enough to actually deplete calcium from the serum. The resulting hypocalcemia then causes a compensatory rise in PTH, which in turn results in increased renal reabsorption and intestinal absorption of calcium (via vitamin D). The elevated PTH levels are merely a normal physiologic response to hypocalcemia. This phenomenon is called the **hungry bone syndrome,** and it may occur after surgical treatment for hyperparathyroidism.

Treatment is calcium supplementation, which hastens the bone recovery. The syndrome is usually a self-limited process that may last several months. Occasional patients may require vitamin D therapy.

Q: What is secondary hyperparathyroidism?

A: **Secondary hyperparathyroidism** occurs in patients with long-standing renal insufficiency. They become hypocalcemic due to their decreased calcium reabsorption, chronic phosphate retention, and diminished production of calcitriol. The chronic hypocalcemia results in elevated PTH levels that have no effect on the kidney, but still have an effect on bone. Chronically elevated PTH can cause bone resorption (renal osteodystrophy), ectopic calcifications, and bone pain. The treatment is restriction of dietary phosphate, and administration of phosphate-binding agents and calcitriol to help increase the serum calcium.

Q: What is tertiary hyperparathyroidism?

A: After years of prolonged hypocalcemia and secondary hyperparathyroidism, autonomous PTH hypersecretion may occur. Eventually, this can result in hypercalcemia due to the effect of PTH on bone. Because hyperplasia has occurred for so long, PTH secretion continues even though the patient is hy-

percalcemic. PTH no longer responds to calcium levels, so the only treatment is near-total parathyroidectomy.

Q: What are the vitamin D-dependent hypercalcemias?

A: **Vitamin D-dependent hypercalcemia** is a result of chronically high vitamin D (typically calcitriol) levels, resulting in enhanced calcium and phosphate absorption from the intestine. One etiology is vitamin D intoxication, which occurs in those taking pharmacologic preparations for calcium disorders (e.g., hypoparathyroidism). Vitamin D intoxication is uncommon with over-the-counter preparations, as their potency is low.

Granulomatous diseases such as tuberculosis, sarcoidosis, berylliosis, and leprosy may also cause this type of disorder. Granuloma cells may possess the 1α-hydroxylase enzyme necessary to convert $25OHD_3$ to $1,25(OH)_2D_3$, resulting in hypercalcemia. Certain malignancies also possess the ability to convert $25OHD_3$ to $1,25(OH)_2D_3$. These include hematologic malignancies such as lymphomas.

Q: What is the treatment of vitamin D-dependent hypercalcemia?

A: Glucocorticoids cause downregulation of calcium receptors in the intestine, and these cause a prompt lowering of calcium levels. In patients with vitamin D toxicity, withdrawal or reduction of medication is necessary. Treatment of any underlying granulomatous disease is also necessary.

Q: What is familial hypocalciuric hypercalcemia?

A: **Familial hypocalciuric hypercalcemia** (FHH) is an uncommon, genetically transmitted disorder, also called familial benign hypercalcemia. It is characterized by mild asymptomatic hypercalcemia, normal or mildly elevated PTH levels, and low fractional excretion of calcium. FHH is a benign disorder and no treatment is necessary. It is commonly mistaken for primary hyperparathyroidism; often FHH patients undergo parathyroidectomy, yet their hypercalcemia persists. As the name implies, calcium excretion is abnormally low, whereas it is high in hyperparathyroidism; the two can be distinguished by calculating the calcium to creatinine clearance ratio, which is low in FHH (< 0.01).

Q: How do lithium and vitamin A intoxication cause hypercalcemia?

A: Lithium appears to alter the "set point" for parathyroid hormone secretion, leading to increased PTH levels. The incidence of hyperparathyroidism is increased, and this appears to be the mechanism of hypercalcemia. Calcium levels should be followed routinely in patients receiving lithium therapy. Lithium must be used with extreme caution in patients with a history of hyperparathyroidism.

Vitamin A excess appears to cause hypercalcemia by enhancing bone resorption, which can be visualized on radiographs of the long bones. It is typically associated with other signs of vitamin A intoxication, such as dermatitis, hepatic dysfunction, and dementia.

Q: What malignancies are most commonly associated with hypercalcemia?

A: The malignancies most commonly associated with hypercalcemia are squamous cell carcinoma, breast carcinoma, renal cell carcinoma, bladder carcinoma, multiple myeloma, and lymphomas. Hypercalcemia is rare in colon and prostate cancer.

Q: How do malignancies produce hypercalcemia?

A: **Humoral hypercalcemia of malignancy** accounts for about 80% of cancer-related hypercalcemia. The tumors typically secrete **PTH-related peptide** (PTH-rP), which acts in a fashion similar to PTH. It is a structurally distinct protein, however, and is not detected by the standard PTH assay; a special PTH-rP test must be done. PTH-rP is present in small amounts in normal persons and appears to be necessary for development of cartilage cells, mammary glands, hair follicles, skin, and regulator of placental calcium transport. Patients with PTH-rP hypersecretion have similar laboratory findings as patients with hyperparathyroidism: hypercalcemia with hypophosphatemia. PTH secretion is inhibited by the hypercalcemia, so PTH levels are low. Although PTH-rP would be expected to increase calcitriol production, instead

the levels are often suppressed; the reason for this is unclear. Native PTH hypersecretion by tumors has been reported, although this is extremely rare.

Local osteolytic hypercalcemia (LOH) accounts for most of the remaining 20% of tumor-associated hypercalcemia cases. This disorder is caused by secretion of osteoclast-activating factors (OAFs), not by direct tumor invasion by bone. These substances include various prostaglandins, interleukins, tumor necrosis factors, and transforming growth factors. Examples include breast carcinoma and hematologic malignancies (e.g., multiple myeloma). Interestingly, the OAF for breast carcinoma appears to be PTH-rP.

Also, certain lymphomas rarely exhibit ectopic calcitriol production, producing a vitamin D-dependent hypercalcemia.

Q: What endocrine disorders can cause hypercalcemia?

A: Hyperthyroidism may lead to increased bone resorption of calcium. This type of hypercalcemia is usually mild, with few or no symptoms, and responds promptly to treatment. Persistence of hypercalcemia after treatment suggests another cause.

Adrenal insufficiency causes upregulation of calcium receptors in the intestine, leading to mild hypercalcemia. This condition is aggravated by the dehydration that normally occurs during adrenal insufficiency. Rehydration and steroid replacement promptly restore calcium levels to normal.

Q: What is the laboratory evaluation of patients with hypercalcemia?

A: The total serum calcium should be corrected if the serum albumin level is abnormal. Alternatively, ionized calcium may be measured to confirm true hypercalcemia. Intact PTH is used to distinguish PTH-dependent from other causes of hypercalcemia. A plot of serum Ca^{2+} versus PTH is useful to distinguish various disorders of calcium metabolism (Fig. 6-8). Serum phosphate is also helpful. PTH-rP and vitamin D levels are useful in certain instances. The differential diagnosis of hypercalcemia is summarized in Table 6-3.

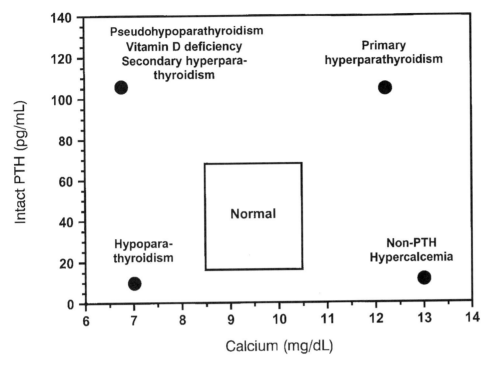

Figure 6-8. PTH levels in various states of hyper- and hypocalcemia.

Q: What is the milk-alkali syndrome?

A: The **milk-alkali syndrome** occurs after ingestion of large amounts of calcium (e.g., milk) and alkali (e.g., sodium bicarbonate), usually taken for peptic ulcer or esophagitis. The metabolic alkalosis results in hypocalciuria and later, hypercalcemia. Renal failure is present. This disorder is uncommon today as the treatment of peptic ulcer disease has been improved. Recently, however, there has been a resurgence in calcium use for prevention of osteoporosis—many patients consume more than the prescribed amount of calcium, which has resulted in more cases of milk-alkali syndrome in recent years.

Q: What is hypercalcemic crisis?

A: **Hypercalcemic crisis** is the end stage of hypercalcemia, and can lead to coma and death. Although any of the above conditions can cause it, it usually is associated with malignancy. Hyperparathyroidism can rarely cause it in cases of parathyroid crisis (acute primary hyperparathyroidism).

Q: What is the treatment of hypercalcemic crisis?

A: The most important first step in treating hypercalcemic crisis is **rehydration** with intravenous fluids, as calcium acts as an osmotic diuretic and causes dehydration. After rehydration has been established, **loop diuretics** (furosemide) promote

TABLE 6-3.   Differential Diagnosis of Hypercalcemia

	Ca^{2+}	PO_4^-	PTH	PTH-rP	$1,25(OH)_2D_3$
Primary hyperparathyroidism	↑	↓	↑	↓	↑
Vitamin D-dependent hypercalcemia	↑	↑	↓	↓	↑
Humoral hypercalcemia of malignancy (HHM)	↑↑	↓	↓	↑	↓ or N
Osteolytic tumors	↑	N	↓	↓	↓

calciuria, and are especially useful in those with renal failure. *Diuretics should never be given before the patient has been rehydrated, as it can worsen the condition.*

Glucocorticoids are useful in the vitamin D-dependent hypercalcemias, hypercalcemia of adrenal insufficiency, and hypercalcemia associated with certain osteolytic tumors, but are of minimal use in other conditions. Humoral hypercalcemia of malignancy is best treated with an antiresorptive agent. These agents include the bisphosphonates (pamidronate and etidronate), which bind irreversibly to bone and prevent its resorption, the antibiotic plicamycin (mithramycin), and gallium nitrate. Salmon calcitonin has mild antiresorptive action and is useful in mild hypercalcemia. After calcium levels have returned to normal, treatment of the underlying disease is indicated.

Q: What are the clinical features of hypocalcemia?

A: The clinical features of hypocalcemia include neuromuscular, cardiac, dental, and gastrointestinal manifestations: paresthesias, hyperventilation, tetany, adrenergic symptoms (tachycardia, diaphoresis), seizures, Chvostek's and Trousseau's signs, QT interval prolongation, hypotension, refractory congestive heart failure, cardiomegaly, abnormalities in dental formation, gastrointestinal malabsorption, and cataracts.

Q: What are Chvostek's and Trousseau's signs?

A: Chvostek's and Trousseau's signs indicate latent tetany in those with hypocalcemia. **Chvostek's sign** is elicited by tapping the face in the area of the facial nerve. A positive response is a spasm of the facial muscles on that side. Many normal persons have a slight Chvostek's sign. **Trousseau's sign** is elicited by inflating a blood pressure cuff around the arm to between systolic and diastolic blood pressures for several minutes; the time to carpal spasm is noted if the sign is positive.

Q: What disorders can cause hypocalcemia?

A: Table 6-4 lists the differential diagnosis of hypocalcemia. Table 6-5 shows the laboratory findings with the various causes of hypocalcemia.

TABLE 6-4.   Differential Diagnosis of Hypocalcemia

Disorders of parathyroid hormone secretion or action
  hypoparathyroidism
  pseudohypoparathyroidism
  hypomagnesemia (functional hypoparathyroidism)

Disorders of vitamin D metabolism
  nutritional
  drugs (anticonvulsants)
  inherited defect in metabolism or receptor

Removal of excess calcium from serum
  EDTA
  pancreatitis
  hyperphosphatemia (rhabdomyolysis, chemotherapy).

Q: Can hypocalcemia occur secondary to dietary deficiency?

A: Dietary deficiency is an unlikely cause of hypocalcemia. The skeleton contains vast amounts of calcium, and this is usually more than adequate to keep calcium levels normal, even in the face of dietary deficiency. The cost of drawing on the skeletal reserve is, however, loss of bone which leads to osteoporosis.

Q: What are the causes of hypoparathyroidism?

A: Most cases of hypoparathyroidism (80%) are a result of extensive neck surgery (e.g., thyroidectomy). Approximately 15% of cases are autoimmune or idiopathic. Functional hypoparathyroidism occurs with severe magnesium (Mg^{2+}) deficiency; function returns after replacement. Infiltrative diseases such as hemochromatosis and amyloidosis rarely can cause hypoparathyroidism.

TABLE 6-5.   Laboratory Studies in Various Causes of Hypocalcemia

	Ca^{2+}	PO_4^-	PTH
Hypoparathyroidism	↓	↑	↓
Pseudohypoparathyroidism	↓	↑	↑
Vitamin D deficiency	↓	↓	↑

Q: What are the laboratory findings in hypoparathyroidism?

A: In hypoparathyroidism, calcium is low, as PTH effects on bone and kidney are diminished. As PTH results in phosphaturia, hypoparathyroidism results in hyperphosphatemia. PTH levels are, of course, diminished.

Q: What is the treatment of hypoparathyroidism?

A: Initial therapy of hypoparathyroidism should treat the acute hypocalcemic symptoms. This is done with intravenous calcium (usually calcium gluconate as an infusion). Currently, it is not possible to replace PTH itself. This means that its effects on the two major sites—kidney and bone— are lost. Its third effect, enhancing calcitriol production, can be mimicked by administering calcitriol itself, which is the most potent of the vitamin D analogs. Current is very fast acting, and onset of action is within 1 to 2 days. Less potent, longer lasting analogs such as dihydrotachysterol and ergocalciferol may also be used, but may be less satisfactory. The latter are less expensive than calcitriol. With sufficient doses and dietary calcium supplementation, serum calcium levels return to normal. Vitamin D also enhances phosphate absorption, but caution must be taken to avoid hyperphosphatemia. Calcium levels are usually kept at the lower level of normal.

Q: What is pseudohypoparathyroidism?

A: **Pseudohypoparathyroidism** (PHP) is a rare condition of target tissue resistance to PTH, producing clinical symptoms of hypoparathyroidism with elevated PTH levels. In addition to the biochemical features of PHP, characteristic somatic abnormalities are often present: short stature, obesity, brachydactyly (short 4th metacarpals), and mental retardation.

Q: What is the treatment of pseudohypoparathyroidism?

A: The treatment of PHP is similar to that of hypoparathyroidism, as the circulating PTH is ineffective. Calcium supplementation plus vitamin D analogs (calcitriol or ergocalciferol) are typically given.

Q: What is pseudo pseudohypoparathyroidism?

A: Patients with **pseudo pseudohypoparathyroidism** have the classic somatic anomalies of PHP but none of the biochemical manifestations (their calcium is normal). No treatment is needed.

Q: What is vitamin D deficiency?

A: **Vitamin D deficiency** is a condition of deficient vitamin D intake or altered metabolism that results in decreased intestinal calcium and phosphate absorption. Dietary deficiency is not common in the United States, but this deficiency may be seen among the elderly or in debilitated patients with poor food intake and sun exposure.

A major step in vitamin D metabolism is conversion to $25OHD_3$ in the liver, so patients with hepatobiliary disease (e.g., hepatitis, cirrhosis) may present with vitamin D deficiency. Patients with intestinal malabsorption of fat-soluble vitamins (e.g., Crohn's disease) may be deficient. It may also occur in protein-wasting conditions (such as various enteropathies or nephrotic syndrome).

Anticonvulsants such as phenytoin and phenobarbital increase the conversion of $25OHD_3$ to inactive metabolites, resulting in vitamin D deficiency. Increased sunlight exposure and vitamin D intake (around 3000 units daily) typically prevents this complication.

Rarely, defects in vitamin D metabolism occur. **Vitamin D-dependent rickets type 1 (VDDR-I)** is caused by defective renal 1α-hydroxylase, resulting in deficient $1,25(OH)_2D_3$ levels. **VDDR type 2** is a result of defective receptors, so there is no response to $1,25(OH)_2D_3$ despite normal or high levels.

Q: What are the laboratory findings in vitamin D deficiency?

A: Vitamin D enhances calcium and phosphate absorption, so these levels are decreased in the deficient state. Because hypocalcemia exists, PTH levels are elevated. The best marker for vitamin D deficiency is calcidiol ($25OHD_3$). Although this metabolite is less active than calcitriol, it serves as a reservoir for production of calcitriol. It is possible to have vitamin D deficiency with low $25OHD_3$ levels but normal $1,25(OH)_2D_3$ levels.

Q: **What is the function of bone?**

A: Bone provides rigid support to extremities and to the body cavities that contain vital organs; it provides effective levers for muscles. It also serves as a large reservoir of ions (calcium, magnesium, phosphorus). There are two major types of bone. **Cortical** or **compact bone** is found in tubular bones (e.g., radius, tibia, etc.). **Trabecular** or **cancellous bone** is found in the vertebrae and axial skeleton.

Bone is a living organ that is constantly being remodeled. Normally, the amount resorbed equals the amount formed. **Osteoblasts** form new bone on the surface and synthesize new **matrix** (collagenous proteins). **Osteocytes** are merely osteoblasts after they are trapped in mineralized matrix. **Osteoclasts** are multinucleated giant cells involved in bone resorption.

Q: **What is osteoporosis?**

A: **Osteoporosis** is the condition of decreased quantity of bone (mineralization + matrix). It is a common medical disorder, and 20% of women have suffered at least one fracture by age 65. The pathogenesis involves uncoupling of normal balance of bone formation and resorption. The bone present is structurally normal. In normal health, the amount formed equals the amount resorbed; in osteoporosis, either too much bone is resorbed (high turnover), or too little is formed (low turnover).

The most common osteoporotic fractures include the femoral neck, vertebral body, and forearm (Colles' fracture).

Q: **What are some risk factors for osteoporosis?**

A: Table 6-6 shows the risk factors for osteoporosis.

Q: **What are the typical causes of osteoporosis?**

A: Osteoporosis most commonly occurs with estrogen deficiency after menopause. Most loss occurs within the first 10 years after natural menopause or oophorectomy; this is a **high turnover** form of osteoporosis (estrogen deficiency enhances bone

TABLE 6-6.   Risk Factors for Osteoporosis

Genetic
Northern Caucasian or Asian race
Small bone mass
Nutritional deficiency (calcium, vitamin D, protein)
Hypogonadism
postmenopausal woman (most common)
hypothalamic amenorrhea (elite athletes, anorexia nervosa)
hypogonadal males (primary or secondary)
Cigarette smoking
Drugs
alcohol
corticosteroids
anticonvulsants
heparin
Renal disease
Hyperparathyroidism
Immobilization and lack of exercise
Gastrointestinal disease
malabsorption
gastric or intestinal resection
hepatic disease

resorption). Not all postmenopausal women develop osteoporosis; bone densitometry is recommended in high-risk individuals so that they can be treated with estrogen as soon as possible. Men with sex hormone deficiency (hypogonadism) also may develop osteoporosis.

Osteoporosis may also occur as a consequence of normal aging ("senile" osteoporosis). Bone mass typically peaks by age 30 in men and women; approximately 25% of this mass is lost over the remainder of the person's lifetime. It is therefore desirable to attain the highest peak bone mass possible. Adequate calcium intake during adolescence has been shown to significantly increase peak bone mass in twin studies.

Q: **What are some secondary causes of osteoporosis?**

A: **Chronic glucocorticoid use** is the most common secondary cause. Corticosteroids inhibit bone formation and produce a **low turnover** form of osteoporosis. Exposure to these drugs should be minimized if possible. Endogenous Cushing's syndrome should be excluded in persons with clinical features of the disorder (e.g., diabetes, truncal obesity, hypertension, striae).

Patients with type 1 diabetes appear to have an increased risk of osteoporosis; the etiology is unclear. Those with type 2 diabetes often have a decreased risk, since obesity is typically associated with a normal or high bone mass. Chronic hyperthyroidism may result in increased bone turnover in osteoporosis. This may result from both endogenous hyperthyroidism (e.g., Graves' disease) and those receiving too much hormone replacement.

Weight bearing is necessary for normal bone remodeling. Obese persons have a decreased risk of osteoporosis, due to the increased stress on their bones. Astronauts who travel into space for long periods of time must exercise to prevent development of osteopenia due to zero gravity. Persons immobilized for long periods (e.g., those with spinal cord injury) show increased bone resorption and may develop osteopenia unless they receive physical therapy. Children with very high bone turnover may even develop immobilization hypercalcemia.

Osteogenesis imperfecta is a rare genetic disorder caused by mutations in a gene that produces collagen for the bone matrix. This disorder is typically associated with juvenile fractures, blue sclerae, and joint laxity. This disease occasionally does not present until adulthood, however. Treatment is supportive. Other genetic disorders of connective tissue associated with osteoporosis include Ehlers-Danlos syndrome, Marfan's syndrome, and homocystinuria.

Q: What is juvenile osteoporosis?

A: This is a rare, self-limited form of osteoporosis that occurs in prepubertal children. The typical patient is a child between ages 8 and 14 years who develops multiple fractures with minimal trauma. Fractures may occur in both the axial and appendicular skeleton. Bone density is low. Surprisingly, this disease almost always goes into remission, often after the onset of puberty; this suggests

that hormonal factors may play a role. Other children have gone into remission before onset of puberty, which places this hypothesis in question. The child typically has no further problems after remission occurs, although he or she may have residual problems from previous fractures. This disorder is distinguished from osteogenesis imperfecta in that the latter does not go into remission.

Q: How is osteoporosis diagnosed?

A: Osteoporosis is a straightforward diagnosis for those with obvious **osteopenia** (radiolucency) on x-ray and pathologic fractures (such as a compression fracture of the spine). Plain x-ray, however, is typically a poor way of diagnosing osteoporosis, as much must be lost before it is detected. Thus, the test of choice is **dual-energy x-ray absorptiometry** (DEXA), which is noninvasive and easy to perform (Fig. 6-9). Other means of measuring bone density exist, but DEXA is the one most widely used.

Bone density is typically measured in the lumbar spine and femoral neck, and plotted on a graph. The patient's values are compared to others in his or her age group and to young adults. It has been found that fracture correlates best when compared to young adults (the "peak" bone mass) than to others of the same age. For example, a 90-year-old woman with a bone density at the 75th percentile for her age still has significant risk of fracture, as

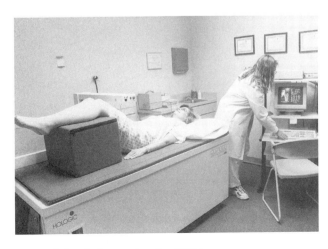

Figure 6-9. Patient undergoing DEXA scan.

practically all persons her age have some osteopenia.

The **Z score** is the standard deviation compared to persons in the same age group. A Z score of 0.00 means the person is right at the mean. Z = +2.00 means that the patient is 2 standard deviations above the mean (~95th percentile); −1.00 is 1 standard deviation below the mean (~25th percentile). As above, this value is not as useful as the **T score,** the value normalized to a reference of young adults.

Persons with a T score of greater than −1.00 (25th percentile) are said to have normal bone density (Fig. 6-10). What is normal is a relative question. Just like not everyone can be tall, not everyone has a high bone density; someone has to be below the mean. Each drop or increase in T score by 1 approximately indicates a doubling or halving of the relative risk of fracture, respectively (compared to the mean). For example, someone with a T of +2.00 is 4 times less likely to have a fracture as someone at the mean; a person with a T of −3.00 is 8 times more likely to have a fracture than someone at the mean. Risk of fracture is also relative; patients with extremely low bone densities may never have fractures if they are sedentary, and those with high densities may fracture if subjected to enough stress (professional football players).

Those with a T score of −1.00 to −2.50 are said to have **osteopenia** or **low bone mass**; those with T < 2.50 are said to have **osteoporosis** (Fig. 6-11).

Q: What laboratory findings are seen in osteoporosis?

A: Laboratory studies are typically normal for osteoporosis. However, screening should be done in all patients to exclude metabolic disease:

- Serum calcium; PTH if calcium is high (exclude hyperparathyroidism)

- Vitamin D levels (especially calcidiol)

- Serum/urine protein electrophoresis (exclude multiple myeloma)

- Liver, renal function tests

- Thyroid function tests (exclude hyperthyroidism)

- Markers of bone turnover (serum osteocalcin, urine collagen cross-links) useful to separate low turnover from high turnover states

- Complete blood count

- Sedimentation rate

Q: What is the treatment of osteoporosis?

A: In postmenopausal or oophorectomized women in whom it is not contraindicated (those with breast cancer or active thromboembolic disease), estro-

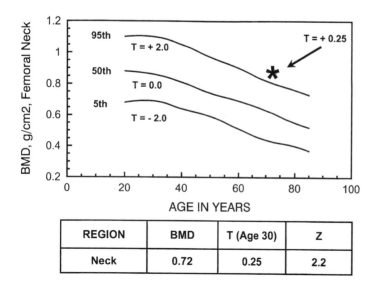

REGION	BMD	T (Age 30)	Z
Neck	0.72	0.25	2.2

Figure 6-10.   Normal bone density (T = +0.25) of femoral neck.

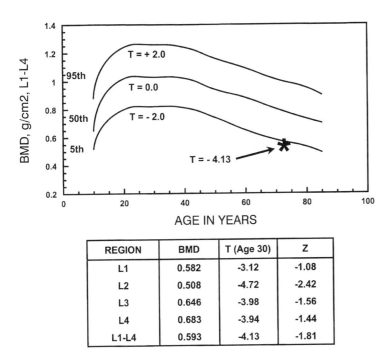

REGION	BMD	T (Age 30)	Z
L1	0.582	-3.12	-1.08
L2	0.508	-4.72	-2.42
L3	0.646	-3.98	-1.56
L4	0.683	-3.94	-1.44
L1-L4	0.593	-4.13	-1.81

Figure 6-11. Osteoporosis (T = −4.13) of lumbar spine.

gen is the best treatment. It is much more effective if it is started soon after menopause or oophorectomy. Men with hypogonadism should receive androgen therapy.

Bisphosphonates (as discussed for treatment of hypercalcemia) are phosphate analogs that bind to bone, thus preventing resorption. They are most useful in high turnover types of osteoporosis (postmenopausal osteoporosis). They also stimulate bone formation to a mild degree. The current agent of choice is alendronate, given once per day.

Salmon calcitonin also inhibits bone resorption and has an analgesic effect. It is available either as a subcutaneous form or as a nasal spray. **Raloxifene** is a synthetic estrogen analog that may be given to certain patients who cannot tolerate estrogen or in whom estrogen is contraindicated (e.g., breast cancer survivors). It has the antiresorptive properties of estrogen but not other hormonal effects, so it is not useful for preventing symptoms such as hot flashes. At this point, raloxifene is indicated for the prevention of osteoporosis in high-risk individuals.

Calcium supplementation is recommended (1500 mg elemental calcium per day). Vitamin D defi-

ciency should also be treated. Risk factors for osteoporosis such as smoking and steroids should be reduced or eliminated if possible.

Q: What is osteomalacia?

A: **Osteomalacia** is a disorder in which the organic matrix of bone does not mineralize properly. It differs from osteoporosis, in which the amount of both matrix and mineralization is deficient. The failure of normal mineralization in children is called **rickets.**

Q: What is the etiology of osteomalacia?

A: The etiologies of osteomalacia include:

- vitamin D deficiency

- malabsorption (GI disease)

- renal disease (impaired calcitriol synthesis)

- phosphate deficiency

- renal tubular phosphate wasting;

- drugs (anticonvulsants that interfere with vitamin D metabolism)

- resistance to vitamin D

- tumor-associated osteomalacia

Q: What is tumor-associated osteomalacia?

A: Certain malignancies appear to secrete a humoral substance that interferes with vitamin D metabolism and causes osteomalacia. This substance has not yet been isolated. Treatment of the tumor improves the condition.

Q: What are the clinical features of osteomalacia?

A: Patients with osteomalacia commonly develop deformities caused by fractures in ribs, vertebrae, and long bones. Often they have a waddling gait, with muscle weakness and diffuse skeletal pain. A classic radiologic finding is the presence of a radiolucent band, often in the long bones, metatarsals, pelvis, and scapula; these lines have been called pseudofractures, Milkman's syndrome, or Looser's zones.

Q: What laboratory features are present in osteomalacia?

A: Vitamin D deficiency often exists in osteomalacia, so hypocalcemia and hypophosphatemia are commonly present. Serum $25OHD_3$ levels are typically low, although $1,25(OH)_2D_3$ levels may be normal. Parathyroid hormone levels are increased if the patient has hypocalcemia. Alkaline phosphatase levels are usually elevated.

Q: What is the treatment of osteomalacia?

A: Treatment of osteomalacia involves active vitamin D metabolites (ergocalciferol, calcitriol) to restore calcium and phosphorus levels to normal, as well as added dietary calcium and phosphate. Malabsorption also should be treated, if it is present. Tumor-associated osteomalacia improves with treatment of the malignancy.

Q: What is Paget's disease of bone?

A: Paget's disease of bone is a localized disorder of bone remodeling in which excessive resorption and formation occur at different sites, resulting in a disorganized mosaic of bone at affected sites. It is a common disorder, affecting as many as 3% of people over age 40 (per autopsy studies). Many cases likely go undiagnosed due to lack of symptoms.

Q: What are the clinical features of Paget's disease?

A: Most patients are asymptomatic and are only discovered incidentally by x-ray, bone scan, or elevated alkaline phosphatase level. Few patients present with pain directly related to the pagetic process. Bowing deformities of the limbs can lead to pain, shortened limbs, and gait abnormalities. The normal side of the body may be affected by the abnormal weight bearing. Osteoarthritis is a common secondary complication, and it may be difficult to separate this from pagetic pain.

Skull involvement may result in an increase in head size with frontal bossing and headache. Hearing loss may occur due to conductive and neurosensory abnormalities; other cranial nerve palsies can also be seen. Facial deformities and dental problems may occur. Vertebral compression fractures may be seen with kyphosis.

Paget's is rarely a serious illness except for in the rare patient (1%) who develops osteosarcoma in a pagetic area. This is the most feared complication and should be excluded in a patient who develops intractable pain in a pagetic joint.

Q: What laboratory abnormalities are present in Paget's disease?

A: The most common laboratory abnormality in a Paget's disease patient is an elevated alkaline phosphatase level, which reflects osteoblastic activity and estimates severity of bone turnover. Degradation products of bone can be measured in the urine; a useful marker is hydroxyproline, found in collagen cross-links. Elevated levels reflect an increase in bone resorption. Serum calcium is typically normal but may be elevated in certain cases (after increased bone resorption or prolonged immobilization).

Q: What radiologic findings are present in these patients?

A: X-rays of Paget's disease of bone may show osteolysis, sclerosis, or both. A typical finding is a V-shaped wedge of resorption. Abnormal bone formation results in characteristic bowing. The skull may be enlarged, with frontal bossing and areas of osteolysis (osteoporosis circumscripta). Radionuclide bone scans often show localization in skull, ribs, spine, pelvis, and femur.

Q: What therapies are available for Paget's disease of bone?

A: Current therapies alter bone remodeling, allowing creation of more uniform bone. Salmon calcitonin, which has been available for many years, decreases bone resorption. It is given by subcutaneous injection.

Bisphosphonates are pyrophosphate analogs that bind irreversibly to bone and prevent resorption. Available oral compounds in the United States are etidronate, alendronate, tiludronate, and risedronate. An intravenous bisphosphonate (pamidronate) may be given for severe exacerbations. The cytotoxic antibiotic mithramycin (plicamycin) also inhibits bone resorption and may be given intravenously until activity subsides. Toxicity may be severe.

Treatment of coexisting osteoarthritis with nonsteroidal anti-inflammatory drugs and orthotics to correct symptoms (e.g., heel lift) is indicated. Surgery is reserved only for those with established or impending fracture. Joint replacement may be difficult, as the underlying bone quality may be low. Neurosurgical intervention may be necessary for spinal cord compression, spinal stenosis, or intracranial lesions.

BIBLIOGRAPHY

Blind E, Nissenson RA, Strewler GJ. Parathyroid hormone-related protein. In: Becker KL, ed. Principles and practice of endocrinology and metabolism. 2nd ed. Philadelphia: Lippincott, 1995:467-472.

Johnston CC, Melton LJ. Bone densitometry. In: Rigss BL, Melton LJ, eds. Osteoporosis: etiology, diagnosis, and management. 2nd ed. Philadelphia: Lippincott-Raven, 1995:275–295.

Massely MJ, Lawrence AM, Brooks M, et al. Hyperparathyroid crisis: successful treatment of ten comatose patients. Surgery 1981;90:741–760.

National Institutes of Health. "Diagnosis and management of asymptomatic primary hyperparathyroidism: consensus development conference statement." Ann Intern Med 1991;114:593–597.

Norton JA, Brennan MF, Wells SA. Surgical management of hyperparathyroidism. In: Bilezikian JP, ed. The parathyroids. Philadelphia: Raven Press, 1994:531–546.

Strewler GJ. Humoral manifestations of malignancy. In: Wilson JD, Foster DW, Kronenberg HM, Larsen PR, eds. Williams' textbook of endocrinology. 9th ed. Philadelphia: W.B. Saunders, 1998:1696–1698.

Strewler GJ. Mineral metabolism & metabolic bone disease. In: Greenspan FS, Strewler GJ, eds. Basic and clinical endocrinology. 5th ed. Stamford, CT: Appleton & Lange, 1997:263–314.

REVIEW QUESTIONS

I. SHORT ANSWER

1. The biologically active form of calcium is called _____ calcium. Approximately ____% travels in this form in serum. The remainder of the calcium is bound to _____ and _____.

2. The most important regulator of calcium metabolism is _____, secreted by the _____. Normally there are _____ of these glands. The stimulus to these glands is a drop in the _____ concentration.

3. Parathyroid hormone (PTH) directly or indirectly acts on three organ systems to increase the serum calcium concentration. These organ systems include the _____, _____, and _____.

4. The main effect of PTH on bone is to increase _____.

5. The effect of PTH on the kidney is to directly increase serum calcium by _____. In addition, PTH increases the excretion of _____. PTH also indirectly increases calcium by stimulating the production of _____, which results in increased _____ and _____ absorption from the small intestine.

6. A weak antagonist of PTH is _____, secreted by the _____. Its role in humans is minimal. Excess of this substance may cause _____.

7. The most common cause of hypercalcemia in the healthy adult population is _____. The most common cause in the ill, hospitalized patient is _____.

8. List five signs or symptoms of hypercalcemia.

9. Primary hyperparathyroidism is caused by _____ in 80% of cases. The remaining 20% of cases are caused by _____. A rare, aggressive cause of hyperparathyroidism is _____.

10. In primary hyperparathyroidism, serum calcium is _____ while phosphate is _____. The best assay for PTH is the _____ assay. Levels of PTH are _____ in hyperparathyroidism. The definitive treatment for primary hyperparathyroidism is _____.

11. A problem that occurs in patients with long-standing renal insufficiency and chronic hypocalcemia is _____. The hypocalcemia occurs because of _____, _____, and _____. Elevated PTH levels can result in _____ and _____.

12. After years of chronic hypocalcemia, PTH hypersecretion may become autonomous and will continue even if serum calcium normalizes. This condition is called _____ and may eventually result in _____.

13. The vitamin D-dependent hypercalcemias result in increased _____ and _____ absorption from the small intestine. Intoxication with large doses of _____ may cause this problem. Tuberculosis and sarcoidosis are _____ diseases that may produce vitamin D-dependent hypercalcemia because these cells possess the enzyme _____. Rarely, certain malig-

nancies such as _____ also may cause this condition. The treatment of choice for vitamin D-dependent hypercalcemia is _____.

14. Most malignancies cause hypercalcemia via secretion of _____. This syndrome is called _____. A less common cause of malignancy-related hypercalcemia is _____ caused by secretion of _____.

15. An endocrine disorder resulting in mild hypercalcemia due to increased calcium resorption from bone is _____. Another disorder that causes hypercalcemia by altering responsiveness of intestinal vitamin D receptors is _____.

16. An uncommon benign genetic disorder often confused with primary hyperparathyroidism is _____. In this, calcium excretion is _____, whereas it is usually _____ in hyperparathyroidism.

17. The most important step in treating hypercalcemic crisis is _____. After this has been done, administration of _____ may enhance calciuresis, especially if renal insufficiency is present.

18. _____ are phosphate analogs that inhibit bone resorption by irreversibly binding to bone. Commonly used agents include _____ and _____. The antibiotic _____ also has antihypercalcemic properties. _____ has moderate antiresorptive properties and is useful in mild hypercalcemia.

19. List five signs or symptoms associated with hypocalcemia.

20. Most cases of hypoparathyroidism are caused by _____. A state of "functional" hypoparathyroidism may occur after prolonged _____ deficiency.

21. Laboratory findings in hypoparathyroidism include decreased serum _____ and increased _____. PTH levels are _____.

22. Chronic treatment of hypoparathyroidism includes administration of _____.

23. Pseudohypoparathyroidism results in hypocalcemia due to end-organ resistance to _____. Phosphate levels are _____, and PTH levels are _____. Treatment involves _____. These patients typically have characteristic somatic abnormalities, such as _____, _____, _____, and _____.

24. Vitamin D deficiency results in decreased _____ and _____ absorption from the small intestine, leading to decreased levels. PTH levels are _____.

25. _____ is a common disorder resulting from decreased quantity of bone. The _____ form occurs when too much bone is resorbed, while _____ results when too little bone is formed. The most common form in women results from _____.

26. The best way of diagnosing osteoporosis is with a _____ test. A patient with a T score (standard deviation normalized for young adults) less than _____ has osteoporosis. One with a T score between _____ and _____ has osteopenia or low bone mass.

27. A condition arising from deficient bone mineralization is _____. It may occur in any disease state interfering with the absorption or metabolism of _____.

28. A localized disorder of bone remodeling resulting in a disorganized mosaic of bone is called _____. A common presentation is the asymptomatic elevation of the enzyme _____.

29. For the following hypercalcemic conditions, fill in the blanks for the laboratory tests indicated (either ↓ or ↑). (PTH = serum parathyroid hormone; PTH-rP = serum parathyroid hormone-related peptide.)

CAUSE OF HYPERCALCEMIA	PHOSPHATE	PTH	PTH-rP
Primary hyperparathyroidism			
Vitamin D-dependent hypercalcemia			
Humoral hypercalcemia of malignancy			

30. For the following hypocalcemic conditions, fill in the blanks for the laboratory tests indicated (either ↓ or ↑). (PTH = serum parathyroid hormone.)

CAUSE OF HYPOCALCEMIA	PHOSPHATE	PTH
Hypoparathyroidism		
Pseudohypoparathyroidism		
Vitamin D deficiency		

II. MULTIPLE CHOICE

Select the one best answer.

31. A 32-year-old male is found to have mild hypercalcemia (10.9 mg/dL; normal: 8.4–10.1). Intact PTH is slightly elevated at 67 pg/mL (normal: 15–65). His father also had mild hypercalcemia that was not improved by parathyroidectomy. The 24-hour urine calcium is 51 mg (normal: 100–250). Which of the following is true about this patient?
    a. He likely has cancer and should undergo a thorough workup.
    b. He should have a parathyroid scan.
    c. No treatment is necessary.
    d. Parathyroid exploration should be done.
    e. He should start taking calcitonin injections.

32. Which one of the following is *not* a metabolic effect of parathyroid hormone?
    a. increased tubular reabsorption of calcium
    b. increased synthesis of $1,25(OH)_2D_3$
    c. increased urinary excretion of cyclic AMP
    d. increased tubular reabsorption of phosphate
    e. increased net release of calcium from bone into extracellular fluid

33. A patient with a total serum calcium of 7.6 mg/dL (normal: 8.4–10.1) has a serum albumin of 2.9 mg/dL (normal: 3.5–4.8). The calcium concentration when corrected for the low serum albumin level is approximately:
    a. 7.2 mg/dL
    b. 8.0 mg/dL
    c. 8.3 mg/dL
    d. 8.5 mg/dL
    e. 8.8 mg/dL

34. A 69-year-old male is admitted after being found on the street, lethargic and stuporous. Laboratory data show a serum calcium of 15.5 mg/dL (normal: = 11). His friend states that he is a heavy smoker, and a chest x-ray shows a large pulmonary mass. Which of the following supports a diagnosis of hypercalcemia from squamous cell carcinoma of the lung?
    a. elevated serum intact PTH, low serum phosphate
    b. high serum PTH related protein, low serum phosphate
    c. elevated serum osteoclast-activating factor, low serum phosphate
    d. elevated serum PTH related protein, elevated serum phosphate
    e. elevated serum $1,25(OH)_2D_3$, low serum PTH-related protein and intact PTH

35. A patient presents to you with mild hypocalcemia. Serum intact PTH level is several times normal. Which one of the following would *not* be a cause of the hypocalcemia?
    a. pseudohypoparathyroidism
    b. osteomalacia
    c. hypoparathyroidism
    d. chronic renal insufficiency
    e. vitamin D deficiency

36. A 47-year-old male presents with numerous vertebral fractures and has osteoporosis demonstrated by DEXA. Which of the following would *not* be a cause of secondary osteoporosis?
    a. ingestion of exogenous glucocorticoids
    b. illicit use of testosterone cypionate
    c. ingestion of exogenous thyroid hormone
    d. panhypopituitarism
    e. Kallmann's syndrome

37. Which one of the following is the best treatment for pseudohypoparathyroidism?
    a. parathyroid hormone, intramuscularly
    b. calcium supplementation, daily
    c. calcitriol $(1,25(OH)_2D_3)$
    d. phosphate, intravenously
    e. mithramycin

38. The most common cause of hypoparathyroidism is:
    a. autoimmune
    b. postsurgical
    c. destruction by hemochromatosis
    d. poor intake of vitamin D
    e. end-organ resistance to PTH

39. The most common presentation of primary hyperparathyroidism is:
    a. band (limbus) keratopathy
    b. proximal muscle weakness
    c. osteoporosis
    d. asymptomatic hypercalcemia
    e. calcium kidney stones

40. Which one of the following statements regarding parathyroid hormone is *not* true?
    a. It stimulates renal synthesis of $1,25(OH)_2D_3$.
    b. It shares biologic activity with PTH-related protein.
    c. It acts directly on the gut to increase calcium absorption.
    d. It promotes reabsorption of calcium from the glomerular filtrate.
    e. Levels are elevated in pseudohypoparathyroidism.

41. A 35-year-old confused male is brought to the hospital from a chemical plant. His serum calcium is 15.0 mg/dL (normal: 8.2–10.6). Serum PTH is 5 pg/mL (normal: 15–65). The serum $1,25(OH)_2D_3$ level is several times normal. You establish hydration and bring the calcium down to normal. A lung lesion is seen on x-ray and biopsied; it demonstrates granulomas. The most likely etiology of the hypercalcemia is:
    a. hyperparathyroidism
    b. mercury poisoning
    c. lung cancer
    d. berylliosis
    e. fluorosis

42. A 63-year-old woman has had lifelong hypocalcemia and hyperphosphatemia. Recent Ca^{2+} values are 5.2 and 5.4 mg/dL (normal: 8.4–10.6). PO_4^- levels are 6.2 and 6.1 mg/dL (normal: 2.5–4.5). She had cataracts removed at age 40. She has mild mental retardation and is rather short (59 inches). Renal function is normal. Serum PTH levels are 123 and 143 pg/mL (normal: 15–65). Her $25OHD_3$ level is normal. This woman has:
    a. vitamin D deficiency
    b. vitamin D-resistant rickets
    c. hypoparathyroidism
    d. pseudohypoparathyroidism
    e. calcitonin-secreting tumor

43. A patient presented with asymptomatic elevation of alkaline phosphatase. A bone scan was

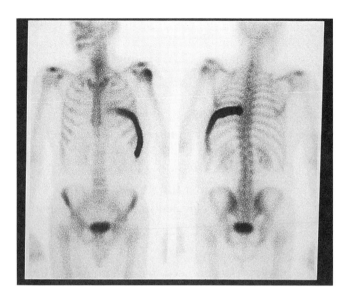

Figure 6-12. Bone scan of patient in question 43.

done, which is shown in Figure 6-12. The most likely diagnosis is:
- a. metastatic cancer
- b. multiple myeloma
- c. Paget's disease of bone
- d. hyperparathyroidism
- e. pseudohypoparathyroidism

44. A 61-year-old male is brought into the intensive care unit for a 2-month history of severe weakness, lethargy, and decreased appetite. He has become increasingly confused at home. He has a long history of chronic obstructive lung disease and has been in poor health for some time. He often complains of stomach pain and keeps a bottle of antacid pills at his bedside. Laboratory studies are as follows:

serum calcium: 16.0 mg/dL (normal: 8.2–10.2)

serum phosphorus: 4.9 mg/dL (normal: 2.5–4.5)

serum creatinine: 5.9 mg/dL (normal: 0.6–1.4)

serum potassium: 5.8 mEq/L (normal: 3.5–5.2)

serum bicarbonate: 33 mEq/L (normal: 18–23)

serum intact PTH: 2 pg/mL (normal: 15–65)

serum intact PTH-related protein: undetectable

The most likely cause of this man's hypercalcemia is:
- a. primary hyperparathyroidism
- b. milk-alkali syndrome
- c. tertiary hyperparathyroidism
- d. malignancy
- e. vitamin D intoxication

45. A 47-year old white male is admitted because of a period of nausea, vomiting, and lethargy that has lasted several days. His past medical history includes type 2 diabetes mellitus, hypertension, and hypercholesterolemia; his medications include insulin, diltiazem, and lovastatin. Physical examination reveals a chronically ill appearing male who is lethargic. His chest demonstrates scattered crackles, and his cardiac and abdominal examinations are normal. The chest x-ray reveals hilar adenopathy, and abdominal CT demonstrates periaortic adenopathy. Laboratory data demonstrate:

serum calcium: 15.0 mg/dL (normal: 8.4–10.2)

serum phosphorus: 5.2 mg/dL (normal: 2.5–4.5)

serum creatinine: 1.3 mg/dL (normal: 0.6–1.6)

serum intact PTH level: 2.3 pg/mL (normal: 15–65)

serum $1,25(OH)_2D_3$ level: 85.2 ng/mL (normal: 15–60).

His serum calcium level improves after rehydration but still remains elevated. The most appropriate definitive treatment at this time should be:
- a. parathyroidectomy
- b. radiation therapy to the lungs
- c. prednisone
- d. furosemide
- e. chemotherapy

46. A 68-year-old male with history of kidney stones is diagnosed with hyperparathyroidism after discovery of elevated serum calcium and PTH levels. He undergoes successful removal of a lower right parathyroid adenoma.

Postoperatively, he develops hypocalcemia (7.2 mg/dL, normal 8.4–10.2) and is asymptomatic. Two weeks later, his calcium is still low (7.4 mg/dL), and the intact PTH level is high at 85 pg/mL (normal: 10–65). Serum alkaline phosphatase is several times normal. Which one of the following statements is correct?

    a. The surgeon has damaged the other glands, resulting in hypoparathyroidism.

    b. He still has hyperparathyroidism and the surgery has failed.

    c. He has "hungry bone" syndrome and should receive calcium supplements.

    d. He has developed resistance to PTH and should receive calcitriol.

    e. The remaining parathyroids are still suppressed from the previous parathyroid adenoma and are not yet functioning sufficiently.

III. TRUE OR FALSE

47. Causes of hypocalcemia associated with a *high* serum parathyroid level include the following:

    ___ a. osteomalacia due to vitamin D deficiency

    ___ b. pseudohypoparathyroidism

    ___ c. chronic renal failure

    ___ d. hypomagnesemia

    ___ e. postsurgical hypoparathyroidism.

48. Characteristics of osteomalacia include the following:

    ___ a. low serum PTH level

    ___ b. pseudofractures or Looser's zones

    ___ c. hypercalcemia

    ___ d. low serum vitamin D level

    ___ e. high serum phosphate level

49. Which of the following statements are true regarding the woman with the bone density in Figure 6-13?

    ___ a. She has osteoporosis.

    ___ b. She likely has hypercalcemia.

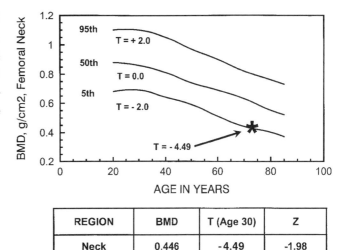

REGION	BMD	T (Age 30)	Z
Neck	0.446	-4.49	-1.98

Figure 6-13. Femoral neck DEXA of patient in question 45.

    ___ c. Vitamin D and calcium supplementation are advised.

    ___ d. She has double the risk of fracture compared to someone at the mean for young adults.

    ___ e. Mithramycin is an approved therapy.

50. A 60-year-old woman has low back pain. Radiographic examination reveals diffuse demineralization and compression fracture of L4. Serum calcium is 12.2 mg/dL (normal: 8.4–10.1). This clinical picture is compatible with which of the following?

    ___ a. osteomalacia

    ___ b. postmenopausal osteoporosis

    ___ c. primary hyperparathyroidism

    ___ d. multiple myeloma

    ___ e. pseudohypoparathyroidism

51. Of the following hypercalcemic conditions, which typically present with hyperphosphatemia?

    ___ a. primary hyperparathyroidism

    ___ b. sarcoidosis

    ___ c. squamous cell lung carcinoma producing PTH-related peptide

    ___ d. milk-alkali syndrome

    ___ e. "tertiary" hyperparathyroidism

52. Treatments for osteoporosis include the following:
    —— a. salmon calcitonin
    —— b. alendronate (a bisphosphonate)
    —— c. gallium nitrate
    —— d. calcium and vitamin D supplementation
    —— e. estrogen (in women)

53. Which of the following are true for PTH-related peptide (PTH-rP)?
    —— a. It cross-reacts with the intact PTH assay.
    —— b. It has similar biologic effects as PTH.
    —— c. It has no physiological purpose in the normal person.
    —— d. Levels are suppressed in hyperparathyroidism.
    —— e. Excess results in increased nephrogenous cyclic AMP.

54. Match the appropriate patient with the correct cause of osteoporosis:

    A. 21-year-old woman with multiple fractures beginning in childhood. Bone density is 4 standard deviations below the mean. Physical examination reveals bluish sclerae.

    B. 54-year old woman with multiple vertebral compression fractures. Recently she has developed severe hypertension and diabetes mellitus. Examination reveals "moon facies," pigmented abdominal striae, and decreased muscle mass.

    C. 17-year-old girl who suffered five fractures of the appendicular skeleton with minimal trauma between ages 8 and 12. She now plays basketball for her school team, and has a normal bone density.

    D. 54-year-old woman with exophthalmos, diffuse goiter, elevated serum T4 level, and undetectable serum TSH level. She stopped having menstrual periods at age 25 for no apparent reason. Examination reveals a thin, nervous woman with tachycardia and diffuse goiter.

    —— a. Graves' disease and premature ovarian failure (type II polyglandular syndrome).
    —— b. Osteogenesis imperfecta.
    —— c. Cushing's syndrome.
    —— d. Juvenile osteoporosis.

ANSWERS

1. ionized; 46; serum proteins, ions (complexed)

2. parathyroid hormone, parathyroid glands; four; ionized calcium

3. bone, kidney, small intestine

4. calcium resorption

5. increasing calcium reabsorption; phosphate; calcitriol $(1,25(OH)_2D_3)$, calcium, phosphate

6. calcitonin, parafollicular or C-cells of the thyroid; vasoactive symptoms (flushing, diarrhea)

7. primary hyperparathyroidism; malignancy

8. List five: dehydration, weight loss, anorexia, pruritus, polydipsia, nausea, vomiting, constipation, fatigue, lethargy, muscle weakness, hyporeflexia, confusion, seizures, psychosis, coma

9. solitary parathyroid adenoma; multi-gland hyperplasia; parathyroid carcinoma

10. increased, decreased; intact PTH; increased; parathyroidectomy

11. secondary hyperparathyroidism; decreased calcitriol, decreased calcium absorption, phosphate retention; ectopic calcifications, renal osteodystrophy

12. tertiary hyperparathyroidism, hypercalcemia

13. calcium, phosphate; vitamin D; granulomatous; 1α-hydroxylase; hematologic malignancies (lymphomas); glucocorticoids

14. parathyroid hormone-related protein (PTH-rP); humoral hypercalcemia of malignancy (HHM); local osteolytic hypercalcemia (LOH), osteoclast-activating factors (OAFs)

15. hyperthyroidism; adrenal insufficiency

16. familial hypocalciuric hypercalcemia (FHH); decreased; elevated

17. rehydration; loop diuretics

18. bisphosphonates; alendronate, etidronate; plicamycin (mithramycin); calcitonin

19. List five: paresthesias, hyperventilation, tetany, adrenergic (tachycardia, diaphoresis, etc.), seizures, Chvostek's and Trousseau's signs, QT interval prolongation, hypotension, refractory congestive heart failure (CHF), cardiomegaly, abnormalities in dental formation, gastrointestinal malabsorption, cataracts

20. surgical resection of parathyroid glands; magnesium

21. calcium, phosphate; decreased

22. vitamin D analogs (calcitriol, ergocalciferol)

23. parathyroid hormone; increased, increased; vitamin D analogs; obesity, mental retardation, short 4th metacarpals (brachydactyly), short stature

24. calcium, phosphate; increased

25. osteoporosis; high turnover, low turnover; estrogen deficiency

26. bone density or DEXA; -2.50; -1.00, -2.50

27. osteomalacia; vitamin D

28. Paget's disease; alkaline phosphatase

29.

CAUSE OF HYPERCALCEMIA	PHOSPHATE	PTH	PTH-rP
Primary hyperparathyroidism	↓	↑	↓
Vitamin D-dependent hypercalcemia	↑	↓	↓
Humoral hypercalcemia of malignancy	↓	↓	↑

30.

CAUSE OF HYPOCALCEMIA	PHOSPHATE	PTH
Hypoparathyroidism	↑	↓
Pseudohypoparathyroidism	↑	↑
Vitamin D deficiency	↓	↑

31. (c). This man has familial hypocalciuric hypercalcemia (FHH), a benign, genetically transmitted disorder. It is often confused with primary hyperparathyroidism. Calcium excretion is usually high in hyperparathyroidism, but low in FHH.

32. (d). PTH causes phosphaturia.

33. (d). Corrected Ca^{2+} = measured Ca^{2+} +

$(0.8)(4 - \text{serum albumin}) = 7.6 + (0.8)(4 - 2.9)$
$= 7.6 + (0.8)(1.1) = 8.48 \approx 8.5 \text{ mg/dL}.$

34. (b). This malignancy typically causes hypercalcemia via secretion of PTH-related protein (PTH-rP). This hormone has similar biologic activity to PTH, and may result in hypophosphatemia (as with hyperparathyroidism). Paradoxically, calcitriol levels are usually low in PTH-rP-related hypercalcemia.

35. (c). PTH levels are low in hypoparathyroidism.

36. (b). Illicit use of sex steroids, while not recommended, may promote a positive bone balance. Drugs such as glucocorticoids (a) and excess thyroid hormone (c) as well as sex steroid deficiency (d, e) are well-known causes of osteoporosis.

37. (c). Vitamin D analogs are the mainstay of treatment. PTH is not commercially available for treatment.

38. (b). Surgery is the most common cause.

39. (d). Band or limbus keratopathy (a) is an uncommon finding in persons with long-standing hypercalcemia, and is seen as a "band" of calcification at 3 and 9 o'clock at the limbus. Osteoporosis (c) and kidney stones (e) occur commonly, but most patients are asymptomatic.

40. (c). The effect of PTH on the gut is indirect, mediated by calcitriol.

41. (d). The presentation is consistent with a vitamin D-dependent hypercalcemia. Berylliosis is a granulomatous disease associated with increased vitamin D production. It is rare and was once associated with certain manufacturing processes. It is treated with glucocorticoids.

42. (d). Hyperphosphatemia, hypocalcemia, and increased PTH along with these physical findings suggest pseudohypoparathyroidism.

43. (c). Asymptomatic elevation of alkaline phosphatase and abnormal uptake on bone scan is suggestive of Paget's disease, and is a common presentation. Metastatic cancer (a) is possible, but not as likely. Multiple myeloma may cause lytic lesions, but these do not typically show up on bone scan. Hyperparathyroidism (d) may cause alkaline phosphatase elevation, but not isolated bone lesions such as this.

44. (b). The history of excessive calcium ingestion, hypercalcemia, metabolic alkalosis, and renal insufficiency is consistent with the milk-alkali syndrome. Hyperparathyroidism (a, c) is excluded by the low PTH level. Hypercalcemia due to malignancy (d) usually presents with elevated PTH-rP levels. Other causes of hypercalcemia in malignancy not related to PTH-rP are possible. Vitamin D intoxication (e) does not typically present with renal failure.

45. (c). The history of hypercalcemia, hyperphosphatemia, elevated calcitriol level, and adenopathy all suggest sarcoidosis as the cause, which responds dramatically to glucocorticoids.

46. (c). In patients with hyperparathyroidism, bone formation often continues even after the source of excess PTH has been removed. This may result in depletion of calcium from serum and hypocalcemia (the hungry bone syndrome). If hypoparathyroidism (a) were present, the PTH level would be low. Although his PTH level is elevated, he does not have hyperparathyroidism (b), as his calcium is low. Resistance to PTH (d) is due to a receptor defect and would not present spontaneously. Hypocalcemia from suppression of the remaining glands (e) would present with a low PTH level.

47. True (a, b, c); False (d, e). All causes of hypocalcemia except hypoparathyroidism result in increased PTH levels. Mg^{2+} deficiency results in a state of functional PTH deficiency that returns to normal after replacement.

48. True (b, d); False (a, c, e). This is typically a result of vitamin D deficiency, with low calcium and phosphate levels. PTH level is elevated.

49. True (a, c); False (b, d, e). The T score is more than 4 standard deviations below the mean for both lumbar spine and femoral neck, indicating osteoporosis. Vitamin D and calcium are advised. Most patients with osteoporosis have normal laboratory studies. The risk of fracture approximately doubles for each standard deviation below the mean; T is approximately -4, so the risk would be $2^4 = 16$ times, not 2 times

(*d*). Mithramycin (*e*) is used for treatment of severe hypercalcemia.

50. True (*c*, *d*); False (*a*, *b*, *e*). Hyperparathyroidism and myeloma may produce hypercalcemia; both predispose the patient to compression fractures. Most patients with typical osteoporosis (*b*) are normocalcemic. Osteomalacia (*a*) and pseudohypoparathyroidism (*e*) may result in hypocalcemia, not hypercalcemia.

51. True (*b*, *d*, *e*); False (*a*, *c*). PTH (*a*) and PTH-rP (*c*) cause phosphaturia and hypophosphatemia. Sarcoidosis (*b*) results in excess calcitriol, and hence increased calcium and phosphorus absorption from the intestine. Milk-alkali syndrome (*d*) may present with azotemia and hence hyperphosphatemia. Tertiary hyperparathyroidism (*e*) only occurs in those patients with long-standing renal failure; these patients eventually develop autonomous PTH secretion even after calcium levels are normalized. They retain phosphate because of their renal failure.

52. True (*a*, *b*, *d*, *e*); False (*c*). Gallium nitrate is used to treat hypercalcemic crisis. The others are accepted treatments for osteoporosis.

53. True (*b*, *d*, *e*); False (*a*, *c*). PTH-rP, although similar in biologic activity to PTH, is different in structure and is not detected in the PTH assay (*a*). It does play a role in the development of certain tissues, such as skin, smooth muscle, cartilage, breast, and placenta. As with all non-PTH-dependent hypercalcemia, PTH levels are suppressed (*d*). PTH and PTH-rP both are peptide hormones that bind to a surface receptor, producing cyclic AMP as a second messenger. Nephrogenous cyclic AMP (cAMP of renal origin) is increased in both hyperparathyroidism and PTH-rP-mediated hypercalcemia.

54. A (*b*); B(*c*); C (*d*); D (*a*). Patient A has the classic clinical features of osteogenesis imperfecta. Patient B likely has Cushing's syndrome. Patient C probably has juvenile osteoporosis; this condition goes into remission, unlike osteogenesis imperfecta. Patient D has hyperthyroidism and premature gonadal failure, both well-recognized causes of osteoporosis.

CHAPTER 7

REPRODUCTIVE ENDOCRINOLOGY

Q: What cells comprise the testes?

A: Sertoli and Leydig cells are the cells of the testes (Fig. 7-1). **Sertoli cells** are the site of spermatogenesis, and also make important proteins, such as inhibin and müllerian inhibitory factor (MIF). These cells are stimulated by the pituitary hormone **follicle-stimulating hormone** (FSH). FSH secretion is stimulated by the testicular hormone **activin** and inhibited by **inhibin,** both produced by the Sertoli cells.

Leydig cells are the major site of **testosterone** synthesis (95%) and are stimulated by **luteinizing hormone** (LH) and inhibited by high levels of **testosterone** (Fig. 7-2). Testosterone is the major androgen of the reproductive system. A small proportion of testosterone in males originates in the adrenal cortex.

Gonadotropins (FSH and LH) are stimulated by the hypothalamic hormone **gonadotropin-hormone releasing hormone** (GnRH), when secreted in a pulsatile fashion (every 90 minutes). If given continuously, GnRH produces paradoxical inhibition of gonadotropin secretion.

Q: What cells are present in the ovary?

A: The ovum is the hormone-producing cell of the female reproductive system. It contains **theca** and **granulosa cells.** Many **follicles** (groups of ova) develop in the ovary, but only one is destined to develop fully, and the others will degenerate. The two main female sex steroids are **estradiol** (Fig. 7-3) and **progesterone** (Fig. 7-4). Approximately 50% of testosterone in women arises from the ovaries; the rest comes from the adrenal cortex and aromatization of steroids in peripheral tissues.

Estradiol is synthesized in several steps (Fig. 7-5). Initially, androgenic precursors (testosterone and androstenedione) are made in the **theca interna cells** under the influence of luteinizing hormone (LH). The androgens then are aromatized to estradiol and estrone in the **granulosa cells** under the influence of follicle-stimulating hormone (FSH). This unique process is called the **"two-cell" concept** of ovarian steroid synthesis.

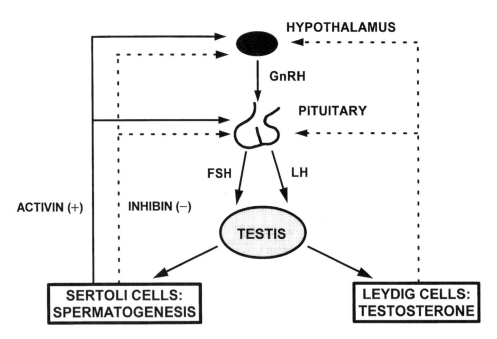

Figure 7-1. Normal male reproductive axis.

Q: How is the female reproductive cycle regulated?

A: The ovarian cycle may be divided into **follicular** (proliferative) and **luteal** (secretory) phases (Fig. 7-6). Early in the follicular phase, FSH secretion predominates, which increases the number of follicles and granulosa cells. Only one of many follicles is destined to become "ripe" for ovulation. LH secretion then increases, leading to theca cell proliferation. As estradiol concentrations increase, this hormone and inhibin serve to decrease FSH secretion. Most follicles regress as the FSH secretion diminishes; one will have enough receptors to remain viable, and this is the one selected to ovulate.

In the viable follicle, estradiol concentrations increase, and, although estrogen normally inhibits LH production, in this instance there is a paradoxical switch from negative to positive feedback, resulting in a pituitary LH surge. This results in ovulation, and the ovum is expelled from the ovary.

Then, the granulosa cells also acquire LH receptors; with the formation of the **corpus luteum,** the cells begin to secrete progesterone (the luteal phase). Progesterone concentrations continue to increase, and estradiol levels remain high. If the ovum is not fertilized, involution of the corpus luteum (luteolysis) occurs.

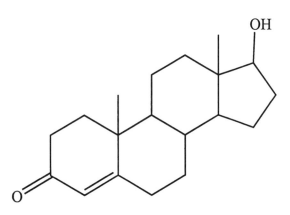

Figure 7-2. Testosterone.

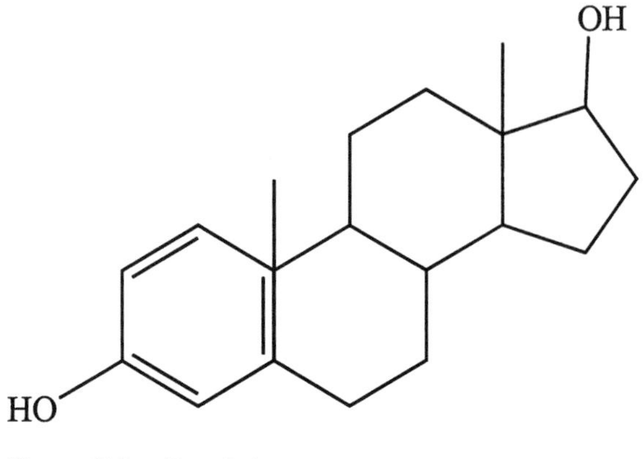

Figure 7-3. Estradiol.

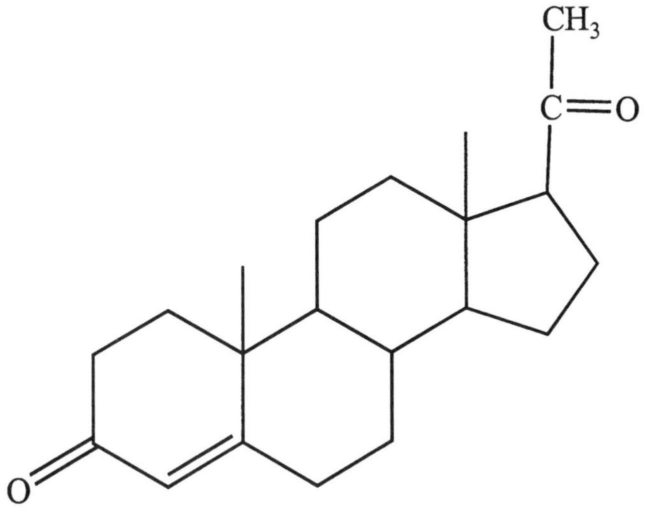

Figure 7-4. Progesterone.

After ovulation, the luteal or secretory phase is facilitated by the progesterone secretion of the corpus luteum. The glands become longer and edematous; the maximum size occurs at day 21. If fertilization does not occur, the ovum regresses and the endometrium is sloughed away (menstruation).

If the ovum is fertilized, the glycoprotein hormone human chorionic gonadotropin (β-hCG) is secreted by the fetoplacental unit. This serves to maintain the hormonal secretion of the corpus luteum. (Pregnancy tests detect hCG either in the blood or the urine.) The elevated estrogen levels suppress FSH, preventing further ovulation.

Q: How do steroids travel in the blood?

A: Sex steroids exist in a protein-bound state (98%), primarily bound to sex hormone-binding globulin (SHBG). Like thyroid hormones, factors that increase or decrease the binding protein concentrations also affect the amount of *total* hormones, without affecting the *free* (unbound) amount.

Q: What are the menstrual changes that take place during this cycle?

A: Menstruation occurs during the first few days of the cycle, preparing the endometrium for a possible pregnancy. During the follicular or proliferative phase, the endometrium thickens and grows in length, mucus is secreted from the cervix, and maturation of vaginal epithelium occurs (due to the effects of estrogens).

Q: What factors increase SHBG?

A: The factors that increase SHBG are estrogens, thyroxine, cirrhosis, and hyperthyroidism.

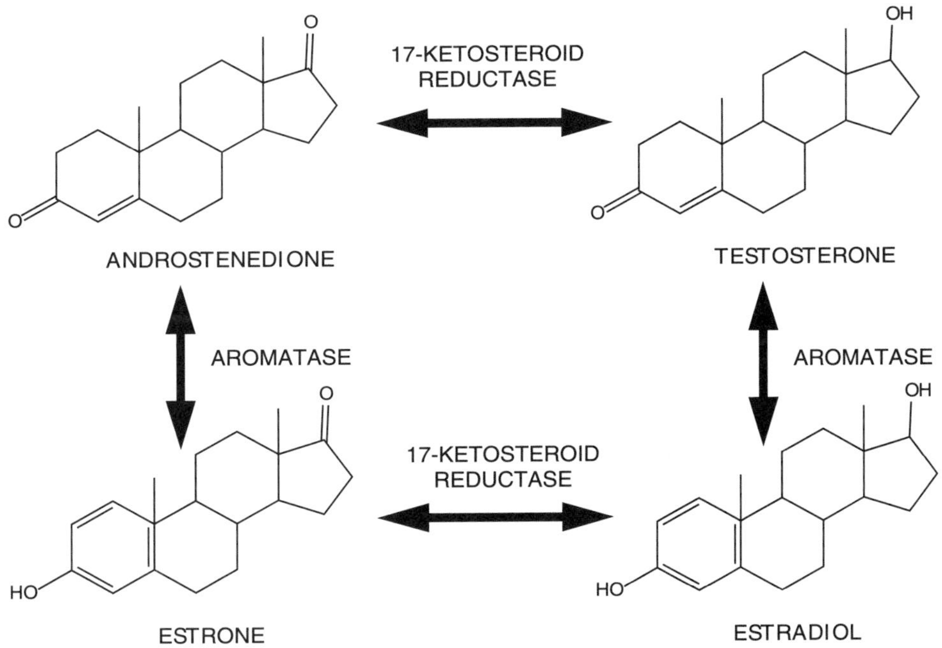

Figure 7-5. Sex steroid aromatization.

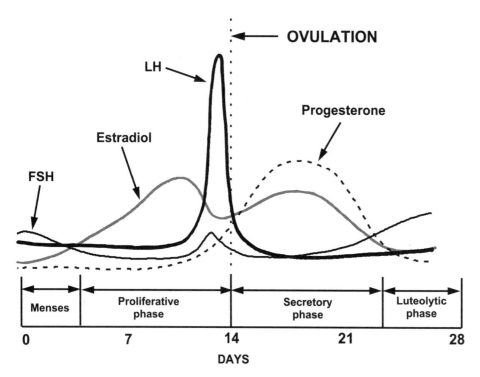

Figure 7-6. Normal female reproductive cycle.

Q: What factors decrease SHBG?

A: The factors that decrease SHBG are androgens, growth hormone, obesity, and hypothyroidism.

Q: How do gonads differentiate?

A: Up to 42 days, the embryonic gonads are indistinguishable (Fig. 7-7). The Y chromosome contains a gene critical for male sexual differentiation, called the **sex-determining region** or SRY. If SRY is present, testis-determining factor (TDF) is secreted, and the primordial gonad becomes a testis. In the absence of SRY, TDF is not secreted and an ovary develops. This is the traditional "female by default" hypothesis. Some experts have challenged this concept, claiming that the X chromosome may play a more active role than was previously believed.

Q: How do the genital ducts and internal structures (such as the uterus, cervix, and vas deferens) develop?

A: The female or **müllerian structures** include the uterus, uterine tubes, cervix, and upper third of the vagina. The male or **wolffian structures** include the epididymis, vas deferens, seminal ves-

icles, and ejaculatory ducts. Both sets of structures are present in the fetus. If a functional testis is present, the Sertoli cells secrete müllerian inhibitory factor (MIF), also called anti-müllerian hormone (AMH), which causes the müllerian structures to involute. In the absence of a testis, müllerian differentiation occurs and wolffian structures involute.

Q: What about the differentiation of external genitalia?

A: Up to 8 weeks, the external genitalia are identical, and they may differentiate into genitalia of either sex. Exposure of the genitalia to dihydrotestosterone (DHT) during the first 8 to 12 weeks of fetal life results in differentiation to male genitalia. Female differentiation occurs in the absence of DHT, which occurs in the presence of ovaries or if no gonad is present.

Q: What are the biologic effects of androgens?

A: Androgens result in differentiation of the internal and external male genital system and the growth of scrotum, epididymis, vas deferens, seminal vesicles, prostate, and penis. They also result in skeletal muscle, laryngeal, and long bone growth.

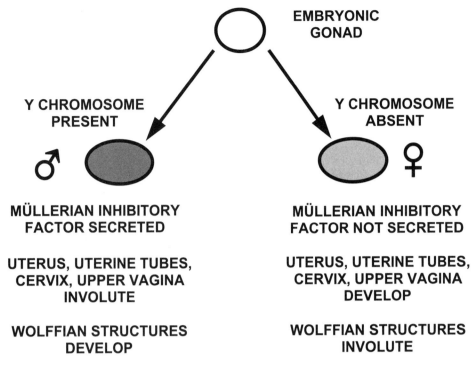

Figure 7-7. Gonadal differentiation.

Q: What are the biologic effects of estrogens?

A: Estrogens cause maturation of the vagina, uterus, and uterine tubes at puberty. They also alter the distribution and type of body fat. **Gynecoid fat** is found on the hips, buttocks, and thighs and is less metabolically active in peripheral steroid conversion than is **android fat,** which is found in the abdomen. Android fat is felt to be more atherogenic due to its increased metabolic activity.

Q: What is the endocrine function of fat?

A: Fat (especially central or android fat) serves as a site for peripheral aromatization of steroids. Specifically, in fat, estrogens (estradiol) are converted to androgens (testosterone) and vice versa. Therefore, hirsutism (excess facial hair in women) is common in obese women. Gynecomastia (excess breast growth in males) is also more common in obese men, as the extra fat may promote conversion of testosterone to estradiol. Android obesity is a recognized risk factor for hyperinsulinism, type 2 diabetes, hyperlipidemia, hypertension, and coronary disease (syndrome X).

Q: What biochemical events occur in puberty?

A: The machinery necessary for going through puberty is present at birth, but is held in check by potent inhibitory mechanisms. The hypothalamic-pituitary axis (HPA) is the governing factor.

In the pre-pubertal state, very small circulating amounts of sex steroids inhibit gonadotropin secretion (Fig. 7-8). At puberty the inhibition decreases, and the hypothalamic hormone gonadotropin-hormone releasing hormone (GnRH) begins secreting in a pulsatile fashion, every 90 minutes (Fig. 7-9). This results in increased gonadotropin secretion and gonadal growth (Fig. 7-10). This onset of gonadal stimulation is termed **gonadarche.** The pulsatile secretion of GnRH is very important—if it is given continuously, LH and FSH secretion is suppressed.

Q: What other hormones are necessary for normal puberty?

A: In addition to sex steroids, adequate growth hormone and thyroid hormone levels are necessary for normal growth.

PRE-PUBERTY

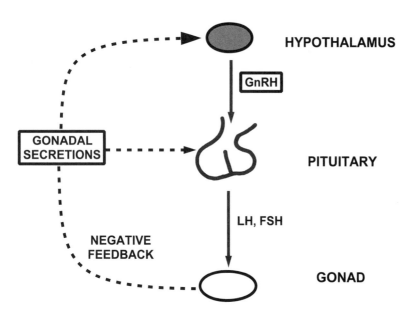

LOW GONADAL STEROID LEVELS RESULT DUE TO SENSITIVITY
OF HYPOTHALAMUS TO VERY LOW CIRCULATING LEVELS

Figure 7-8. Pre-pubertal gonadal axis.

INITIATION OF PUBERTY

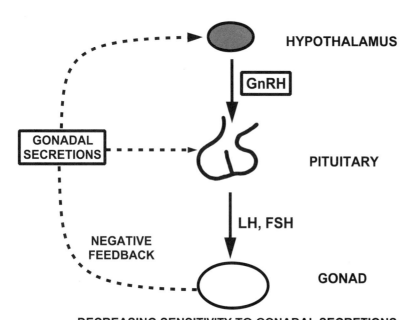

DECREASING SENSITIVITY TO GONADAL SECRETIONS
RESULTS IN INCREASED PULSATILE SECRETION OF GnRH

Figure 7-9. Initiation of puberty.

ADULT

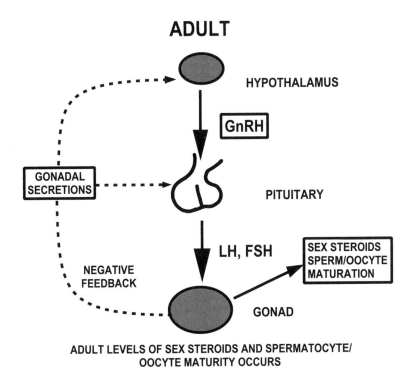

Figure 7-10. Adult gonadal axis.

Q: What is the normal age for pubertal onset?

A: In females, 99% will begin puberty between ages 8 and 13. In males, 99% begin puberty between ages 9 and 14. Those who do not have onset of puberty by age 13 (females) or 14 (males) are said to have **delayed puberty.** Those with onset of puberty before age 8 (females) or 9 (males) are said to have **precocious puberty.**

Q: What changes in body composition are seen during puberty?

A: Males and females start with equal lean body mass. Because of the effects of testosterone, males end up on average with 1.5 times as much muscle mass and 0.5 times as much fat as females. Increasing androgen secretion (males and females) results in deepening voice and acne. Sex steroids and growth hormone result in increased bone density, with peak values occurring in the mid-twenties.

Sex steroids result in an initial increase in growth velocity, and eventually result in closing of the epiphyseal plates of long bones and cessation of growth. As puberty begins earlier in girls than boys, the epiphyseal plates close sooner, and girls are typically shorter than boys (other things being equal).

The **Tanner stages** refer to specific developmental milestones that occur in puberty. The stages are numbered 1 through 5; 1 is prepubertal, and 5 is adult development. Girls typically start puberty sooner; the initial sign of puberty in a girl is **breast budding.** The growth spurt starts earlier in girls, and ends sooner. The first physical sign of puberty in a boy is **testicular enlargement.** Tanner stages are shown in Figures 7-11 (boys) and 7-12 (girls).

Q: What is adrenarche?

A: **Adrenarche** (also referred to as **pubarche**) is the onset of adrenal androgen secretion. Adrenarche usually starts 1 to 2 years earlier than gonadarche in boys, and often occurs after gonadarche in girls. It is responsible for a major portion of androgen secretion (25% to 50%) in the female. The age of onset is typically 8 to 11. It is responsible for much of the terminal (dark, pigmented) hairs in the axillary and pubic areas, and for the development of sweat glands in those areas (resulting in characteristic adult body odor).

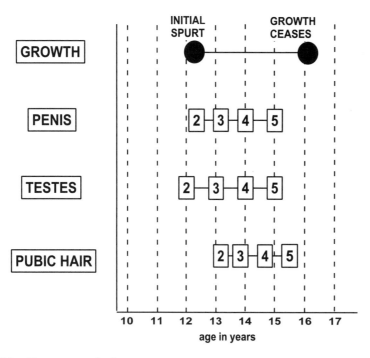

Figure 7-11. Tanner stages for boys.

Q: What is terminal hair?

A: **Terminal hair** is coarse, pigmented, and has a greater potential for growth than **vellus hair,** which is fine and unpigmented. Terminal hairs occur on the scalp, eyebrows, and to varying de-

grees on the body, depending on the amount of circulating androgens and genetic differences in hair sensitivity. Vellus hairs will transform into terminal hairs given sufficient androgen concentrations. This accounts for the typical heavy termi-

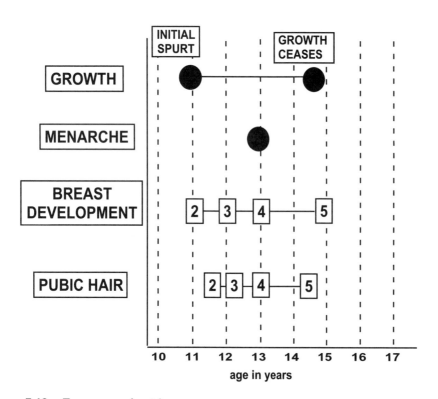

Figure 7-12. Tanner stages for girls.

nal hair growth on the face, chest, and extremities of males. Pubic and axillary hairs appear to require lower androgen concentrations than other hairs for transformation. Increased adrenal androgen production is the hallmark of adrenarche, which results in increased testosterone secretion, development of pubic and axillary hair, and acne.

Q: What biochemical events control adrenarche?

A: The control of adrenarche is unknown. It does not appear to be controlled by the gonadotropins or prolactin. It appears to be a separate process from gonadarche, as individuals whose gonadarche is suppressed (as in those treated for central precocious puberty) may go through adrenarche normally.

Q: What is delayed puberty?

A: Delayed puberty is the absence of *any* pubertal development in a boy of 14 or girl of 13.

Q: What is the most common cause of delayed puberty?

A: Constitutional delay is the most common cause of delayed puberty; such individuals simply tend to develop later than normal, but do eventually go through puberty normally and reach a normal adult height. There is typically a positive family history in parents and siblings. It is important to distinguish those with constitutional delay from those with organic disease (e.g., growth hormone deficiency). Delayed puberty growth charts demonstrate early short stature, with eventual increase into the normal range; the chart has been "shifted to the right" a few years but otherwise is normal (Figs. 7-13, 7-14).

Q: What is a bone age study?

A: **Bone** or **skeletal age** (BA) is found by comparing an x-ray of the wrist bones to a standard (Greulich-Pyle) atlas of standards. Bones characteristically change with age, until the epiphyses fuse. Typically, bone age (BA) equals chronologic age (CA). In those with delayed puberty, the full effect of sex steroids have not been realized, and the bone age is delayed (BA < CA). In those with precocious puberty, the reverse is true (BA > CA). Bone age is therefore an estimate of a child's remaining growth.

Q: What other conditions can result in delayed puberty?

A: Hypopituitarism (growth hormone deficiency), hypothyroidism, and chromosomal abnormalities can all be causes of delayed puberty.

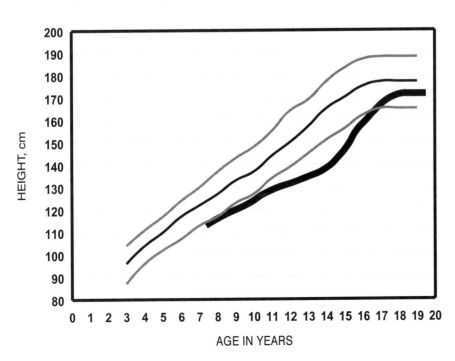

Figure 7-13. Growth of child with constitutional delay of puberty.

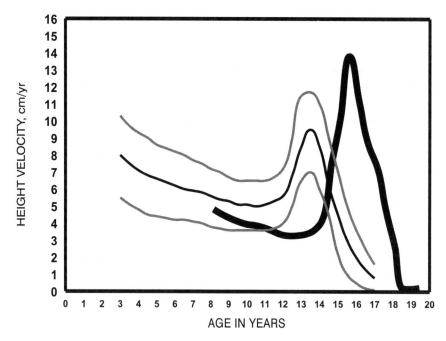

Figure 7-14. Growth velocity of child with constitutional delay of puberty.

Q: Can puberty occur earlier than normal?

A: **Precocious puberty** (PP) is defined as the onset of secondary sexual development in a female before age 8 and a male before age 9. Precocious development consistent with genetic sex is termed **isosexual** PP; if characteristics are of the opposite sex, it is called **heterosexual** PP.

Most commonly, precocious puberty is **central** (complete or true), meaning that puberty occurs via premature activation of the hypothalamic-pituitary axis (HPA). It is called "true" because it occurs by the same mechanism as normal puberty, except at an earlier age. **Peripheral** (incomplete) precocious puberty is caused by abnormal gonadotropin and/or sex steroid secretion, rather than by premature activation of the HPA.

Q: Why does central precocious puberty occur?

A: The potential for going through puberty is present at birth, but is held in check by strong inhibitory mechanisms. If these are disturbed, puberty commences and sexual maturation and fertility achieved. Any central nervous system lesion that disrupts the normal inhibitory responses can cause this (e.g., hydrocephalus and central nervous system tumors). Central precocious puberty may also be idiopathic, and no obvious cause may be found.

Q: What are some causes of incomplete or peripheral precocious puberty?

A: Any condition that results in increased gonadotropin and/or sex steroid secretion can cause peripheral precocious puberty:

Exogenous steroids

Premature adrenarche

Congenital adrenal hyperplasia (feminizing or virilizing)

Steroid-secreting adrenal tumors

Steroid-secreting ovarian/testicular tumors

Testotoxicosis

Gonadotropin-secreting tumors

β-hCG-secreting tumors

Severe hypothyroidism (mechanism: ? TRH stimulation of gonadotropins)

McCune-Albright syndrome (precocious puberty associated with café au lait spots, polyostotic fibrous dysplasia, and other endocrine disorders)

Q: Can "normal" puberty occur at an earlier age than average?

A: Like constitutionally delayed puberty, a child may have constitutional early puberty. There is typically a family history of such and often these children are overweight. These children are large for their age but stop growing early at a normal adult height. Their growth curve appears normal but is "shifted to the left" 2 or 3 years (the opposite of constitutional delay).

Q: How can complete and incomplete precocious puberty be distinguished?

A: To distinguish between complete and incomplete precocious puberty, a GnRH (gonadotropin-hormone releasing hormone) test is done. GnRH is infused, and LH and FSH are measured at 30-minute intervals. Prepubertal patients have a typical flat response, because of the potent inhibitory mechanisms in place. Those with complete (central) precocious puberty have a pubertal LH/FSH response to GnRH. Those with peripheral or incomplete precocious puberty usually have a flat response as the gonadotropins are usually suppressed from ectopic secretion of steroids.

Q: What is the outcome of untreated precocious puberty?

A: Sex steroid secretion occurs at an early age, so precocious puberty causes premature skeletal growth and epiphyseal closure, resulting in early tall stature and eventual short adult stature. Early sexual development may also be psychologically devastating to the child.

Q: What is the treatment of precocious puberty?

A: The treatment for central precocious puberty is to "shut off" the hypothalamic-pituitary axis (HPA). This is best done by the administration of GnRH analogs (e.g., leuprolide), which, when given in a continuous fashion, cause paradoxical gonadotropin suppression. These drugs may be given either intramuscularly or intranasally. At the appropriate age, the agent is withdrawn, allowing the child to go through puberty normally.

Treatment for peripheral precocious puberty involves location of the site of steroid excess (e.g., the tumor or congenital adrenal enzyme defect) and treating it through surgical removal or medical therapy.

Q: What is premature thelarche?

A: **Premature thelarche** is a benign disorder in which breast development occurs without other signs of puberty. The bone age and growth are normal, and it requires no treatment.

Q: What is premature adrenarche?

A: **Premature adrenarche** is the premature appearance of terminal (sexual) hair in children, without other signs of sexual development. Adrenal androgen (DHEA and DHEA sulfate) levels are increased. It is a variation of normal puberty and requires no treatment.

Q: What is hypogonadism?

A: **Hypogonadism** (HG) is the condition of sex steroid deficiency. It may be primary, caused by a gonadal defect; this is termed **hypergonadotropic** hypogonadism because gonadotropin levels are elevated. The secondary (lack of gonadotropin secretion) or tertiary (lack of GnRH) forms of hypogonadism are called **hypogonadotropic**.

Q: What should the physical examination of hypogonadal patients include?

A: The physical examination of a hypogonadal patient should include measurement of body proportions (arm span; height; upper to lower segment ratio). The patient's height and weight should be plotted on standard growth charts and compared to normal persons.

The external genitalia should be also be examined. In males, testicular size is best measured with an **orchidometer,** a series of successive ellipsoids that represent testicular size (Fig. 7-15). Normal adult testes measure 25 mL each. A vaginal and bimanual examination should be done in females.

The sense of smell should be assessed to exclude anosmia (seen in Kallmann's syndrome). The patient is asked to smell several common odors (e.g., coffee, mouthwash, fruit extract). These may be gradually diluted if greater accuracy is desired.

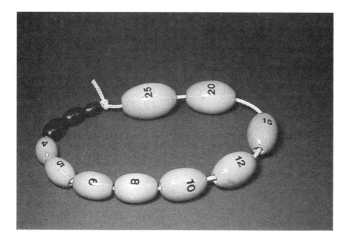

Figure 7-15. Prader orchidometer.

The amount of body hair (axillary, pubic, beard, chest) should also be recorded.

Q: What are hypogonadal proportions?

A: **Hypogonadal** or **eunuchoidal proportions** are a result of hypogonadism during adolescence. In a normal person, sex steroid secretion during puberty results in epiphyseal fusion and cessation of long bone growth; the arm span approximates height, and the upper and lower body segment measurements are equal (Fig. 7-16). In hypogonadal persons, the long bones continue to grow out of proportion to the axial skeleton, resulting in long extremities and taller stature than if hypogonadism were not present (Fig. 7-17). These persons have an arm span that exceeds linear height, and a lower body segment that is longer than the

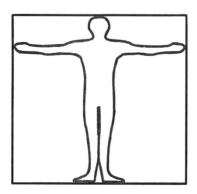

NORMAL BODY PROPORTIONS
ARM SPAN = HEIGHT
UPPER = LOWER BODY SEGMENT

Figure 7-16. Normal proportions.

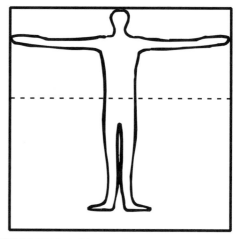

HYPOGONADAL OR EUNUCHOIDAL PROPORTIONS
ARM SPAN > HEIGHT
UPPER < LOWER BODY SEGMENT

Figure 7-17. Eunuchoidal proportions.

upper body segment. Individuals with onset of hypogonadism in adulthood have normal proportions, as their skeleton has already finished growing.

Q: What is hypogonadotropic hypogonadism?

A: **Hypogonadotropic hypogonadism** is hypogonadism caused by a defect in GnRH or LH/FSH secretion. The end organ (gonad) is intact, yet is hypofunctional due to decreased stimulation. LH and FSH levels are low.

Q: What are the causes of hypogonadotropic hypogonadism?

A: The most common cause of hypogonadotropic hypogonadism is **Kallmann's syndrome,** a disorder of GnRH secretion associated with **anosmia** (olfactory lobe hypoplasia). Other midline defects, such as cleft palate, may be seen. It can be inherited and is much more common in males. Any condition that results in GnRH and/or gonadotropin deficiency can also cause hypogonadotropic hypogonadism:

Pituitary or hypothalamic tumors

Idiopathic

Acquired (radiation therapy, developmental defects, etc.)

Congenital syndromes (often with mental retardation): Prader-Willi, Laurence-Moon-Biedl

Anorexia nervosa (women)

Hypothalamic amenorrhea (women)

Chronic disease and malnutrition

Q: What is the treatment of hypogonadotropic hypogonadism?

A: If fertility is not desired, hypogonadotropic hypogonadism is treated by testosterone (male) or estrogen (female) replacement. Cyclic progestin is also given to females to prevent endometrial hyperplasia.

If fertility is desired, gonadal stimulation can be induced by administration of gonadotropins. The glycoprotein β-hCG (human chorionic gonadotropin) has LH-like activity and is given along with FSH (human menopausal gonadotropins, hMG). Synthetic FSH of recombinant DNA origin is now available. This only works in those with hypothalamic disease; an intact pituitary gland must be present. Fertility can be induced in both sexes, but is more difficult in women.

Alternatively, GnRH may be given in pulsatile fashion by a subcutaneous infusion pump, which induces LH and FSH secretion by the pituitary. It must be given in pulses every 90 minutes, as continuous therapy results in paradoxical suppression of the pituitary.

Q: What is hypergonadotropic hypogonadism?

A: **Hypergonadotropic hypogonadism** is caused by defective gonads, resulting in hypogonadism and high gonadotropin levels (as the hypothalamus and pituitary function normally).

Q: What are the causes of hypergonadotropic hypogonadism?

A: These most commonly are a result of chromosomal abnormalities. In males, the most common cause is Klinefelter's syndrome, occurring in 1 in 1000 males. In females, the most common cause is Turner's syndrome (incidence 1 in 3000 girls). Other causes are less common and include congenital anorchia, cryptorchidism, gonadal damage (from chemotherapy or radiation therapy), gonadectomy, and mumps orchitis.

Q: What are the features of Klinefelter's syndrome?

A: Individuals with **Klinefelter's syndrome** typically have a 47,XXY karyotype, although some are mosaics (46,XY/47,XXY) and others may have more than two X chromosomes (e.g., 48,XXXY). Spermatogenesis is absent, and there is seminiferous tubule hyalinization. Testes are usually small and hard. Because the testosterone levels are deficient, eunuchoidal proportions develop. Gynecomastia is common, and these individuals have a higher incidence of breast carcinoma. Behavioral problems are also common, although mental retardation is rare.

Q: What is congenital anorchia?

A: **Congenital anorchia** or **vanishing testis syndrome** occurs in males in whom functional testicular tissue is present during the first 14 to 16 weeks of embryonic development. Normal wolffian duct growth and müllerian duct regression occurs, and external genitalia differentiates among male lines. If testicular destruction occurs after 16 weeks of gestation (as a result of trauma, vascular insufficiency, infection, or torsion), the testes are absent at birth, although the child is an otherwise normal phenotypic male—hence the term "vanishing testis syndrome." Cell karyotype is normal. Because the testes are absent, testosterone therapy is required for normal secondary sexual development.

Q: What is 5α-reductase deficiency?

A: Certain tissues in the male (prostate, male genital ducts, and external genitalia) require **dihydrotestosterone** (DHT) for proper development (Fig. 7-18). Testosterone is converted to DHT by the

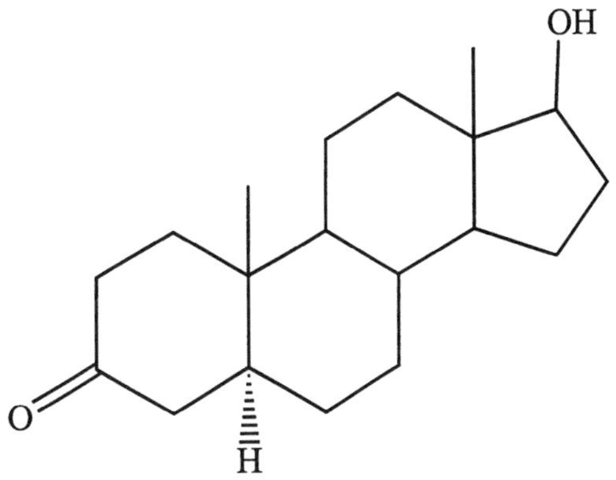

Figure 7-18. Dihydrotestosterone (DHT).

enzyme **5α-reductase.** Its deficiency is an autosomal recessive trait, and in this disorder, the dependent structures do not develop, leading to ambiguous genitalia with a clitoris-like penis. At puberty, pubertal amounts of testosterone are produced, leading to masculinization of other, non-DHT dependent parts of the body (such as body hair, skeletal muscle, and the larynx). DHT does have an effect on these tissues, but they differentiate with testosterone alone. Gynecomastia does not result, as testosterone levels are normal.

In many cases, 5α-reductase deficiency has resulted in a male child being reared as a female until puberty occurs, when the dramatic masculinization of other tissues and "gender change" take place. Reconstructive surgery may be required for the penis. DHT may be applied locally, preferably as soon as the diagnosis is known.

Q: How is testosterone administered?

A: Testosterone is well absorbed by the gut but is rapidly degraded in the liver by the first-pass effect. Testosterone may be esterified at the 17β position of the D ring, producing long-lasting compounds that may be given intramuscularly. The traditional method is to inject these esters (cypionate, enanthate, or propionate) every 2 weeks to 1 month. Transdermal testosterone is available, and is administered as a once-daily patch.

Testosterone may be synthetically alkylated at the 17α position, resulting in a compound that resists hepatic degradation. Examples of 17α-alkylated derivatives include fluoxymesterone, methyltestosterone, and oxandrolone. These derivatives are well known to cause hepatotoxicity. *For this reason, their use cannot be recommended.*

Q: What changes in gonadal function take place in the adult male?

A: Men undergo a gradual decline in testicular function as they age, unlike women who undergo an abrupt decline in ovarian function at menopause. Some have proposed the concept of an "andropause," in which male hormone levels abruptly decline, but there is little evidence to support this.

Testosterone levels decline approximately 1% to 2% each year after age 30, due to a gradual decrease in Leydig cell mass. Gonadotropins increase somewhat, but often do not become elevated. Older men with low testosterone levels often have LH and FSH levels that are in the middle to upper normal range and not elevated. This again is in contrast to women, who usually have elevated gonadotropin levels. The reason for this phenomenon is unclear; it may be because of the gradual onset of the hypogonadism.

Adult hypogonadal men lose muscle mass, bone mass, and libido. These improve after testosterone therapy. Many men with erectile dysfunction have improvement after treatment.

Q: What is amenorrhea?

A: **Amenorrhea** is the absence of menses. It is classified as two types: **primary,** in which menses have never occurred, or **secondary,** in which menses have occurred before but have now stopped.

Q: What are the causes of primary amenorrhea?

A: The most common cause of primary amenorrhea is Turner's syndrome, followed by müllerian agenesis and androgen resistance (testicular feminization). Other causes include outflow tract obstruction and hypogonadotropic hypogonadism.

Q: What is Turner's syndrome?

A: **Turner's syndrome** is a type of gonadal dysgenesis in which the gonads do not develop properly, associated with a variety of somatic abnormalities. It is relatively common (1 in 3000 girls) and is associated with absence of an X chromosome (45,X). Some are mosaics (45,X/46,XX) and may appear relatively normal. The gonads are small and have streaks ('streak' gonads). Intelligence is usually normal. The characteristic somatic abnormalities are shown in Table 7-1. Other types of gonadal dysgenesis exist with other cell karyotypes (e.g., 46,XX, and 46,XY) but these are not properly termed Turner's syndrome unless the somatic abnormalities are present.

Q: What is the treatment of Turner's syndrome?

A: In treating Turner's syndrome, estrogen is given to promote development of secondary sex characteristics and to prevent long-term sequelae of prolonged hypogonadism (e.g., osteoporosis). Cyclic

TABLE 7-1.   Clinical Features of Turner's Syndrome

Short stature—cause unknown, as GH secretion is normal
"Webbed" neck
Congenital organ abnormalities (heart, kidney)
Coarctation of aorta
Cubitus valgus
Micrognathia

Other associated diseases
   Hypothyroidism
   Diabetes mellitus
   Obesity
   Rheumatoid arthritis
   Inflammatory bowel disease

progestin also is given to promote menstrual bleeding. Human growth hormone (GH) therapy has been shown to improve short stature and is an approved indication for therapy. Patients should be evaluated for associated diseases and organ abnormalities. Because the gonads are abnormal, fertility is not possible. Patients with other forms of gonadal dysgenesis with a Y chromosome (46,XY gonadal dysgenesis) have a much higher incidence of ovarian malignancy, so the ovaries should be removed.

Q: **What is müllerian agenesis?**

A: **Müllerian agenesis** (Mayer-Rokitansky-Kuster-Hauser syndrome) is the second most common cause of primary amenorrhea. As the name implies, it is associated with absent müllerian structures. As the patient has no uterus, menses cannot occur. The ovaries are normal, however, so secondary sex characteristics are normal.

Q: **What is pseudohermaphrodism?**

A: **Pseudohermaphrodism** is a condition in which the phenotype is opposite that of the genetic sex; for example, a female pseudohermaphrodite has a 46,XX karyotype but appears male. The most common cause in females is the 21-hydroxylase variant of congenital adrenal hyperplasia. Causes in

males include the feminizing forms of congenital adrenal hyperplasia and testicular feminization.

Q: **What is true hermaphrodism?**

A: **True hermaphrodism** is an extremely rare condition in which both ovarian and testicular tissue is found in the same individual. The differentiation of external and internal genitalia is highly variable; most often, ambiguous external genitalia are present.

Q: **What is testicular feminization?**

A: The syndrome of complete **androgen resistance, or testicular feminization,** is the third most common cause of primary amenorrhea in girls (Fig. 7-19). These patients are genetic males (46,XY) who lack testosterone receptors, resulting in end-organ insensitivity to androgen. Because testosterone has no effect, wolffian structures are primordial; müllerian structures (uterus, uterine tubes, upper vagina) are absent because the testes make müllerian inhibitory factor. In the *complete* form, testicular feminization results in complete lack of masculinization (lack of terminal hair except on scalp and eyebrows) and a strikingly normal female appearance. This is a rare disorder affecting 1:20,000 to 1:60,000 genetic males. In the *incomplete* form, varying degrees of masculinization occur, sometimes with ambiguous genitalia.

Girls with complete testicular feminization have only vellus hairs except on non-androgen-dependent areas (the scalp and eyebrows). Because of decreased androgen effect, they may not suffer from acne and their voices may be higher-pitched than normal girls.

Q: **Because they lack ovaries, how can patients with androgen resistance have sufficient estrogen levels to permit feminization?**

A: Testosterone of testicular origin is aromatized to estradiol in the peripheral compartment (fat). Thus, levels are in the normal female range.

Q: **How is testicular feminization treated?**

A: Individuals with testicular feminization have a normal female appearance and therefore are raised as such. Their cryptorchid testes are at higher risk for malignancy and should be removed at adult-

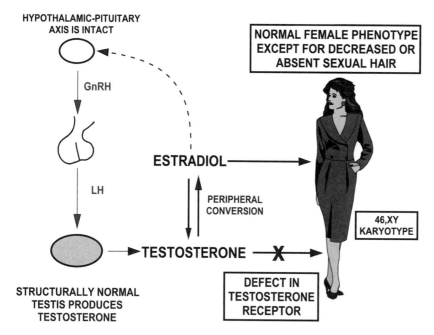

HYPOTHALAMIC-PITUITARY
AXIS IS INTACT

GnRH

LH

STRUCTURALLY NORMAL
TESTIS PRODUCES
TESTOSTERONE

ESTRADIOL

PERIPHERAL
CONVERSION

TESTOSTERONE —— X ——

DEFECT IN
TESTOSTERONE
RECEPTOR

NORMAL FEMALE PHENOTYPE
EXCEPT FOR DECREASED OR
ABSENT SEXUAL HAIR

46,XY
KARYOTYPE

Figure 7-19.   Testicular feminization.

hood. Supplemental estrogen must then be given, as their source of estrogen is gone. Because they have no uterus, menses cannot occur. Only the lower portion of the vagina is present, and it ends in a blind pouch. Usually, a vagina long enough to permit intercourse is achievable by slowly introducing larger forms to stretch it. In severe cases, reconstructive surgery may be done. Psychological counseling may be necessary for some patients.

Q: What is secondary amenorrhea?

A: **Secondary amenorrhea** is a condition in which menses occurred previously but have ceased. The causes include anovulation (most common), ovarian failure, hypothalamic amenorrhea, hypopituitarism, hyperprolactinemia, and uterine outflow obstruction.

Q: How is secondary amenorrhea evaluated?

A: In evaluating secondary amenorrhea, the first goal is to determine if the ovaries are producing estrogen. Although estradiol levels can be measured, the best way of determining adequate estrogenization is a **progestin challenge.** In this test, a synthetic progestin (medroxyprogesterone) is given for several days. If **withdrawal bleeding** occurs after the progestin is stopped, this confirms adequate estrogenization and means that there is in-

adequate progesterone secretion (usually due to anovulation).

If there is no withdrawal bleeding after progestin, a combination of estrogen and progestin is given (estrogen for the first 25 days of the month, progestin for the last 10 days). If a withdrawal bleed occurs, it suggests inadequate estrogenization (ovarian failure, hypothalamic amenorrhea, etc.). If there is no bleeding with combination therapy, there is either an outflow obstruction or absence of the uterus.

Q: What is hypothalamic amenorrhea?

A: **Hypothalamic amenorrhea** is a functional abnormality in GnRH secretion resulting in low gonadotropin levels and secondary amenorrhea. It is common in young women with increased psychological stress (e.g., going away to college or starting new job). It typically is a self-limited disorder.

Q: How is hypothalamic amenorrhea distinguished from ovarian failure?

A: In hypothalamic amenorrhea and other forms of hypogonadotropic hypogonadism, LH/FSH levels are low. With ovarian failure, gonadotropins are elevated. The differential diagnosis of amenorrhea is illustrated in Table 7-2.

TABLE 7-2.   Differential Diagnosis of Amenorrhea

	WB: P ONLY	WB: P + E	LH, FSH	ESTRADIOL
Anovulation	Yes	Yes	↑ LH/FSH ratio	normal to ↑
Hypogonadotropic (hypopituitarism, hypothalamic amenorrhea)	No	Yes	↓	↓
Turner's syndrome	No	Yes	↑	↓
Müllerian agenesis	No	No	Normal	Normal
Outflow defect	No	No	Normal	Normal
Testicular feminization	No	No	Normal	Normal

WB = withdrawal bleed; P = progestin; E = estrogen

Q: **What are the consequences of estrogen deficiency?**

A: Early deficiency of estrogen leads to vaginal atrophy and dyspareunia (painful intercourse). A decrease in estrogen levels leads to stimulation of central thermoregulatory centers, with resultant **vasomotor** or **hot flashes.** The mechanism is unknown. Women who have a sudden decrease in estrogen (e.g., after oophorectomy) experience hot flashes to a greater degree than those with a slower decrease (e.g., natural menopause). It has been postulated that surges of GnRH cause the vasomotor flashes, but administration of long-acting GnRH agonists does not improve them. Women with absence of LH (hypothalamic or pituitary dysfunction) still have hot flashes.

In the long term, estrogen deficiency results in decreased bone mass and osteoporosis in susceptible persons. This is a high-turnover form of osteoporosis, and most of the bone is lost within the first 10 to 15 years after menopause. It is therefore most beneficial to replace estrogen as soon as possible after menopause.

Estrogen also has beneficial cardiovascular effects, including increasing HDL cholesterol and decreasing LDL cholesterol. Estrogen deficiency also leads to increase in android (central) obesity, which is more atherogenic than gynecoid obesity. Menopausal women who do not receive replacement lose these beneficial effects.

Q: **How is estrogen replacement given?**

A: Like testosterone, estradiol is well absorbed orally but rapidly degraded by the first-pass phenomenon. Micronized estradiol, however, produces satisfactory plasma levels. Conjugated estrogens can be synthesized or prepared from the urine of pregnant mares. Other compounds include esterified estrogens, estropipate, and ethinyl estradiol.

Women without a uterus may take continuous estrogen alone. Progestin (medroxyprogesterone) should be added for women who still have a uterus. One method is to give the estrogen for the first part of the month and add progestin to the last week of the month, with withdrawal of both drugs for several days. This results in withdrawal menses similar to that of natural menses. This ensures that the uterine lining is sloughed each month; unopposed estrogen stimulation leads to endometrial buildup which can result in endometrial carcinoma. Another method is to administer the estrogen and progestin continuously. This also decreases endometrial buildup and results in less bleeding than in those treated with intermittent therapy.

As with testosterone, estrogen can also be given transdermally. The lipid-lowering effect is less when given by this route, because less estrogen passes through the liver (the site of lipoprotein synthesis). Those with a uterus are also given continuous progestin.

Estrogen generally should be avoided in women with a history of breast cancer, as estrogen may stimulate tumor growth. Estrogen administration also results in a very small increase in breast cancer, so women with a strong family history may not wish to take it. Estrogen should be avoided in those with active thromboembolic disease (e.g., women with a recent pulmonary embolism on anticoagulant therapy).

Estrogen receptor modulators such as raloxifene appear to have protective effects against osteoporosis without the risk of breast cancer or thromboembolic disease. These drugs do not help with vasomotor flashes, however.

Q: What can cause uterine outflow tract obstruction?

A: Destruction of the endometrium (Asherman's syndrome) may cause secondary amenorrhea and is usually a result of excessive postpartum curettage. A hysterogram (x-ray study in which contrast is injected into the uterus) demonstrates numerous adhesions. Ovarian function is normal.

Q: What is gynecomastia?

A: **Gynecomastia** is the presence of abnormal breast tissue in the male.

Q: What are the causes of gynecomastia?

A: Gynecomastia occurs whenever there is a decrease in the androgen to estrogen (A:E) ratio. This may occur either with androgen deficiency or estrogen excess. The most common cause is **pubertal gynecomastia:** stimulation of the testes by high amounts of gonadotropins tends to alter steroidogenesis to favor estrogen secretion. The high levels of LH early in puberty may lead to higher estrogen levels, and decreased A:E ratio. As puberty ceases, steroid synthesis favors androgen production, and pubertal gynecomastia disappears in most cases.

Obese boys tend to have higher estrogen levels due to the peripheral conversion of androgen to estrogen in fat; their incidence of gynecomastia is higher. One must distinguish **lipomastia** (increased fat in the breast area) from true gynecomastia; often, the large breast appearance is simply fat.

Hypogonadism may cause gynecomastia by decreasing the A:E ratio. It is common in Klinefelter's syndrome. Adults may develop gynecomastia

if hypogonadism occurs (e.g., men undergoing orchiectomy for prostate cancer).

Several drugs may cause gynecomastia by interfering with androgen production, blocking androgen receptors, or boosting the estrogen to androgen ratio. These include amphetamines, antihypertensives (methyldopa, reserpine), androgens, antineoplastics (alkylating agents), cimetidine, penicillamine, digitalis, estrogens, INH, ketoconazole, marijuana, phenothiazines, phenytoin, spironolactone, sulindac, theophylline, and tricyclic antidepressants.

Steroid-producing (adrenal, testis) or β-hCG-producing (testis, lung) neoplasms can cause gynecomastia. Acromegaly results in soft tissue growth and can be another cause; it may also be associated with hypogonadism and/or hyperprolactinemia.

Hepatic failure and cirrhosis may lead to gynecomastia via decreased clearance of estrogen. Gynecomastia has also been associated with hyperthyroidism, which increases peripheral aromatization of steroids, resulting in decreased A:E ratio.

Hyperprolactinemia may produce hypogonadism via suppression of LH/FSH secretion; drugs such as phenothiazines cause gynecomastia by this effect. Severe hypothyroidism may also cause gynecomastia by increasing prolactin secretion and producing hypogonadism.

Q: What is the treatment of gynecomastia?

A: Pubertal gynecomastia is typically self-limited. Underlying disorders (such as hypogonadism or germ cell tumors) should be treated. If significant gynecomastia has occurred, however, complete regression is unlikely to occur. If the problem causes psychological distress, reduction mammoplasty may be done. Patients with Klinefelter's syndrome have a higher incidence of breast carcinoma and should be checked regularly. The aromatase inhibitor testolactone decreases peripheral conversion and may be useful in some cases.

Q: What is hirsutism?

A: **Hirsutism,** a term derived from the Latin word *hirsutus,* meaning coarse or stiff, refers to females having terminal hair in male distribution—on the face, chest, and other areas (Fig. 7-20). Vellus

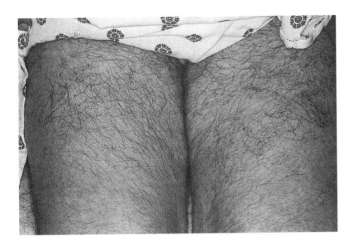

Figure 7-20. Woman with severe hirsutism on legs.

hairs, which are soft, fine, and unpigmented, transform into terminal (coarse, pigmented) hair after stimulation by androgen. Terminal hairs are androgen-dependent except on the scalp and eyebrows; in these areas, androgens have the opposite effect. In many men, the terminal hairs on the scalp are sensitive to androgen, causing reverse transformation to vellus hair: **male pattern baldness.** Male pattern baldness can also occur in women if androgen levels and/or hair sensitivity to androgen is high enough.

Women normally have terminal hair only on the scalp, eyebrows, and adrenarchal areas (the axilla and pubic area). There is a marked genetic difference in the amount of terminal hair expressed due to variability in androgen sensitivity; androgen levels are similar among all ethnic groups. The goal is to rule out serious underlying disease.

One must distinguish hirsutism (presence of excess terminal hair) from **virilization,** the development of other masculine qualities such as increased muscle mass, deepening of the voice, and baldness. Virilization is much more suggestive of endocrine disease than is simple hirsutism.

Q: What causes hirsutism?

A: Hirsutism results either from increased sensitivity to "normal" amounts of androgen (familial or idiopathic hirsutism) or an increase in the androgen to estrogen (A:E) ratio (via increase in androgen or decrease in estrogen).

In normal women, approximately 50% of androgen production is from the ovary, 25% from the adrenal, and 25% from peripheral conversion of estrogen to androgen. Android fat (around the middle) is more metabolically active in aromatizing steroids than is gynecoid fat (around the hips). Therefore, obese women have a higher incidence of hirsutism. Any endocrine disorder resulting in increased A:E ratio may result in hirsutism:

Cushing's syndrome

Polycystic ovary syndrome

Congenital adrenal hyperplasia (typically non-classical 21-hydroxylase deficiency)

Ovarian hyperthecosis

Androgen-producing ovarian neoplasms (arrhenoblastomas), hilar cell (lipoid) tumors

Virilizing adrenal tumors (adenoma or carcinoma)

Medications (steroids, anticonvulsants)

Q: What sex-steroid-producing cells arise in the ovary?

A: **Arrhenoblastomas** (Sertoli-Leydig cell tumors or androblastomas) are benign tumors that present with androgen excess: hirsutism, acne, breast atrophy, and clitoral hypertrophy. Tumor removal results in complete or partial reverse of virilization. They rarely may produce estrogen, resulting in isosexual precocity in the female.

Hilar cell (lipoid) tumors may cause severe masculinization, and occur most often in elderly women. On microscopic examination, they contain Reinke crystalloids (usually found in testicular cells). **Granulosa-theca cell tumors** usually result in hyperestrogenemia and result in isosexual precocity in girls.

Q: Do any biochemical markers distinguish virilizing gonadal from virilizing adrenal tumors?

A: The adrenal gland possesses the sulfatase to convert the weak androgen dehydroepiandrosterone (DHEA) to dehydroepiandrosterone sulfate (DHEA-SO$_4$). Therefore, virilizing adrenal tumors usually have markedly elevated DHEA-SO$_4$ levels, while those of ovarian origin have low levels. Interestingly, DHEA-SO$_4$ levels may be mildly elevated in patients with the polycystic ovary syndrome, despite the ovarian origin of the hyperandrogenism. DHEA-SO$_4$ levels are much lower in polycystic ovary syndrome than in virilizing adrenal tumors, however.

Q: What is the evaluation of patients with hirsutism?

A: The evaluation of patients with hirsutism should include measurement of total and free testosterone and DHEA-SO$_4$ levels. Baseline and stimulated 17-hydroxyprogesterone are also recommended to exclude nonclassical 21-hydroxylase deficiency. Patients with severe hypertension and/or virilization should be evaluated for Cushing's syndrome and virilizing ovarian or adrenal tumors. Some women have idiopathic increased 5α-reductase activity; elevation of serum androstanediol glucuronide helps identify these patients.

In many cases, no biochemical defect can be found (idiopathic hirsutism). Most women with hirsutism due to polycystic ovary syndrome will have normal or minimal elevation of testosterone. Those with total testosterone levels over 200 ng/dL should be evaluated for more serious disease.

Q: What is the treatment of hirsutism?

A: Treatment of hirsutism includes treatment of underlying disorders.

Antiandrogens (spironolactone, cyproterone acetate, and flutamide) block the effect of testosterone on the receptor. The diuretic spironolactone, most widely used for this purpose, also inhibits 5α-reductase. Cyproterone is not yet approved for the use in the United States.

Oral contraceptives decrease the A:E ratio by increasing estrogen levels. They also increase SHBG, which binds more free testosterone, thus decreasing free levels. (This is one instance where changing the total protein level does alter the free level.) In those with masculinizing forms of congenital adrenal hyperplasia, glucocorticoids are used.

GnRH analogs (e.g., leuprolide) suppress endogenous steroid production from the ovary and reduce steroid secretion. The 5α-reductase inhibitors (finasteride) inhibit DHT production with reduction in terminal hair.

Cosmetic treatments include simple shaving or bleaching the hair. Electrolysis permanently destroys the hair follicle and is the best long-term solution for those with hirsutism over a limited area; many treatments may be required.

Q: What is the polycystic ovary syndrome?

A: **Polycystic ovary syndrome** (PCOS) is a common condition, occurring in 5% of women. It is a disorder of chronic anovulation leading to increased estrogen production and infertility.

In the ovary, there is a two-cell concept of steroidogenesis (Fig. 7-21). LH primarily stimulates the *theca* cells, which synthesize androgen from cholesterol. Androgens, in turn, are aromatized to estrogen in the *granulosa* cells under the influence of FSH. In PCOS, ovulation does not occur, so the increased LH pulse amplitude leads to a vicious cycle of stimulation and further ovarian steroidogenesis (theca cell) (Fig. 7-22). Without ovulation, FSH levels are lower and androgen secretion predominates.

Q: What are the features of polycystic ovary syndrome?

A: The characteristic woman with PCOS has chronic anovulation, android obesity, hyperinsulinism, and hyperandrogenism with sequelae: hirsutism, acne, and male pattern baldness. These components occur in varying degrees; not all women are obese, for example. Some have only minimal hirsutism, whereas in many it is quite severe.

Q: What is the relationship of obesity and hyperinsulinism to PCOS?

A: Android obesity often results in hyperinsulinemia (insulin resistance) due to defective insulin receptor action, and it can lead to glucose intolerance and type 2 diabetes mellitus (Fig. 7-23). Because insulin binding to the insulin receptor is defective, it may bind to IGF-I receptors, which enhance the theca cell response to LH, increasing androgen production. In the absence of ovulation, the thecal cell response predominates, and hyperandrogenism results.

Android fat is also metabolically active in aromatizing estrogen to androgen, and this also plays a role. Hyperandrogenism itself can impair insulin

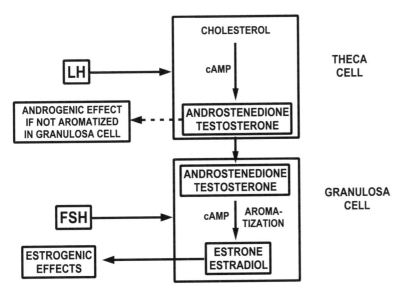

Figure 7-21. Two-cell concept of ovarian steroidogenesis.

action, which perpetuates the vicious cycle so predominant in PCOS.

Q: What is the treatment of PCOS?

A: Treatment of PCOS depends on the desired result. If the woman wants to have children, ovulation must be induced. This is typically done with the estrogen agonist **clomiphene citrate.** This compound effectively inhibits the effects of stronger estrogens and allows gonadotropins to be secreted normally, allowing for ovulation.

If clomiphene fails, a common next step is to attempt ovulation with human menopausal gonadotropins (hMG), a preparation made from the

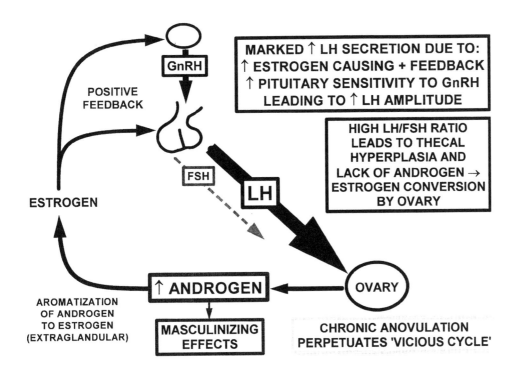

Figure 7-22. Polycystic ovary syndrome.

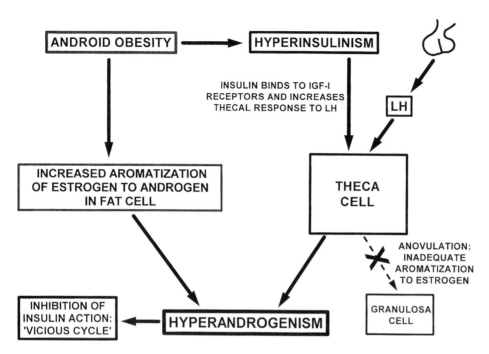

Figure 7-23. Hyperinsulinism and hyperandrogenism.

urine of menopausal women (which contains high concentrations of FSH). Insulin-sensitizing agents (e.g., troglitazone, metformin) may theoretically be useful.

A third approach is to stop the abnormal LH secretion by administering a long-acting GnRH analog (leuprolide), which produces hypogonadotropic hypogonadism. After this, hMG (FSH) and hCG (LH analog) are given to simulate the normal events of ovulation (while leuprolide inhibits the abnormal ovarian-HPA mechanisms). Alternatively, pulsatile GnRH can be given instead of gonadotropins.

Laparoscopic ovulation induction, producing small burns in the ovary with a laser, is a last resort after the chemical therapies fail. The final treatment if all else fails is in vitro fertilization, in which the ovum is fertilized outside the body, then re-implanted.

If fertility is not desired, progestin is given at the end of the month to induce withdrawal bleeding. This is necessary because the endometrium is hyperplastic and is at higher risk for transforming into endometrial carcinoma if it is not sloughed regularly. Hirsutism may be treated with the methods above. Weight loss may decrease hyperinsulinism and improve symptoms in obese women.

Q: What is hyperthecosis?

A: **Hyperthecosis** is a non-neoplastic ovarian lesion, characterized by islands of luteinized thecal cells in the ovarian stroma that produce hyperandrogenism. These patients appear very similar to those with PCOS, but several features are distinct. The degree of hyperandrogenism is greater in hyperthecosis, and the elevated LH/FSH ratio is usually not seen. Unlike in PCOS, the patient fails to ovulate with medical therapy (clomiphene). The islands of luteinized theca cells of hyperthecosis are not present in PCOS patients.

Hyperthecosis is more of a primary ovarian disorder than a vicious cycle of ovarian-HPA dysfunction like PCOS. As with PCOS, obesity and hyperinsulinism are commonly present, usually to a higher degree in hyperthecosis. The treatment of ovarian hyperthecosis is oophorectomy.

Q: Can neoplastic disorders cause hyperandrogenism?

A: Any tumor that can produce androgen can cause hirsutism and virilization. These include adrenocortical carcinomas (which also may produce Cushing's syndrome and hyperaldosteronism), and virilizing ovarian tumors. Treatment is surgical resection of the tumor.

BIBLIOGRAPHY

Conte FA, Grumbach MM. Abnormalities of sexual determination and differentiation. In: Greenspan FS, Strewler GJ, eds. Basic and clinical endocrinology. 5th ed. Stamford, CT: Appleton & Lange, 1997:487–517.

Griffin JE, Wilson JD. Disorders of the testes and the male reproductive tract. In: Wilson JD, Foster DW, Kronenbert HM, Larsen PR, eds. Williams' textbook of endocrinology. 9th ed. Philadelphia: W.B. Saunders, 1998:819–870.

Horton R. Testicular steroid transport, metabolism, and effects. In: Becker KL, ed. Principles and practice of endocrinology and metabolism. 2nd ed. Philadelphia: Lippincott, 1995:1042–1047.

Speroff L, Glass RH, Kase NG. Anovulation and the polycystic ovary. In: Speroff L, Glass RH, Kase NG, eds. Clinical gynecologic endocrinology and infertility. 5th ed. Baltimore: Williams & Wilkins, 1994:457–458.

Speroff L, Glass RH, Kase NG. Hirsutism. In: Speroff L, Glass RH, Kase NG, eds. Clinical gynecologic endocrinology and infertility. 5th ed. Baltimore: Williams & Wilkins, 1994:483–512.

Styne DM. Normal and abnormal sexual development and puberty. In: Besser GM, Thorner MO, eds., Clinical endocrinology. 2nd ed. St. Louis: Mosby-Wolfe, 1994:13.2–13.14.

Tenover LJ. Male hormone replacement therapy including "andropause." Endo Metab Clin North Am 1998;27:969–981.

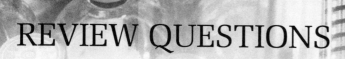

REVIEW QUESTIONS

I. SHORT ANSWER

1. The testis contains two major cell types, _____ and _____ cells. _____ cells are the site of spermatogenesis and are stimulated by the anterior pituitary hormone _____. This hormone's secretion is stimulated by _____ and inhibited by _____. _____ cells produce testosterone.

2. FSH and LH secretion are stimulated by the hypothalamic hormone _____ when it is secreted in a _____ fashion. When this same hormone is given continuously, _____ of gonadotropin secretion occurs.

3. The hormone-producing cells of the ovum are the _____ and _____ cells. Many groups of ova, or _____, develop, but only one will develop fully. The major female sex steroids are _____ and _____.

4. The ovarian cycle is divided into _____ and _____ phases. In the first phase, _____ secretion predominates. Later, _____ secretion leads to theca cell proliferation and estradiol increase, which causes paradoxical _____ feedback on the pituitary to increase its secretion.

5. Granulosa cells acquire LH receptors and secrete the hormone _____ with formation of the _____. If the ovum is not fertilized, _____ of this structure occurs.

6. In the first phase of the ovarian cycle, estrogen results in endometrial _____. Under the influence of progesterone, the endometrial glands become longer and edematous in what is called the _____ phase. If pregnancy does not occur, _____ occurs as the ovum regresses.

7. If the ovum is fertilized, the hormonal milieu is maintained by the glycoprotein hormone _____.

8. Sex steroids travel in serum primarily attached to _____. Estrogen and hyperthyroidism are known to _____ its concentration, while testosterone and obesity can _____ its levels.

9. If a _____ chromosome is present, _____ is secreted, resulting in differentiation of primordial gonads to become testes. This chromosome contains a gene called _____. If this area is not present, the gonads become _____.

10. If a functional testis is present, the male or _____ structures develop to become the epididymis, vas deferens, seminal vesicles, and ejaculatory ducts. If no testis is present, the _____ structures develop to become the uterus, uterine tubes, cervix, and upper vagina.

11. If no gonad is present, the external genitalia will be _____ at birth. In the presence of a functional testis, _____ secretion results in _____ external genitalia.

12. _____ is an important ancillary endocrine organ because of its ability to aromatize steroids. The most metabolically active type is _____.

13. Although the "machinery" for going through puberty is present at birth, it normally does not occur because of potent _____ mechanisms. At the onset of puberty or _____, _____ secretion increases in a pulsatile fashion, increasing the _____ levels.

14. The onset of adrenal androgen secretion is called _____ and is responsible for _____ and _____ development in the axillary and pubic areas.

15. Absence of any pubertal development in a boy of 14 or girl of 13 is termed _____. The most common cause is _____, where there is often a strong family history.

16. A useful study for determining the amount of remaining growth is the _____. In those with delayed puberty, it is _____; in precocious puberty, it is _____.

17. Onset of puberty in a girl under age 8 or boy under age 9 is called _____. The complete or "true" form occurs via premature activation of the _____. The peripheral or "incomplete" form occurs by ectopic secretion of _____ or _____. These conditions will result in early _____ stature as a child, but eventual _____ stature as an adult.

18. Sex steroid deficiency in a child or adolescent results in _____ growth of the long bones relative to the axial skeleton. This results in a disproportionate body habitus known as _____.

19. The most common cause of hypogonadotropic hypogonadism is _____, a disorder of _____ secretion. It is associated with _____.

20. If fertility is not desired, hypogonadotropic hypogonadism is treated with _____. If fertility is desired, it can be accomplished by administration of _____ via injections or _____ via a pump that provides pulsatile secretion.

21. The most common cause of hypergonadotropic hypogonadism occurs in males and is called _____. It is associated with a typical _____ cell karyotype. The most common cause in females is _____; these patients have a typical _____ karyotype.

22. Certain parts of the body (e.g., prostate and penis) require _____ for proper development, which is a product of _____ conversion. Deficiency of the enzyme _____ produces a syndrome in which _____ genitalia are present at birth but masculinization of other tissues occurs at puberty.

23. Testosterone is degraded when given orally but may be given by _____ or _____. Synthetic, orally absorbed derivatives may cause _____ and are not recommended.

24. Unlike testosterone, certain forms of estrogen may be given _____. Estrogen may also be given _____. Menopausal women who do not take estrogen are at higher risk of developing _____ and _____.

25. Menopausal women who do not take estrogen often experience a centrally mediated phenomenon called _____.

26. The absence of menses is called _____.
If menses have never occurred, it is termed
_____; if they were present pre-
viously but have now stopped, it is called
_____.

27. The most common cause of primary amenorrhea is _____. This occurs in approximately 1 in 3000 girls and is usually associated
with the cell karyotype _____. Treatment is administration of _____ and
_____. _____ may be given
to treat short stature, although secretion is
normal.

28. The second most common cause of primary
amenorrhea is _____. Menses cannot
occur because there is no uterus. Sex steroid replacement is unnecessary because the
_____ are normal.

29. The condition in which the phenotypic sex is
opposite that of the genotypic sex is called
_____. The _____ form oc-
curs when a genetic male appears female; the
_____ form occurs when a genetic female appears male. _____ is an extremely rare condition in which both ovarian
and testicular tissue is found in the same individual.

30. Genetic males who have defects in the testosterone receptor and androgen resistance have the
syndrome of _____. These individuals appear as _____ and the typical
presenting complaint is _____.

31. Fine, nonpigmented hairs that have limited
growth are called _____ hairs. Darker,
thicker hairs with greater potential for growth are
called _____ hairs. Except on the scalp
and eyebrows, the latter hairs are dependent on
_____ for growth. Upon stimulation
by these hormones, _____ hairs transform into _____ hairs on most parts of
the body. In many men, the reverse happens on
the scalp, resulting in _____.

32. Women who have menstruated in the past but
do not any longer have _____. The
most common cause in non-menopausal
women is _____. A functional test to
evaluate the cause is the withdrawal bleed challenge. If the woman has menses after administration of progestin, this means that adequate
_____ is present. If menses occur after giving estrogen and progestin, the problem
is due to _____ deficiency, from various causes. If no menses occurs after estrogen
and progestin are given, there is likely a problem with _____ of the uterus.

33. A functional abnormality in GnRH secretion
occurring in women under severe physical or
psychological stress is _____. Withdrawal menses would occur after administration of _____. It can be distinguished
from premature ovarian failure by measurement of _____ levels.

34. The presence of abnormal breast tissue in the
male is called _____. It occurs whenever there is a decrease in the _____ ratio.
It most commonly occurs during _____
due to high LH and increased estrogen levels; it is
usually self-limited. Males with _____
and decreased sex steroid production may have
this problem, as do those who take certain
_____.

35. Women with excess terminal hair in a male distribution have _____. It should be
distinguished from _____, in which
true male secondary sex characteristics develop. It results from an increase in the
_____ ratio.

36. A condition of chronic anovulation leading to
increased LH levels and hyperandrogenemia is
the _____. LH results in increased androgen synthesis in the _____ cells;

_____ levels are low, resulting in decreased aromatization of androgens to estrogens in the _____ cells.

37. Patients with polycystic ovary syndrome (PCOS) are often obese, which may cause elevated serum _____ levels. This in turn may potentiate LH and result in increased androgen synthesis in the _____ cells. Increased androgen levels in turn may inhibit _____ action, potentiating a vicious cycle. These patients are at risk for developing _____.

38. Treatment of PCOS may involve ovulation induction. This is typically done with the estrogen agonist _____, which inhibits the effects of endogenous estrogen and allows for normal gonadotropin secretion. If fertility is not desired, _____ is given every month to induce withdrawal menses.

39. A non-neoplastic disorder of ovarian androgen hypersecretion is _____. Unlike PCOS, it is not a dysfunction of the ovarian-HPA system. Androgen levels and virilization are typically _____ than with PCOS.

40. Complete the following table.

Cause of Amenorrhea	Progestin Withdrawal Bleed (+ or −)	Estrogen and Progestin Withdrawal Bleed (+ or −)	LH and FSH Levels (↓ or ↑)	Estrogen Levels (↓ or ↑)
Polycystic ovary syndrome			N/A	
Turner's syndrome				
Testicular feminization			N/A	N/A
Hypopituitarism				

II. MULTIPLE CHOICE

Select the one best answer.

41. In the absence of any gonads in a fetus, the external genitalia will be:
    a. absent
    b. ambiguous
    c. male
    d. female
    e. The fetus will be stillborn.

42. Which statement is true of Kallmann's syndrome?
    a. Gonadotropin releasing hormone (GnRH) secretion is impaired.
    b. Formation of dihydrotestosterone from testosterone is impaired.
    c. LH and FSH levels are elevated.
    d. It is an acquired condition.
    e. There is an increase in prolactin secretion.

43. A 19-year-old sexually active woman has not had menses for the last 3 months and has gained 12 pounds. Her serum prolactin is twice normal. The next best test to order would be (choose one):
    a. MRI of pituitary gland
    b. CT of pituitary gland
    c. serum pregnancy test
    d. cell karyotype
    e. serum LH and FSH

44. An 18-year-old male is brought to you for evaluation of hypogonadism. He has minimal development of secondary sexual characteristics (minimal pubic hair, beard, high voice, etc.). His height is 71 inches. He has done poorly in school and has had numerous behavior problems. Crown-to-pubic measurement is 33 inches. The testes are small and hard. Laboratory values demonstrate:

    Serum total testosterone: 101 ng/dL (normal: 300–900)

    Serum LH: 46 mU/mL (normal: 4–18)

Serum FSH: 37 mU/mL (normal: 2–17)

Serum prolactin: 3.4 ng/mL (normal: 4.3–19.2)

The next step in his evaluation should be:

    a. serum T_4 and TSH levels

    b. bone age determination

    c. cell karyotype

    d. GnRH level

    e. MRI of the pituitary gland

45. A 16-year-old girl presents with primary amenorrhea. Secondary sexual characteristics are normal. Pubic and axillary hair are normal. Her height is 5 feet 9 inches (175 cm). Pelvic examination reveals normal external female genitalia but no cervix or uterus. Normal appearing ovaries are seen on ultrasound examination. Which one of the following is the most likely finding in this patient?

    a. serum prolactin of 200 ng/mL (normal: 4–20)

    b. 45,X cell karyotype

    c. serum TSH of 0.03 μU/mL (normal: 0.35–5.00)

    d. 46,XX cell karyotype

    e. 46,XY cell karyotype

46. In girls, what is the first physical sign of pubertal change?

    a. onset of menses (menarche)

    b. breast development (thelarche)

    c. pubic hair development

    d. acne

47. In boys, what is the first physical sign of pubertal change?

    a. pubic hair

    b. increase in penile length

    c. increase in testicular size

    d. beard growth

48. Determination bone or skeletal age may be used as:

    a. a factor in prediction of adult height.

    b. an indicator of level of physical maturation.

    c. a factor in growth potential.

    d. a factor in the prediction of onset of adolescent development.

    e. all of the above.

49. A 34-year-old woman has noticed the absence of menses for the last 4 months. The pregnancy test is negative. Serum LH and FSH are elevated, and the serum estradiol level is low. The most likely cause of the amenorrhea is (choose one):

    a. congenital adrenal hyperplasia

    b. premature menopause

    c. exogenous estrogen administration

    d. panhypopituitarism

    e. polycystic ovarian syndrome

50. A 17-year-old girl presents with secondary amenorrhea. Serum prolactin is three times normal. She feels tired and has a small goiter on physical examination. The next test that should be ordered is:

    a. MRI of the pituitary gland

    b. serum pregnancy test

    c. serum FSH and LH

    d. serum TSH

    e. ovarian ultrasound

51. A 14-year-old male had ambiguous genitalia at birth and was raised as female. He is now developing male secondary sexual characteristics (beard, deepening voice, increased muscle mass, etc.). His genitalia remain small and primordial. This patient has:

    a. 5α-reductase deficiency.

    b. testicular feminization.

    c. Klinefelter's syndrome.

    d. Kallmann's syndrome.

    e. 21-hydroxylase deficiency.

52. A 45-year-old woman presents with secondary amenorrhea. The laboratory workup demonstrates LH and FSH levels that are several times normal; prolactin is slightly elevated at 39 ng/mL (normal: 2.0–21.0). Serum TSH and T4 are normal. Galactorrhea is absent. MRI

scan of the sella turcica is normal. Which would be the best management at this time?

    a. bromocriptine

    b. transsphenoidal hypophysectomy

    c. estrogen

    d. levothyroxine

    e. cabergoline

53. A 16-year-old male has not yet begun puberty and is very anxious. Both his brother and father had late onset of puberty. Examination is normal for a prepubertal male. Laboratory measurements of testosterone and gonadotropins are low. Bone age is approximately 3 years less than chronologic age. Which of the following is most appropriate at this time?

    a. cell karyotype determination

    b. administration of human growth hormone and testosterone

    c. reassurance and monitoring to see if puberty commences soon (the "tincture of time")

    d. administration of human chorionic gonadotropin

    e. sellar MRI, because he likely has a pituitary tumor

54. A 19-year-old male is seen for delayed sexual development. As far as he knows, he has never had testes; he was given medication to help descend them, to no avail. Linear growth has been normal. The penis looks structurally normal, but is small. He has a normal scrotum, but no testes can be felt. His arm span is greater than height, and facial and body hair is sparse. This male most likely has:

    a. testicular feminization

    b. congenital anorchia

    c. 5α-reductase deficiency

    d. 21-hydroxylase deficiency

    e. Klinefelter's syndrome

55. A 20-year-old male is referred for delayed sexual development. Linear growth has been normal, and cognitive function is normal. Examination reveals a male of above average height, with increased arm span and small testes. The baseline LH and FSH levels are low, but they increase after GnRH infusion. TSH and ACTH responses to TRH and CRH are normal. He is unable to detect certain odors. This male most likely has:

    a. constitutional delay of puberty

    b. Klinefelter's syndrome

    c. mumps orchitis

    d. Kallmann's syndrome

    e. craniopharyngioma

56. A 22-year-old college endurance runner has secondary amenorrhea. Withdrawal menses occur after administration of medroxyprogesterone. Examination reveals a normal appearing female; height is 56 inches, weight 127 pounds. There is no hirsutism or virilization. The LH level is the upper limits of normal, and FSH is low normal. The most likely cause of the secondary amenorrhea is:

    a. hypothalamic amenorrhea

    b. polycystic ovary syndrome

    c. Turner's syndrome

    d. 21-hydroxylase deficiency

    e. premature ovarian failure

III. TRUE OR FALSE

57. Women with which condition(s) should experience withdrawal menses with administration of estrogen and progestin?

    ___ a. polycystic ovary syndrome

    ___ b. testicular feminization

    ___ c. müllerian agenesis

    ___ d. Turner's syndrome

    ___ e. hypothalamic amenorrhea

58. Conditions or substances that can result in gynecomastia include:

    ___ a. acromegaly

    ___ b. hypothyroidism

    ___ c. marijuana

    ___ d. cigarette smoking

    ___ e. illicit use of testosterone

59. A 7-year-old girl is noted to have Tanner stage IV breast development and onset of menses. Axillary and pubic hair are sparse. Which of the following support a diagnosis of central rather than peripheral precocious puberty?

— a. rise in LH and FSH levels to pubertal levels after administration of a GnRH bolus

— b. pubertal levels of estradiol

— c. ovarian mass on ultrasound

— d. regression of pubertal changes after treatment with leuprolide (a long-acting GnRH agonist

— e. elevated levels of cortisol and DHEA-SO$_4$

60. Findings in patients with Turner's syndrome include:

— a. chromatin positive buccal smear

— b. lack of breast development

— c. normal ovaries

— d. amenorrhea

— e. higher incidence of hypothyroidism

61. Which of the following are true of estrogen deficiency in women?

— a. Estrogen should be combined with progestin in hysterectomized women.

— b. Estrogen results in decreased HDL and increased LDL cholesterol.

— c. Most bone loss occurs within the first decade after menopause.

— d. Those with a history of breast cancer should not take estrogen.

— e. Transdermal estrogen provides a more favorable lipid profile than oral estrogen.

62. The biological effects of androgens include the following:

— a. stimulates skeletal muscle and laryngeal growth

— b. decreases tendency for acne vulgaris

— c. increases binding proteins such as SHBG and thyroid-binding globulin

— d. causes transformation of terminal (coarse, pigmented) hair to vellus (soft, fine) hair on the face, chest, and extremities

— e. may increase insulin resistance in susceptible individuals

63. A 22-year-old woman has moderate hirsutism and irregular menses. Possible causes of the hirsutism include:

— a. testicular feminization

— b. "cryptic" or "nonclassical" 21-hydroxylase deficiency

— c. hyperprolactinemia

— d. polycystic ovary syndrome

— e. Cushing's syndrome

64. Which of the following patients with hypogonadism would you expect to have hypogonadal or "eunuchoidal" proportions?

— a. 19-year-old male with Kallmann's syndrome

— b. 53-year-old male with testicular failure due to mumps orchitis suffered at age 23

— c. 34-year-old female with secondary amenorrhea due to a prolactinoma

— d. 16-year-old female with testicular feminization

— e. 21-year-old female with hypothalamic amenorrhea due to stress at college

65. A 31-year-old male failed medical therapy for acromegaly and subsequently underwent tumor resection and postoperative radiotherapy. He subsequently develops hypopituitarism and is given oral hydrocortisone and levothyroxine. He and his wife want to have children. Regimens that might successfully induce fertility in this man include:

— a. intramuscular testosterone cypionate every 2 weeks

— b. transdermal testosterone

___ c. β-hCG (human chorionic gonado-
        tropin) injections

___ d. β-hCG and hMG (FSH) injections

___ e. GnRH, infused every 90 minutes by
        a special pump

66. A 67-year-old woman has developed severe hir-
    sutism and masculinization. Test results that
    would help distinguish an arrhenoblastoma
    (Sertoli-Leydig cell tumor) from a virilizing ad-
    renal tumor include:

    ___ a. low serum LH and FSH levels

    ___ b. increased urinary 17-ketosteroid
            levels

    ___ c. low dehydroepiandrosterone sulfate
            levels

    ___ d. ovarian tumor present on ultrasound

    ___ e. regression with GnRH agonist
            (leuprolide) therapy

67. Which of the following are true of female ovar-
    ian function?

    ___ a. Late in the proliferative phase, in-
            creasing estrogen levels lead to a
            surge of FSH and ovulation.

    ___ b. In the "two-cell" concept, LH drives
            androgen production by theca cells,
            which are aromatized to estrogens in
            the granulosa cells under the influ-
            ence of FSH.

    ___ c. In the secretory phase, estradiol is se-
            creted by the corpus luteum.

    ___ d. Chronic anovulation may lead to in-
            creased LH levels and hyperandro-
            genism.

    ___ e. After conception, progesterone inhib-
            its FSH and further ovulation.

ANSWERS

1. Sertoli, Leydig; Sertoli; FSH; activin, inhibin; Leydig

2. GnRH, pulsatile; inhibition

3. theca, granulosa; follicles; estrogen, progesterone

4. follicular (proliferative), luteal (secretory); FSH; LH, positive

5. progesterone, corpus luteum; involution (luteolysis)

6. proliferation; secretory; menstruation

7. human chorionic gonadotropin (β-hCG)

8. sex hormone-binding globulin (SHBG); increase, decrease

9. Y, testis-determining factor (TDF); sex-determining region (SRY); ovaries

10. wolffian; müllerian

11. female; testosterone, male

12. fat; central (android) fat

13. inhibitory; gonadarche, GnRH, gonadotropin (FSH and LH)

14. adrenarche (pubarche), terminal hair, sweat gland

15. delayed puberty; constitutional delay

16. skeletal or bone age; delayed; advanced

17. precocious puberty; hypothalamic-pituitary axis (HPA); gonadotropins, sex steroids; tall, short

18. increased; hypogonadal or eunuchoidal proportions

19. Kallmann's syndrome, GnRH; anosmia

20. sex steroids; gonadotropins, GnRH

21. Klinefelter's syndrome; 47,XXY; Turner's; 45,X

22. dihydrotestosterone, testosterone; 5α-reductase, ambiguous

23. injection, transdermal preparation (patch); hepatotoxicity

24. orally; transdermally; osteoporosis, cardiovascular disease

25. menopausal (hot) flashes

26. amenorrhea; primary; secondary

27. Turner's syndrome; 45,X; estrogen, progestin; growth hormone

28. müllerian agenesis (Mayer-Rokitansky-Kuster-Hauser syndrome); ovaries

29. pseudohermaphrodism; male; female; hermaphrodism

30. testicular feminization; normal females, primary amenorrhea

31. vellus; terminal; androgen; vellus, terminal; male pattern baldness

32. secondary amenorrhea; anovulation; estrogen; estrogen; outflow tract obstruction

33. hypothalamic amenorrhea; estrogen and progestin; gonadotropin (FSH and LH)

34. gynecomastia; androgen/estrogen; puberty; hypogonadism; drugs

35. hirsutism; virilization; androgen/estrogen

36. polycystic ovary syndrome; theca; FSH, granulosa

37. insulin; theca; insulin; diabetes mellitus

38. clomiphene citrate; progestin

39. hyperthecosis; higher

40.

Cause of Amenorrhea	Progestin Withdrawal Bleed (+ or −)	Estrogen and Progestin Withdrawal Bleed (+ or −)	LH and FSH Levels (↓ or ↑)	Estrogen Levels (↓ or ↑)
Polycystic ovary syndrome	+	+	N/A	↑
Turner's syndrome	−	+	↑	↓
Testicular feminization	−	−	N/A	N/A
Hypopituitarism	−	+	↓	↓

41. (d). External genitalia develop along female lines with the absence of a functional testis (the "female by default" theory). Therefore, presence of an ovary is not required. Ambigu-

ous genitalia (*b*) only occur in the presence of excess testosterone in a female, or deficient testosterone in a male (both usually due to abnormal adrenal enzyme synthesis). Gonads are not required for life (*e*).

42. (*a*). Kallmann's syndrome is an isolated disorder of GnRH secretion.

43. (*c*). The most likely cause of secondary amenorrhea in a sexually active woman with weight gain is pregnancy. Prolactin normally increases during pregnancy to prepare for lactation.

44. (*c*). The most likely presentation in this male with small testes and elevated gonadotropin levels is Klinefelter's syndrome. A cell karyotype would confirm the diagnosis.

45. (*d*). The absence of müllerian structures with normal ovaries, secondary sex characteristics, and external genitalia suggests müllerian agenesis (Mayer-Rokitansky-Kuster-Hauser syndrome). Although she could have a prolactinoma (*a*), it is unlikely and not the cause of the amenorrhea. Turner's (*b*) is ruled out by absence of müllerian structures, normal ovaries, and normal height. Hyperthyroidism (*c*) would not cause primary amenorrhea. Patients with testicular feminization (*e*) do not have ovaries, and have diminished terminal hair.

46. (*b*).

47. (*c*).

48. (*e*).

49. (*b*). Elevated gonadotropin levels in the absence of pregnancy are suggestive of premature ovarian failure. This is defined as primary ovarian failure in women under age 40.

50. (*d*). Primary hypothyroidism may be a cause of hyperprolactinemia, and should be excluded before other tests are ordered.

51. (*a*). Certain tissues (e.g., penis, prostate) depend on dihydrotestosterone (DHT) for proper development. Testosterone is converted to DHT via the enzyme 5α-reductase. With 5α-reductase deficiency, the DHT-dependent structures do not develop properly. This leads to ambiguous genitalia at birth. Because testosterone levels are low during childhood, the non-DHT-dependent structures (terminal hair, muscle mass, etc.) remain pubertal, occasionally allowing a female sex to be assigned. As testosterone levels rise during puberty, these non-DHT-dependent structures develop, and the patient acquires male secondary sexual characteristics, although the genitalia remain undeveloped. This may rarely lead to a change in phenotype from female to male.

Patients with testicular feminization (*b*) have a normal female phenotype without ambiguous genitalia. There is no change after puberty. Those with Klinefelter's or Kallmann's syndromes (*c* and *d*) have small, but clearly male, external genitalia. There is no change during puberty. A 21-hydroxylase deficiency (*e*) would lead to virilization.

52. (*c*). The elevated LH and FSH levels mean that her ovaries have failed and she has gone through natural menopause. There is no treatment for this other than estrogen replacement. The prolactin is moderately elevated and she could have a small microadenoma not visible on MRI. However, this is not the cause of the amenorrhea because the gonadotropins are elevated, not low as would be expected with hyperprolactinemia (which causes *hypo*gonadotropic hypogonadism). This is merely a coincidental finding, and normalization of the prolactin will have no effect on the amenorrhea. It should be monitored, however.

53. (*c*). This boy probably has constitutional delay of puberty given the history. Gonadotropin and testosterone measurements are appropriately low in a prepubertal child.

54. (*b*). This male has the vanishing testis syndrome (congenital anorchia). Testes are present in utero long enough to allow for wolffian structure development and differentiation of external genitalia into male structures. After that, however, the testes involute and are not present at birth. This results in delayed pubertal development, and eunuchoidal body proportions. Therapy is replacement of testosterone. Testicular feminization (*a*) usually results in phenotypic females or persons with ambiguous genitalia (incomplete form). Those with 5α-

reductase deficiency (*c*) have normal testes and ambiguous genitalia. Females with 21-hydroxylase deficiency (*d*) often have ambiguous genitalia and virilization; males with this disorder are excessively virilized. Males with Klinefelter's syndrome (*e*) have small testes, not anorchia.

55. (*d*). Hypogonadotropic hypogonadism with anosmia suggests Kallmann's syndrome. Persons with constitutional delay of puberty (*a*) are usually delayed in growth as well as sexual development. Klinefelter's syndrome (*b*) and mumps orchitis (*c*) are both primary testicular disorders, and gonadotropin levels would be elevated. Craniopharyngioma (*e*) would result in panhypopituitarism.

56. (*b*). This woman is anovulatory as menses occur with progestin alone. This confirms a state of adequate estrogenization. The most common cause is the polycystic ovary syndrome. Although many with this disorder are obese and hirsute, not all are. Hypothalamic amenorrhea (*c*) may occur in young women athletes, but these persons have low gonadotropin levels and do not menstruate with progestin. Turner's syndrome (*c*) is a cause of primary amenorrhea. Congenital adrenal hyperplasia (*d*) may result in secondary amenorrhea, but is much less common than PCOS. Those with premature ovarian failure (*e*) would have elevated gonadotropin levels and would not withdraw with progestin alone.

57. True (*a, d, e*); False (*b, c*). All patients with an intact uterus (without outflow tract obstruction) should menstruate with combination therapy. Those with PCOS (*a*) would be expected also to menstruate with progestin only, although it will happen if both estrogen and progestin are given. Patients with müllerian agenesis and testicular feminization (*b, c*) lack a uterus and therefore cannot menstruate.

58. True (*a, c, e*); False (*b, d*). Growth hormone excess (acromegaly) may cause proliferation of tissues, including breast. Marijuana (*c*) is known to cause gynecomastia via its hCG-like actions. Testosterone (*e*) in large amounts may cause gynecomastia via peripheral aromatization to

estradiol. Hyperthyroidism, not hypothyroidism (*b*) may cause gynecomastia. Cigarette smoking (*d*) does not cause gynecomastia.

59. True (*a, d*); False (*b, c, e*). Central, or true, precocious puberty results from premature activation of the hypothalamic-pituitary axis (HPA). Gonadotropin levels typically are in the pubertal range and characteristically rise after a GnRH bolus. Constant administration of GnRH or a long-lasting analog (*d*) result in regression of symptoms. Pubertal estradiol levels (*b*) would be seen in both central and peripheral PP. An ovarian mass (*c*) suggests peripheral PP. Elevated cortisol and DHEA-SO$_4$ levels suggest peripheral PP due to a functioning adrenal tumor.

60. True (*b, d, e*); False (*a, c*). Two or more X chromosomes are necessary to have a chromatin-positive buccal smear (Barr body). Ovaries are abnormal in Turner's syndrome. Patients lack breast development and menses and have a higher incidence of hypothyroidism.

61. True (*c, d*); False (*a, b, e*). Only women with an intact uterus need take progestin to prevent endometrial hyperplasia. Estrogen results in increased HDL and decreased LDL cholesterol. Estrogen is contraindicated in most patients with breast cancer (*d*). Transdermal estrogen (*e*) has a less pronounced effect on the lipid profile than does oral estrogen. This is because oral estrogen passes through the liver, where endogenous lipoproteins are made, and thus has a greater effect on their metabolism.

62. True (*a, e*); False (*b, c, d*). Androgens result in an increase in acne vulgaris, common in puberty (*b*). Androgens decrease serum binding proteins; estrogens increase them (*c*). Androgens result in terminal hair proliferation on the face and body. The opposite effect occurs on the scalp in susceptible males, resulting in transformation to vellus hair (male pattern baldness). Hyperandrogenism is linked to insulin resistance in certain persons (e.g., women with polycystic ovary syndrome).

63. True (*b, d, e*); False (*a, c*). Polycystic ovary syndrome (*c*) is the most common pathological cause of hirsutism. The nonclassical or cryptic

form of 21-hydroxylase deficiency (*b*) may result in hirsutism; this is the most common autosomal recessive disorder. 3β-hydroxysteroid dehydrogenase deficiency also results in hirsutism. Cushing's syndrome (*e*) is an uncommon cause of hirsutism. Patients with testicular feminization (*a*) typically have decreased body hair, and they cannot menstruate because they have no uterus. Hyperprolactinemia (*c*) does not itself cause hirsutism, although many with polycystic ovary syndrome have hyperprolactinemia. The cause appears to be estrogenic stimulation of the pituitary.

64. True (*a*); False (*b, c, d, e*). Hypogonadal proportions occur if the person goes through puberty without normal levels of sex steroids, resulting in delayed long bone fusion and disproportionately long arms and legs. Of those listed, the only disorder resulting in sex steroid deficiency during puberty is Kallmann's syndrome (*a*). The girl with testicular feminization (*d*) has normal estrogen levels and therefore would be proportioned normally. The others are acquired disorders that would have no effect on skeletal growth.

65. True (*d*); False (*a, b, c, d*). Exogenous testosterone alone (*a, b*) will not result in spermatogene-sis. The LH analog β-hCG will result in testicular enlargement and testosterone production, but not spermatogenesis. LH (β-hCG) and FSH (or hMG) must both be given (*d*) for this to occur. GnRH would not be effective in persons with panhypopituitarism, because the gonadotropin response would be inadequate. Pulsatile GnRH works for persons with deficient hypothalamic GnRH secretion (e.g., Kallmann's syndrome) if the pituitary is intact.

66. True (*c, d*); False (*a, b, e*). Both types of tumors would result in low gonadotropin levels (due to feedback inhibition) and increased 17-KS levels. DHEA-SO$_4$ levels are expected to be low with virilizing ovarian tumors, and high with adrenal tumors. The presence of ovarian tumor on ultrasound or CT is suggestive of arrhenoblastoma. Neither tumor would be affected by GnRH agonist (leuprolide) therapy; this would only benefit centrally mediated processes, such as central precocious puberty.

67. True (*b, d*); False (*a, c, e*). Ovulation occurs after increased estradiol levels cause an LH, not FSH, surge (*a*). Progesterone, not estradiol, is secreted by the corpus luteum (*c*). Increased estrogen levels, not progesterone (*e*), inhibit FSH levels and further ovulation.

CHAPTER 8

LIPID METABOLISM

Q: What is the function of lipids in humans?

A: Lipids provide energy by placing a great deal of energy into a small package. The body's immediate energy needs can be met by liver and muscle glycogen, which are broken down to glucose. Average glycogen stores are only about 0.2 kg, and with a caloric density of 4 kcal/gram, it is clear that this cannot meet long-term needs. The average person has about 10 to 15 kg of adipose tissue, however, with a caloric density of 9 kcal/gram. Thus, fat is available for energy after glycogen stores are depleted (about 12 hours in the average person). Triglycerides are the main storage fuel and are denser than glycogen, thereby occupying less space.

Lipids are also important structural parts of cell membranes (e.g., sphingomyelin). Cholesterol is necessary for synthesis of steroid hormones. Bile acids act as detergents and help make nonpolar molecules soluble.

Q: What are lipoproteins?

A: Lipoproteins are lipid-protein complexes that transport hydrophobic lipid molecules in plasma. They consist of a nonpolar lipid (triglycerides and cholesterol esters) core with an outer shell of more polar molecules (cholesterol, phospholipids, and apolipoproteins).

The four major lipoproteins in humans include chylomicrons, very low-density lipoproteins (VLDL), low-density lipoproteins (LDL), and high-density lipoproteins (HDL) (Fig. 8-1). Others include intermediate-density lipoproteins (IDL) and lipoprotein(a).

Chylomicrons are the largest and least dense particles, consisting chiefly of triglycerides (90%). They transport dietary triglyceride from the gut into the lymphatics. They float to the top of plasma, forming a whitish "cream" layer. Triglycerides are removed from the chylomicrons by the enzyme **lipoprotein lipase,** which yields triglyceride plus chylomicron **remnants.** Deficiency in lipoprotein lipase results in severe hypertriglyceridemia.

Very low-density lipoproteins (VLDL), also called pre-β-lipoproteins for their pattern on electrophoresis, are next in size. They consist chiefly of

LIPOPROTEIN ELECTROPHORESIS

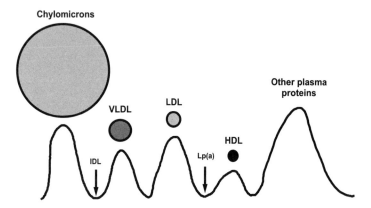

Figure 8-1. Lipoproteins.

triglycerides and are important in the endogenous triglyceride pathway, transporting triglycerides made in the liver. As with chylomicrons, lipoprotein lipase removes triglyceride from VLDL, resulting in triglyceride plus intermediate-density lipoprotein (IDL). Another enzyme, **hepatic-triglyceride lipase** (HTGL), converts IDL to LDL (low-density lipoprotein), which is taken up by LDL receptors.

Low-density lipoproteins (LDL), also called the β-lipoproteins, are rich in cholesterol and result from the degradation of VLDL. As opposed to chylomicrons and VLDL, which transport triglycerides to lymphatics for energy, LDL transports cholesterol to peripheral tissues. They are taken up by LDL receptors. Increased LDL cholesterol is associated with premature atherosclerosis.

High-density lipoproteins (HDL), also called the α-lipoproteins, are smallest in size and contain only 20% cholesterol, the rest being phospholipid and apolipoproteins. They are needed for the activation of lipoprotein lipase and lecithin-cholesterol acyltransferase (LCAT). They are important in removing excess cholesterol from peripheral tissues. Increased levels are associated with decreased atherosclerosis, and decreased levels with increased atherosclerosis.

Q: What are apolipoproteins?

A: **Apolipoproteins** are protein components that are important in lipoprotein structure and metabolism. Some act as ligands (binding sites) for receptors; others act as enzyme cofactors. Others provide structural integrity to the lipoprotein. Five classes exist in humans: A, B, C, D, and E.

The **apo-A** class is a major component of HDL and, to a lesser degree, chylomicrons and VLDL. The major subtype is apo A-I, which is a cofactor in LCAT, which esterifies cholesterol on HDL.

The **apo-B** class is found in all lipoproteins except HDL. The major protein is apo B-100, which is the ligand for LDL to its receptor. B-100 also plays a structural role in VLDL and LDL. Lipoproteins containing B-100 are felt to be atherogenic; HDL, which does not contain apo-B, is antiatherogenic. Another type is apo B-48, a structural component of chylomicrons.

The **apo-C** proteins are primary constituents of VLDL and chylomicrons. C-II is a cofactor for lipoprotein lipase, which removes triglyceride from these proteins. Apo C-I, however, is found in HDL and also is a cofactor for LCAT (as is apo A-I).

Apo-D is found only in HDL and is also called cholesterol ester transfer protein (CETP). In the reverse cholesterol pathway, CETP facilitates transfer of cholesterol from HDL to apo-B rich lipoproteins (LDL, VLDL, chylomicron remnants) in exchange for triglyceride. The cholesterol is then taken to the liver where it is disposed.

The **apo-E** class consists of apo E-II, E-III, and E-IV. They are receptor ligands for VLDL, chylomicron remnants, and IDL. LDL contains little apo-E, and apo B-100 is its receptor ligand.

Q: How are lipoproteins eliminated?

A: LDL is eliminated by the LDL receptor. LDL receptors also bind other lipoproteins that contain apo-B (VLDL, IDL). Some apo-E-containing lipoproteins are also taken up by the LDL receptor. All cells contain the LDL receptor, although most are in the liver.

Apo-E receptors bind to apo-E containing lipoproteins (mainly HDL but also VLDL and chylomicron remnants). They are found only in the liver. "Scavenger" receptors are found in macrophages and bind to oxidized LDL.

Q: What is lipoprotein(a)?

A: **Lipoprotein(a),** or Lp(a), is LDL (low-density lipoprotein) attached to a protein, apoprotein(a), which is very similar to plasminogen, which normally breaks down fibrin. Lp(a) appears to inhibit thrombus dissolution and is atherogenic. High levels are clearly linked to premature atherosclerotic disease. Individuals with increased Lp(a) often respond poorly to drug therapy; nicotinic acid appears to be the best therapy.

Q: How are triglycerides and cholesterol obtained by the body?

A: Triglycerides and cholesterol may be obtained either from diet or degradation of lipid-rich lipoproteins. In addition, cholesterol can be synthesized from acetate.

In the **exogenous lipid pathway** (Fig. 8-2), dietary cholesterol is absorbed into the intestinal mucosa, and incorporated as *cholesterol esters* into chylomicrons, which are made chiefly of triglyceride. Chylomicrons then go into the lymphatic system and then the bloodstream, where the enzyme *lipoprotein lipase* cleaves the chylomicron into triglyceride and a *chylomicron remnant*, which contains cholesterol ester. The liver then assimilates the chylomicron remnant where free cholesterol is isolated.

In the **endogenous pathway** (Fig. 8-3), triglyceride- and cholesterol ester-rich VLDL is secreted by the liver, which is converted to triglyceride and IDL again by *lipoprotein lipase*. HDL is also involved in this process. IDL is then converted by hepatic-triglyceride lipase (HTGL, hepatic lipase) to LDL, which is taken up by tissues with an LDL receptor. Triglyceride may also be removed from LDL by HTGL.

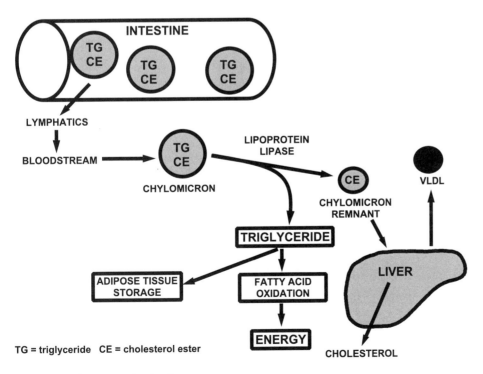

Figure 8-2. Exogenous lipid pathway.

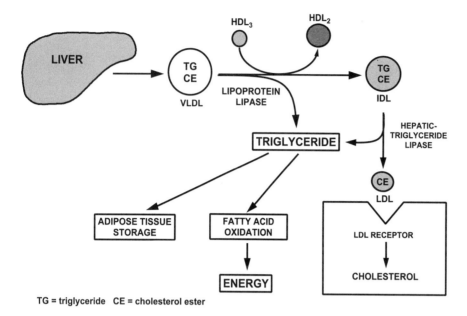

Figure 8-3. Endogenous lipid pathway.

Cholesterol is synthesized from acetate via a complex series of reactions (Fig. 8-4). Two acetyl-CoA (coenzyme A) molecules form acetoacetyl CoA; a third acetyl CoA is added to form **3-hydroxy-3-methylglutaryl CoA** (HMG-CoA). The next, **rate-limiting** step is the conversion of HMG-CoA to **mevalonate** by the enzyme **HMG-CoA reductase.**

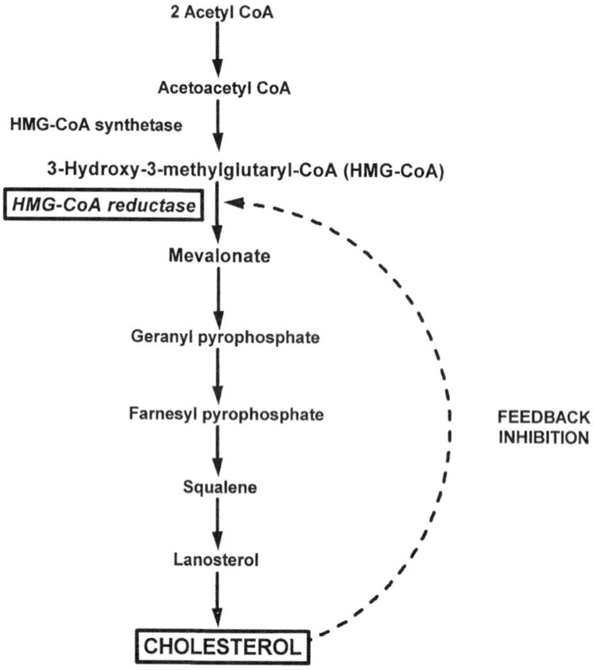

Mevalonate is condensed to squalene, lanosterol, and finally cholesterol in a series of reactions.

Cholesterol synthesis in humans is tightly regulated. Increased cholesterol levels result in feedback inhibition of HMG-CoA reductase, thus decreasing synthesis.

Q: What is the role of HDL?

A: HDL cholesterol is important in the **reverse cholesterol pathway** (Fig. 8-5). Small, immature, disc-shaped HDL particles (*nascent* HDL) are secreted by the liver and intestines. Apolipoproteins bind to nascent HDL, and free cholesterol is acquired from cells, forming a small, cholesterol-poor, spherical HDL (HDL$_3$). Cholesterol is then **esterified** by **lecithin-cholesterol acyltransferase** (LCAT). The cholesterol molecules become more nonpolar, resulting to migration to the core and enlargement of the particle. This, along with transfer of apolipoprotein, cholesterol, and phospholipid from the delipidation of VLDL, results in a "mature" HDL particle (HDL$_2$). Delipidation of VLDL also yields triglyceride (used for energy) and IDL. The excess cholesterol is then transferred to the apo-B-rich lipoproteins (LDL, VLDL, IDL, and chylomicron remnants) by means of **cholesterol ester transfer protein** (CETP). These lipoproteins then dispose of cholesterol in the liver, with

2 Acetyl CoA

Acetoacetyl CoA

HMG-CoA synthetase

3-Hydroxy-3-methylglutaryl-CoA (HMG-CoA)

HMG-CoA reductase

Mevalonate

Geranyl pyrophosphate

Farnesyl pyrophosphate   FEEDBACK
                                          INHIBITION

Squalene

Lanosterol

CHOLESTEROL

Figure 8-4. Cholesterol synthesis.

REVERSE CHOLESTEROL PATHWAY

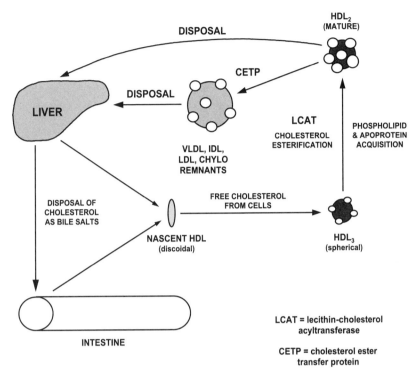

Figure 8-5. Reverse cholesterol pathway.

excretion of the excess cholesterol as bile salts. Patients with low HDL levels therefore have decreased cholesterol removal and are at risk for atherosclerosis.

Q: How are lipid disorders classified?

A: **Dyslipidemias** may be classified as primary or secondary. **Primary dyslipidemias** are inherited, either as a specific gene mutation (e.g., primary hypercholesterolemia) or a polygenic disorder (e.g., familial combined hyperlipidemia). In the past, primary hyperlipidemias were classified according to the **Fredrickson scheme,** which groups lipid disorders into separate phenotypes according to the appearance of serum in a test tube after centrifugation (Fig. 8-6, Tables 8-1, 8-2). The current classification assigns names to the primary dyslipidemias rather than Fredrickson numbers, which can be difficult to remember.

Secondary dyslipidemias are caused by diseases interfering with lipoprotein metabolism. All six Fredrickson subtypes are encountered (Table 8-3). For example, a common presentation is type IV hyperlipidemia associated with insulin resistance

and type 2 diabetes mellitus. Hypothyroidism is also very common and may result in significant LDL elevation (IIa).

Q: What is the Friedewald equation?

A: Not to be confused with the Fredrickson classification, the **Friedewald equation** allows the estimation of LDL cholesterol, which is difficult to measure directly. Total cholesterol is composed of LDL, VLDL, and HDL cholesterol. VLDL cholesterol is triglyceride-rich, and VLDL cholesterol is equal to the triglyceride level divided by 5, assuming the TG concentration is less than 400 mg/dL. Over 400 mg/dL, this relationship does not hold.

$$LDL\text{-}C = Total\ C - HDL\text{-}C - TG/5$$

This equation depends on three different variables, and error in any one measurement confounds the result. Fortunately, many laboratories can now measure LDL cholesterol directly, obviating the need for such cumbersome equations. LDL cholesterol also has a long half-life in serum, and thus can be measured in the nonfasting state, unlike triglycerides.

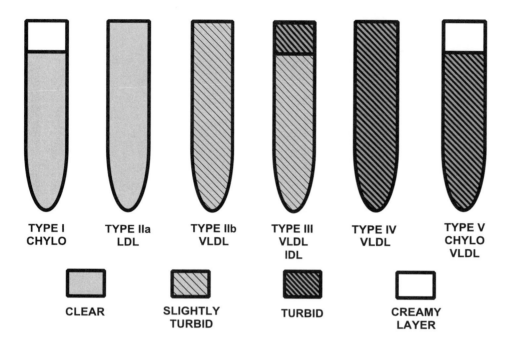

Figure 8-6. Appearance of plasma in hyperlipidemia.

Q: What is familial lipoprotein lipase deficiency?

A: **Familial lipoprotein lipase deficiency,** also called type I hyperlipidemia or primary chylomicronemia, results from defective lipoprotein lipase (LPL) activity, with resultant increase in triglyceride and chylomicron levels. It may occur with deficiency of LPL itself or apo C-II, a cofactor necessary for LDL activity. Severe hypertriglyceridemia often presents in childhood, with eruptive xanthomas, lipemia retinalis, and attacks of pancreatitis.

Q: What is familial hypercholesterolemia?

A: **Familial hypercholesterolemia** (Fredrickson phenotype IIa) is an autosomal codominant disease. It is caused by a defect in the LDL receptor, resulting in increased LDL and incidence of atherosclerosis. The heterozygous state is most common (1 in 500), resulting in LDL levels of 250 or more and onset of coronary artery disease, typically between ages 40 and 50. The homozygous state occurs in 1 per 1,000,000 patients; LDL levels often exceed 500 mg/dL and coronary disease often begins between

TABLE 8-1.   Appearance of Plasma in Hyperlipidemia

TYPE	PARTICLES	PLASMA APPEARANCE
I	Chylomicrons	Turbid "cream" layer on top of clear to slightly turbid infranatant
IIa	LDL	Clear
IIb	VLDL, LDL	Slightly turbid without top layer
III	VLDL, IDL	Slightly turbid with smaller more turbid layer on top
IV	VLDL	Very turbid, opaque without top layer
V	VLDL, chylomicrons	Cream layer on top of turbid infranatant

TABLE 8-2.   Fredrickson and Current Classification of the Primary Hyperlipidemias

FREDRICKSON CLASSIFICATION	CURRENT CLASSIFICATION	FEATURES
Type I (rare)	**Familial lipoprotein lipase deficiency**	**Laboratory** TG ↑↑↑↑, Chol ↑ Chylomicronemia Secondary decrease in HDL due to TG ↑↑↑↑ Electrophoresis shows dense band at origin (chylomicrons) **Pathogenesis** Apo-C-II deficiency Lipoprotein lipase deficiency **Clinical presentation** Severe pancreatitis, eruptive xanthomas, hepatomegaly, splenomegaly, lipemia retinalis
Type IIa (common)	**Familial hypercholesterolemia**	**Heterozygote:** 1:500 incidence **Laboratory** Chol ↑↑↑, TG normal Frequent cardiovascular disease by age 50 **Pathogenesis:** 50% absence of LDL receptors **Homozygote:** 1:1,000,000 incidence Almost no functioning LDL receptors Coronary disease by age 20 in most cases Total cholesterol > 600 **Clinical presentation** Premature corneal arcus, tendinous xanthomas, coronary artery disease
Type IIb (common)	**Familial combined hyperlipidemia**	**Laboratory** Chol ↑, TG ↑ Most common primary dyslipidemia (1 per 300 persons) Autosomal codominant Different family members may have different phenotypes (IIa, IIb, IV) May progress within patient (e.g., IIb → IV) **Pathogenesis:** Increased VLDL–apo-B synthesis **Clinical presentation** Rare xanthomas, premature coronary artery disease
Type III (rare)	**Familial dysbetalipoproteinemia (broad beta disease)**	**Laboratory** Chol ↑↑, TG ↑↑ Electrophoresis shows broad beta, "floating" beta, beta-VLDL **Pathogenesis** Absence or deficiency of apo-E Defective apo-E receptors **Clinical presentation** Increased risk of CAD, palmar xanthomas (diagnostic), tuberous xanthomas

TABLE 8-2.   (Continued)

FREDRICKSON CLASSIFICATION	CURRENT CLASSIFICATION	FEATURES
Type IV (common)	Familial hypertriglyceridemia	**Laboratory** Chol ↑, TG ↑↑↑ **Pathogenesis** Increased VLDL production Familial hypercholesterolemia with type IV phenotype Apo-A-I defect **Clinical presentation** Xanthomas uncommon, obesity, diabetes mellitus common
Type V (rare)	Familial chylomicronemia	**Laboratory** Chol ↑, TG ↑↑↑↑ Elevated band at origin (chylomicrons) and pre-beta **Pathogenesis** Absence of lipoprotein lipase or apo-C-II **Clinical presentation** Hepatomegaly, splenomegaly, obesity, hyperuricemia, hyperglycemia, chylomicronemia; may have dry mouth, arthralgias, arthritis

TABLE 8-3.   Secondary Dyslipidemias

TYPE I	TYPE IIA AND IIB	TYPE III	TYPE IV AND IV
Diabetes mellitus	Anorexia nervosa	Diabetes mellitus	Ethanol
Dysproteinemia	Cushing's syndrome	Dysproteinemia	Cushing's syndrome
Pancreatitis	Dysproteinemia	Hypothyroidism	Diabetes mellitus
Systemic lupus erythematosus	Hyperparathyroidism	Lupus	Dysproteinemia
	Hypothyroidism	Obesity	Glycogen storage diseases
	Nephrotic syndrome		Hypothyroidism
	Obesity		Nephrotic syndrome
			Pregnancy
			Renal failure
			Drugs Estrogens Glucocorticoids Thiazides Beta-blockers

ages 10 and 20. The most common secondary cause of type IIa hyperlipidemia is hypothyroidism.

Reductase inhibitors are very effective for those with heterozygous disease. Nicotinic acid and resins may be useful in combination therapy. Homozygotes respond poorly to drug therapy, as there are few LDL receptors. Liver transplantation provides LDL receptors and offers the best hope in these individuals.

Familial defective apo-B is a similar disorder characterized by a gene coding for abnormal apo-B-100. Because this is the ligand for the LDL receptor, LDL particles with this abnormal B-100 are not cleared adequately, also resulting in a type IIa phenotype and premature atherosclerosis. This has an incidence of approximately 1 in 700.

Q: What is familial combined hyperlipidemia?

A: **Familial combined hyperlipidemia,** or type IIb hyperlipidemia, is the most common primary dyslipidemia and occurs in 1 in 300 persons. This disease is inherited as autosomal dominant and is characterized by overabundance of apo-B-containing lipoproteins (VLDL and LDL). It is typically characterized by moderate elevations of both triglyceride (VLDL) and LDL cholesterol. Incidence of atherogenesis is increased.

Q: What is familial dysbetalipoproteinemia?

A: **Familial dysbetalipoproteinemia,** also called type III hyperlipidemia, remnant disease, or broad beta disease, is a disorder of the apoprotein-E gene, resulting in an abnormal apo-E (E-II). This results in delayed removal of VLDL remnants and IDL (pre-beta lipoprotein). These lipoproteins are atherogenic and are associated with coronary artery and peripheral vascular disease.

Patients have comparable elevation of both cholesterol and triglyceride. Palmar xanthomas (yellowish lipid deposits on the lines of the palm) are virtually diagnostic. Tuberous xanthomas may also be seen. This disorder may be difficult to detect by conventional lipoprotein assays as they cannot distinguish the pre-beta IDL from LDL. This is one condition in which a lipoprotein electrophoresis is recommended.

Q: What is familial hypertriglyceridemia?

A: **Familial hypertriglyceridemia,** also called type IV hyperlipidemia, is a common disorder affecting approximately 1% of persons. This is a disorder of increased VLDL resulting in moderate to severe hypertriglyceridemia. Unlike type IIb, in type IV the apo-B synthesis appears to be normal; VLDL particles are normal in number but contain increased amount of triglyceride. These patients have a lower susceptibility to atherogenesis than those with type IIb.

The most common secondary disorder associated with type IV is type 2 diabetes mellitus. Insulin plays a role in triglyceride removal, and impaired insulin action results in decreased clearance and hypertriglyceridemia.

Q: What is type V hyperlipidemia?

A: **Chylomicronemia syndrome,** also called type V hyperlipidemia, results from increased accumulation of both VLDL and chylomicrons, with consequent severe hypertriglyceridemia. It is unusual as a primary lipid disorder; usually it is associated with a secondary cause. As with type IV, type V is often associated with poorly controlled type 2 diabetes and insulin resistance. Patients may present with eruptive xanthomas, lipemia retinalis, and pancreatitis.

Q: Do lipoprotein phenotypes always stay the same?

A: Lipoprotein phenotypes may shift from one to another. For example, persons with poorly controlled diabetes often shift from type IV to V and back again after the diabetes is controlled.

Q: What physical signs are seen in patients with dyslipidemia?

A: Patients with large elevations in LDL cholesterol (typically familial hypercholesterolemia) may have **tendon xanthomas**—areas of tendon thickening—in the extensor tendons of the hand, patellar, and Achilles areas.

Eruptive xanthomas are hallmarks of severe hypertriglyceridemia (Fig. 8-7). These occur on the buttocks and over extensor surfaces of the arms and legs. They are pustular lesions that wax and wane with the hypertriglyceridemia.

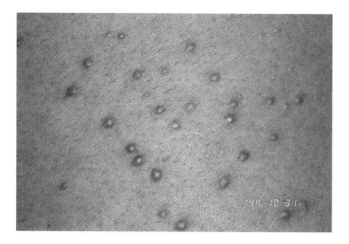

Figure 8-7. Eruptive xanthomas.

Corneal arcus is a whitish band on the outer cornea of the eye near the limbus. It is normal in elderly individuals but may indicate hypercholesterolemia in younger patients.

Xanthelasma are yellowish plaques seen near the eyelids. They are commonly seen in hypercholesterolemia but are nonspecific, as many patients with this finding have no lipid disorder.

Lipemia retinalis is seen in patients with severe hypertriglyceridemia (usually 3000 mg/dL or greater). It is a whitish discoloration of the retinal vessels due to lipemic blood.

Patients with type III dyslipidemia (dysbetalipoproteinemia) may have a pathognomonic lesion, **palmar xanthomas.** These are yellowish deposits along the palm creases.

Tuberous xanthomas are depositions of cholesterol in soft tissues (e.g., knees and elbows, not tendons) and are seen in familial hypercholesterolemia (IIa) and dysbetalipoproteinemia (III).

Q: What other disorders result from abnormalities in LDL metabolism?

A: Familial hypercholesterolemia and defective apo-B are the most common (discussed above). **Familial hypobetalipoproteinemia** is a genetic disorder associated with extremely low concentrations of LDL, apolipoprotein B, and total cholesterol. These patients have an abnormal B-100 gene; apo B-100 is the major lipoprotein of LDL and the ligand for the LDL receptor. With inadequate apo B-100 levels, LDL levels decrease. Heterozygotes

with this disorder may have some protection against atherosclerosis due to the low LDL levels. This disorder must be distinguished from familial defective apo-B, in which apo-B is made but is defective; in this case, LDL is indeed made but cannot be cleared adequately because of the abnormal ligand for the LDL receptor. Homozygotes for hypobetalipoproteinemia may have some of the same symptoms as those with abetalipoproteinemia. Heterozygotes are asymptomatic.

Abetalipoproteinemia is an autosomal recessive disorder characterized by the complete absence of apo-B, resulting in absence of not only LDL, but VLDL and chylomicrons. Triglyceride and cholesterol levels are low. These patients also may develop fat-soluble vitamin deficiency, retinitis pigmentosa, anemia, and neurologic disease. Treatment includes fat-soluble vitamins and tocopherol (vitamin E) at very high doses, which appears to limit the progressive neurologic degeneration.

Q: What disorders result from abnormalities in HDL metabolism?

A: Deficiency of HDL is seen in **Tangier disease,** a rare genetic disorder associated with very low HDL levels and excess cholesterol accumulation. Patients have large, orange-colored tonsils, corneal opacities, and polyneuropathy. Even though HDL levels are low, premature atherosclerosis is not seen because LDL levels are also low.

Familial hypoalphalipoproteinemia is a condition associated with low HDL levels and premature CAD. **Familial hyperalphalipoproteinemia** is a syndrome of HDL excess associated with longevity and low CAD risk.

LCAT deficiency is extremely rare and results in markedly decreased HDL fractions. It is often associated with renal insufficiency, anemia, and hemolytic anemia, and corneal opacities. **Fish-eye disease** is rarer still and associated with absent LCAT activity in HDL fractions. Corneal opacities are present and account for its name. The other findings of LCAT deficiency are not seen. In both, VLDL levels (and hence, triglyceride levels) are increased.

Q: What are the consequences of hypertriglyceridemia?

A: Severe hypertriglyceridemia (> 1000 mg/dL) may result in acute pancreatitis, with severe nausea, vomiting, and abdominal pain. Repeated attacks may result in chronic pancreatitis, pancreatic insufficiency, and even death. Eruptive xanthomas may be seen on the buttocks and extensor areas (elbows and knees). Lipemia retinalis (whitish appearance of retinal vessels) may be seen on examination. Retinal vein occlusion and blindness may occur.

The significance of mild hypertriglyceridemia (250–500 mg/dL) is less clear. In the past, it was believed that isolated hypertriglyceridemia was not a risk factor for cardiovascular disease. But hypertriglyceridemia does lower HDL levels, thus potentiating cardiac risk in this fashion. It is now recognized that persons with hypertriglyceridemia have denser, more atherogenic forms of low-density lipoprotein (LDL); normalization of triglycerides decreases its concentration. It is now recommended that triglyceride levels be normalized if possible through diet or medication.

Q: How does hypertriglyceridemia affect laboratory measurements?

A: Extreme elevations in triglyceride levels (i.e., > 1000 mg/dL) falsely lower plasma measurements of many substances. Triglycerides are quite hydrophobic and do not mix with plasma; these increase the total blood volume, although the plasma volume stays the same. Because the increased lipid volume effectively dilutes the quantity of the measured item (e.g., sodium), the measured amount is lower even though the actual amount is normal (i.e., a pseudohyponatremia). Some enzymes (such as amylase) are inhibited by triglyceride-containing lipoproteins, and falsely low values may be seen in patients with severe hypertriglyceridemia.

Q: What are the guidelines for cholesterol screening?

A: The National Cholesterol Education Program (NCEP) guidelines are as follows:

   1. Check total cholesterol and HDL-C levels in adults over age 20. If total cholesterol is high or HDL low, recheck level.

   2. Do lipid profile if:

   History of coronary artery disease (CAD) or atherosclerotic disease is present.

   Total cholesterol is > 240.

   Total cholesterol > 200 plus two risk factors and HDL < 35.

   3. Assess risks for coronary artery disease:

   Age > 45 (men); > 55 (women)

   Positive family history

   Smoking

   Hypertension

   HDL < 35

   Diabetes mellitus

   Premature menopause without estrogen replacement

Q: What are the guidelines for treatment of hypercholesterolemia?

A: Treatment goals are based on risk factors and LDL and triglyceride levels (Tables 8-4, 8-5). Therapy should never be initiated based on an isolated cholesterol level. A lipoprotein profile should be obtained to identify specific abnormalities. Cholesterol may be elevated because of elevated LDL, VLDL, or even HDL. For example, LDL elevation may be treated with reductase inhibitors, but patients with VLDL cholesterol elevation present with hypertriglyceridemia, for which reductase inhibitors usually are not first-line agents.

A lipid profile should be obtained after a 12-hour fast. Dietary chylomicrons must be cleared from plasma by fasting. Other lipids (VLDL) have short half-lives and are also dependent on diet. LDL direct cholesterol can be measured in the nonfasting state because of its long half-life.

Lipoprotein electrophoresis is seldom necessary except in type III hyperlipidemia (dysbetalipoproteinemia), which can be difficult to diagnose by conventional laboratory methods.

Q: What is the dietary therapy of dyslipidemia?

A: Diet is a cornerstone of therapy, but unfortunately may be quite difficult for the patient. Many persons who are willing to take a lipid-lowering

TABLE 8-4.   Treatment Based on LDL Cholesterol (NCEP Guidelines)

RISK FACTORS	DIET (mg/dL)	DIET AND DRUG (mg/dL)	GOAL (mg/dL)
< 2 risk factors No AVD	> 160	> 190	< 160
≥ 2 risk factors No AVD	> 130	> 160	< 130
AVD	> 100	> 130	< 100

Negative risk factor for CAD: HDL > 60 mg/dL (subtract one risk factor)
AVD = atherosclerotic vascular disease

medication are unwilling to make dietary modifications. The step 1 diet is started first, with the step 2 diet added later if goals are not met (Table 8-6). Consultation with a registered dietitian is recommended to help meal planning. This service should be provided at a hospital or lipid clinic.

Q: What are reductase inhibitors?

A: **HMG-CoA reductase inhibitors** (often called "statins") are competitive inhibitors of HMG-CoA reductase, the rate-limiting step in cholesterol biosynthesis (Fig. 8-4). These compounds, which are derivatives of fungal fermentation products, inhibit the conversion of HMG-CoA to mevalonate. They are extremely effective at reducing LDL cholesterol and are often first-line agents as they are easily taken and are well tolerated. They are not as useful as fibrates or niacin for the treatment of hypertriglyceridemia, with the exception of atorvastatin, which has moderate triglyceride-lowering properties.

Potentially serious side effects of these drugs include hepatotoxicity and myositis, but fortunately both are rare. Gastrointestinal complaints (diarrhea, nausea, flatulence) are occasionally seen.

Q: What are fibric acid derivatives?

A: **Fibric acid derivatives** are agents primarily used in the treatment of hypertriglyceridemia. These drugs appear to act by increasing VLDL and chylomicron clearance and inhibiting VLDL production. The three agents currently available in the United States are gemfibrozil, clofibrate, and fenofibrate. Clofibrate was the first agent used, but it is no longer favored because of clinical studies showing increased mortality with its use. In addition to lowering triglyceride levels, HDL levels are increased. It may cause SIADH, and may be used in the treatment of partial central diabetes insipidus.

Gemfibrozil has been available for many years, is effective, and is well tolerated. Fenofibrate, which was recently introduced into the United States, appears to be at least as effective. Side effects are rare and include mild gastrointestinal symptoms (nausea), myositis, and hepatotoxicity. Gemfi-

TABLE 8-5.   Treatment Based on Triglycerides (NCEP Guidelines)

CATEGORY	TRIGLYCERIDE LEVEL (mg/dL)	ADVERSE EFFECTS
Desirable	< 200	
Borderline	200–400	? CAD risk (low HDL, dense LDL)
High	400–1000	? pancreatitis risk
Very high	> 1000	pancreatitis risk

TABLE 8-6.   Diet Therapy in Hyperlipidemia

DIETARY COMPONENT	STEP 1 DIET	STEP 2 DIET
Total fat	< 30% total calories	< 30% total calories
Saturated fatty acids	8–10% total calories	< 7% total calories
Polyunsaturated fatty acids	< 10% total calories	< 10% total calories
Monounsaturated fatty acids	10–15% total calories	10–15% total calories
Carbohydrates	50–60% total calories	50–60% total calories
Protein	10–20% total calories	10–20% total calories
Cholesterol	< 300 mg/day	< 200 mg/day

brozil may potentiate the action of warfarin, so dosages should be adjusted accordingly.

Fibric acid derivatives also cause a modest reduction in LDL-cholesterol, possibly by inhibiting HMG-CoA reductase. They are not usually used as monotherapy for isolated LDL elevation.

Q: What are bile acid sequestrants?

A: **Bile acid sequestrants,** also called "resins," are molecules that bind bile acids in the intestine, thus decreasing the enterohepatic circulation of cholesterol (much bodily cholesterol is obtained from recirculation of bile acids rather than synthesis). The bile acid-resin complex is then excreted. These drugs are useful for mild to moderate LDL elevation and are the preferred agents in children as they are not systemically absorbed. Common side effects include constipation and bloating. They should not be taken with other medications, as their absorption may be impaired. They may exacerbate hypertriglyceridemia and should be used with caution in these patients.

Q: What is nicotinic acid?

A: **Nicotinic acid** (niacin, vitamin B_3) is required for normal metabolism but has potent lipid-lowering characteristics in supraphysiologic doses. It acts by inhibiting VLDL and LDL synthesis. It has been used for many years without permanent long-term toxicity and is an excellent treatment for both LDL cholesterol elevation and hypertriglyceridemia. Modest elevation of HDL levels also occurs.

The most frequent side effect of niacin is cutaneous flushing, similar to the menopausal hot flash. This reaction is prostaglandin-mediated and often can be averted by giving aspirin or a non-steroidal inflammatory agent such as ibuprofen before the dose. Administration with a cold liquid is often helpful. Niacin should never be taken with hot liquids or alcohol. Niacin is available as both the crystalline form (immediate release) and sustained-release forms. The sustained-release forms have a lower incidence of flushing.

Hepatotoxicity may be seen with niacin but is rare. The incidence increases with very high doses (i.e., > 4000 mg/day). The sustained-release forms appear to have a higher incidence of hepatotoxicity at very high doses. Increased uric acid levels may result, so niacin should be avoided in patients with gout.

Niacin may raise blood glucose and must be used with caution in individuals with impaired glucose tolerance or diabetes mellitus. Unfortunately, these individuals frequently have severe hypertriglyceridemia that requires therapy with niacin. Niacin is not recommended in diabetics unless no other agent is effective, in which case the benefits outweigh the risks. Increased dosages of insulin and/or oral agents may be required.

Q: What are omega-3 fatty acids?

A: **Omega-3 fatty acids,** found in marine (fish) oils, significantly lower VLDL cholesterol (and there-

TABLE 8-7.   Lipid-Lowering Medications

DRUG	BILE ACID SEQUESTRANTS (RESINS)	HMG-COA REDUCTASE INHIBITORS	NICOTINIC ACID	FIBRATES	ANTIOXIDANT	MARINE (FISH) OILS
Mechanism	Bind bile acids in gut, decreasing enterohepatic circulation of bile acids; ↑LDL receptor activity	Competitive inhibitor of HMG-CoA reductase, decreasing cholesterol biosynthesis	Inhibits VLDL production; increases activity of lipoprotein lipase; decreases cholesterol synthesis	Decreased VLDL production; increase VLDL and chylomicron removal	↑LDL clearance; ↓HDL synthesis	Decreases hepatic VLDL production and triglycerides
Primary effect	↓Chol	↓↓Chol, ↓TG	↓↓Chol, ↓↓↓TG	↓Chol, ↓↓TG	↓Chol	↓TG
Examples	Cholestyramine, colestipol	Lovastatin, pravastatin, simvastatin, fluvastatin, atorvastatin, cerivastatin	Crystalline (short-acting) and various long-acting preparations	Gemfibrozil, clofibrate, fenofibrate	Probucol	Omega-3 fatty acids
Side effects	Constipation, bloating, may interfere with absorption of other drugs	GI symptoms; myositis, hepatitis	Flushing, diarrhea, nausea, vomiting, hyperglycemia, hepatotoxicity, hyperuricemia	GI symptoms; hepatitis, myopathy; potentiates warfarin action	GI symptoms; prolongation of QT interval; lowers HDL	May aggravate diabetes control; increased bleeding time
Cost	Moderate	Moderate to high	Low	Moderate to high	Moderate	Low
Compliance	Fair	Good	Fair to poor	Good	Good	Good
Uses	Mild LDL elevation	Moderate to severe LDL elevation	Moderate to severe LDL or TG elevation	Moderate TG elevation	Mild LDL elevation	Refractory TG elevation

fore triglyceride) levels in hyperlipidemic patients. Little or no change occurs in those with normal lipids or with isolated cholesterol elevation. Omega-3 fatty acids also appear to have antiatherogenic effects that are independent of the lipid-lowering effects, possible due to their effect on prostaglandin metabolism. They may be of use in patients with severe hypertriglyceridemia refractory to fibrates and/or nicotinic acid. They increase hepatic glucose production and must be used with caution in diabetics. They also have antiplatelet activity and thus should be avoided in patients with bleeding disorders.

Q: What is probucol?

A: **Probucol** is an antioxidant that causes modest LDL cholesterol reduction via increased clearance. Unfortunately, this drug also reduces HDL cholesterol. Although in theory antioxidants may prevent atherogenesis, this has not been demonstrated in clinical studies. Probucol is only rarely used and is not a good first-line agent for hyperlipidemia.

Q: What is the treatment of elevated LDL cholesterol?

A: Secondary causes such as hypothyroidism should be excluded. Dietary management should be tried initially. Reductase inhibitors are very well tolerated, very effective, and often are the initial agents of choice. Side effects such as myositis and hepatotoxicity are rare. Bile acid sequestrants (resins) are useful for mild LDL elevations and may be used as a first-line agent or if reductase inhibitors cannot be tolerated. Constipation and bloating are common with resins. Because they are not absorbed into the bloodstream, systemic effects do not occur. Resins are the only agent approved for use in children (i.e., with familial hypercholesterolemia).

Nicotinic acid is extremely effective, but its use can be limited by its side effects (nausea, flushing, and diarrhea). However, with proper education, the majority of patients can tolerate it.

If one agent is not sufficient, combination therapy may be indicated (e.g., reductase inhibitor and resin, reductase inhibitor and niacin). Both niacin and reductase inhibitors are potentially hepatotoxic, and the incidence is increased slightly when combined.

Q: What is the treatment of hypertriglyceridemia?

A: Hypertriglyceridemia is often very responsive to diet therapy. Secondary causes such as diabetes must also be evaluated and treated. The first-line medication is typically a fibric acid derivative (e.g., gemfibrozil). Reductase inhibitors are typically not very effective, with the exception of atorvastatin. Resins can actually exacerbate hypertriglyceridemia and should be avoided. Niacin has potent triglyceride-lowering actions but its use is limited by its side effects. Omega-3 fatty acids may be useful in severe cases.

Q: What is the evidence that hyperlipidemia causes atherogenesis, and that treatment improves outcomes?

A: Numerous clinical studies have implicated lipoproteins in the development of atherosclerotic disease. They are summarized in Table 8-8.

TABLE 8-8.   Some Major Clinical Trials of Hyperlipidemia and Atherosclerosis

STUDY	RESULT
Framingham Study	Cholesterol levels are linked with long-term cardiovascular mortality in persons under age 50
Lipid Research Clinics—Coronary Primary Prevention Trial I (LRC-CPPT)	Patients treated with cholestyramine for several years had decrease in death from coronary disease and decrease in nonfatal myocardial infarction
Helsinki Heart Study	Gemfibrozil reduced the incidence of coronary disease in men with hyperlipidemia
Familial Atherosclerosis Treatment Study	Reduction in LDL cholesterol in men resulted in decreased progression of coronary disease and incidence of cardiac events in high-risk men receiving lovastatin + colestipol or niacin + colestipol
St. Thomas Atherosclerosis Regression Study (STARS)	Diet alone or diet + cholestyramine slowed progression and increased regression of coronary artery disease
Monitored Atherosclerosis Regression Study (MARS)	Lovastatin + diet decreased progression of coronary lesions in patients with coronary disease
Scandinavian Simvastatin Survival Study	Simvastatin decreased the relative risk for death in patients with CAD
Long-Term Intervention with Pravastatin in Ischemic Disease (LIPID)	Pravastatin reduced the risk of coronary events in patients with CAD
Cholesterol Lowering Atherosclerosis Study	Nonprogression and regression of coronary lesions in those treated with colestipol + niacin

BIBLIOGRAPHY

Chait A, Brunzell JD. Acquired hyperlipidemia (secondary dyslipoproteinemias). Endocr Metab Clin North Am 1990;19:259–274.

Chait A, Brunzell JD. Lipids and lipoproteins. In: Besser GM, Thorner MO, eds. Clinical endocrinology. 2nd ed. St. Louis: Mosby-Wolfe, 1994:6.2–6.16.

Galton D, Krone W. The chemistry of lipids. In: Galton D, Krone W. Hyperlipidemia in practice. New York: Gower Medical Publishing, 1991:1–17.

Heinonen OP, Huttunen JK, Manninen V, Manttari M, et al. The Helsinki heart study: coronary heart disease incidence during an extended follow-up. J Intern Med 1994;235:41–49.

Julian DG. Treatment for survivors of acute myocardial infarction: what have we learned from large intervention trials? Cardiovasc Drugs Ther 1995; 9(suppl 3):495–502.

Oberman A, Kreisbert RA, Henkin Y. Lipoprotein transport. In: Oberman A, Kreisbert RA, Henkin Y. Principles and management of lipid disorders: a primary care approach. Baltimore: Williams & Wilkins, 1992:88–101.

Prevention of cardiovascular events and death with pravastatin in patients with coronary heart disease and a broad range of initial cholesterol levels: the long-term intervention with pravastatin in ischaemic disease (LIPID) study group. N Engl J Med 1998;339:1349–1357.

Summary of the second report of the National Cholesterol Education Program (NCEP) Expert Panel on Detection, Evaluation, and Treatment of High Blood Cholesterol in Adults (Adult Treatment Panel II). JAMA 1993;269:3015–3023.

REVIEW QUESTIONS

I. SHORT ANSWER

1. List three important functions of lipids in humans.

2. List the four major lipoproteins in humans.

3. The largest and least dense lipoprotein class is _____, which is made chiefly of _____. Its role is to transfer _____ from the _____ to the circulation.

4. The second least dense lipoprotein subtype is _____, which is made mainly of _____. It transports _____ made in the liver to peripheral sites.

5. _____ is formed from the delipidation of VLDL and is rich in _____, which is transported to peripheral tissues.

6. _____ is the densest lipoprotein class. It is important in removal of _____ from peripheral tissues for disposal.

7. _____ are special proteins important in lipoprotein structure and function. They may serve as _____ to receptors, act as enzyme _____, or provide _____ to the lipoprotein.

8. The major subtype of the apolipoprotein A class is _____, which is a cofactor for the enzyme _____. One of the C apolipoproteins that is also important as a cofactor for the same enzyme is _____. Another apo-C protein, _____, is a cofactor for the en-

zyme _____, important in removal of triglyceride from chylomicrons and VLDL.

9. The major B apolipoprotein is _____; it is the binding site for _____ to its receptor. Lipoproteins rich in this are considered _____.

10. LDL may be modified by attachment of a plasminogen-like protein, resulting in a protein called _____. This lipoprotein is very _____.

11. Triglycerides are used as fuel by the body. They may be obtained from dietary sources via the _____ pathway. They also may be synthesized in the liver and transported to cells by the _____ pathway.

12. In the exogenous lipid pathway, triglyceride-rich _____ are absorbed from the intestine into the lymphatic system. In the bloodstream, these lipoproteins are degraded to _____ by the enzyme _____ with release of energy-rich _____ for oxidation or storage.

13. In the endogenous lipid pathway, the lipoprotein _____ is secreted by the liver, and is rich in _____ and _____. The enzyme _____ promotes the removal of _____ with formation of _____. This lipoprotein is then converted to _____ by the action of _____.

14. The rate-limiting step in cholesterol biosynthesis is the conversion of _____ to _____ by the enzyme _____.

15. The primary lipoprotein in the reverse cholesterol pathway is _____. It is first secreted as the discoidal _____, which acquires free cholesterol to produce the small, spherical particle _____. Under the influence of _____, cholesterol is esterified to form the mature, larger _____. Cholesterol esters are later transferred to apo-B rich lipoproteins by the enzyme _____, which are then taken to the _____ for disposal or recirculation as bile acids in the _____.

16. Hyperlipidemias may be classified as _____ or _____. The classical way of describing the former is by the _____ classification, in which each disorder corresponds to a characteristic appearance of plasma.

17. A turbid, creamy layer on top of a clear infranatant represents an excess of _____ and type ____ hyperlipidemia. _____ levels are markedly elevated. This disorder is also called _____.

18. If the creamy layer is also associated with a turbid infranatant, this represents excess of both _____ and _____ and corresponds to type ____ hyperlipidemia. This is also termed _____. Levels of _____ are again markedly elevated.

19. The only primary hyperlipidemia with clear plasma is type ____ or _____. This is due to an excess of the lipoprotein _____.

20. Slightly turbid plasma without a creamy layer is termed type ____ hyperlipidemia or _____. It is due to elevation of both _____ and _____ lipoproteins, and hence _____ and _____.

21. Type ____ hyperlipidemia is associated with very turbid plasma without a creamy layer.

This is due to an excess of the lipoprotein _____. Levels of _____ are quite elevated.

22. _____ hyperlipidemias are due to diseases that interfere with lipoprotein metabolism. A common cause of secondary hyperlipidemia is hypertriglyceridemia due to _____.

23. _____ is due to a defect in the LDL receptor and occurs in approximately 1 in 500 individuals (heterozygotes). These persons have a markedly increased risk of _____. Another familial disorder resulting in this lipoprotein phenotype is _____, in which the ligand for the LDL receptor is abnormal.

24. The most common primary dyslipidemia is type ____ or _____. It is manifested by elevations of _____, _____, or both.

25. A disorder of the apo-E gene resulting in increased IDL levels is called type ____ dyslipidemia or _____. These patients may have characteristic yellow deposits on the palm called _____.

26. A common disorder resulting from increased triglyceride accumulation in VLDL particles is _____ or type _____ hyperlipidemia. A common secondary cause is _____.

27. Accumulation of both VLDL and chylomicrons is seen in the chylomicronemia syndrome or type ____ hyperlipidemia. _____ levels are markedly elevated. Patients may present with attacks of abdominal pain due to _____.

28. Persons with elevated LDL cholesterol may develop thickening of tendons over extensor ar-

eas; this is called _____. _____ are pustular lesions occurring over the buttocks and extensor surfaces of persons with severe hypertriglyceridemia. These patients also may have a whitish discoloration of the retinal vessels known as _____. Yellowish deposits in the palm creases are called _____; these are virtually pathognomonic for _____. Deposits of cholesterol in soft tissues (not tendons) are called

_____.

29. A condition resulting from deficient apo B-100 and decreased LDL levels is known as _____. Heterozygotes may have a _____ risk of atherogenesis. A condition resulting in the complete deficiency of LDL associated with fat-soluble vitamin deficiency, retinitis pigmentosa, anemia, and neurologic disease is _____.

30. A deficiency of HDL leading to large orange-colored tonsils and excess cholesterol accumulation is _____. Another disorder leading to low HDL levels and premature atherosclerosis is _____. A syndrome of HDL excess leading to increased longevity is _____.

31. In most cases, the first step in management of a lipid disorder should be _____.

32. Potent lipid-lowering agents that inhibit the rate-limiting step of cholesterol biosynthesis are _____. They are very effective at lowering _____ with a lesser effect on _____. Rare side effects include _____ and _____.

33. _____ are useful in the treatment of hypertriglyceridemia because they increase VLDL and chylomicron clearance, and inhibit VLDL production. _____ is not routinely recommended because of adverse outcomes in some clinical trials. _____ is the most

widely used agent. A drug recently introduced into the United States is _____.

34. _____ bind bile acids in the intestine, decreasing _____ of bile acids and decreasing the size of the pool, resulting in decreased _____ levels. Common side effects include _____.

35. A vitamin that has potent lipid-lowering properties at high doses is _____. It is a good treatment for elevations of both _____ and _____. A common side effect, _____, is mediated by _____. It should be used with caution in diabetics as it may worsen _____.

36. _____ are found in fish oil and are useful in patients with refractory _____. As with niacin, they may worsen _____ and should be used cautiously in diabetics. They should be avoided in those with _____.

II. MULTIPLE CHOICE

Select the one best answer.

37. The most common familial lipid disorder is:
    a. familial hypertriglyceridemia
    b. familial hypercholesterolemia
    c. familial apoprotein C-II deficiency
    d. familial lipoprotein lipase deficiency
    e. familial combined hyperlipidemia

38. A patient has a total cholesterol of 245 mg/dL, triglycerides of 250 mg/dL, and HDL cholesterol of 45 mg/dL. The calculated LDL cholesterol is:
    a. 125 mg/dL
    b. 140 mg/dL
    c. 150 mg/dL
    d. 170 mg/dL
    e. 185 mg/dL

39. The lipoprotein richest in triglycerides is:
    a. LDL
    b. chylomicrons
    c. VLDL
    d. Lp(a)
    e. HDL

40. The rate-limiting step in cholesterol biosynthesis is the conversion of:
    a. acetyl CoA to acetoacetyl CoA
    b. lanosterol to cholesterol
    c. mevalonate to 5-pyrophosphomevalonate
    d. geranyl pyrophosphate to farnesyl pyrophosphate
    e. 3-hydroxy-3-methylglutaryl CoA to mevalonate

41. The function of LDL is to:
    a. supply cholesterol to tissues.
    b. supply triglyceride to tissues.
    c. transport triglyceride from the intestine to the circulation.
    d. remove cholesterol from cells.
    e. serve as a precursor of chylomicrons.

42. A 37-year-old white male presents to the emergency room with an acute inferior myocardial infarction. His father died of a myocardial infarction at age 38. On physical examination you note tendon xanthomas over the Achilles area. His total cholesterol is 455 and triglycerides are 95 mg/dL. This patient most likely has:
    a. familial hypercholesterolemia, type IIa
    b. familial combined hyperlipidemia, type IIb
    c. dysbetalipoproteinemia, type III
    d. familial apo CII deficiency, type V
    e. familial hypertriglyceridemia, type IV

43. Proven positive risk factors for coronary artery disease include all of the following except:
    a. male > 45 years of age
    b. HDL levels > 45 mg/dL
    c. diabetes mellitus
    d. positive family history of coronary artery disease
    e. hypertension

44. A 45-year-old female with poorly controlled type 2 diabetes mellitus presents with acute onset of nausea, vomiting, and severe abdominal pain radiating to the back. On examination you note small orange-red papules on her buttocks and on her back. The triglyceride level is 7400 mg/dL. The most likely cause of her abdominal pain is:
    a. acute pancreatitis
    b. perforated peptic ulcer
    c. acute cholecystitis
    d. diabetic ketoacidosis
    e. cholelithiasis

45. Consequences of hypertriglyceridemia may include all but which one of the following?
    a. pancreatitis
    b. increased atherogenesis due to increased density of LDL particles
    c. elevation in serum HDL level
    d. false lowering of certain ion and enzyme measurements
    e. eruptive xanthomas

46. Which of the following drugs is *not* useful in the treatment of hypertriglyceridemia?
    a. atorvastatin
    b. nicotinic acid
    c. cholestyramine
    d. fenofibrate
    e. omega-3 fatty acids

47. A 35-year-old male has known history of coronary artery disease. Several other family members had atherosclerotic disease at an early age. His lipid profile shows abnormally low HDL cholesterol of 5 mg/dL (normal: 35–50 mg/dL). LDL cholesterol is 145 mg/dL (normal: 130–160 mg/dL). Physical examination is unremarkable. This man most likely has:
    a. Tangier disease
    b. hypoalphalipoproteinemia
    c. familial hypercholesterolemia
    d. hypobetalipoproteinemia
    e. familial defective apo-B

48. A 21-year-old male is found to have renal insufficiency, hemolytic anemia, and corneal opacities. His HDL levels are extremely low, and triglyceride levels are elevated. He most likely has:
    a. fish-eye disease
    b. familial combined hyperlipidemia
    c. familial hypertriglyceridemia
    d. abetalipoproteinemia
    e. LCAT deficiency

49. Which drug has *not* been shown by clinical trials to result in improvement in coronary lesions and/or coronary event risk?
    a. lovastatin
    b. nicotinic acid
    c. gemfibrozil
    d. probucol
    e. cholestyramine

III. TRUE OR FALSE

50. Hepatic transaminase levels should be monitored in persons receiving which medications?
    — a. nicotinic acid
    — b. lovastatin
    — c. gemfibrozil
    — d. colestipol
    — e. pravastatin.

51. A whitish, creamy layer is seen in which of the following Frederickson phenotypes?
    — a. type I
    — b. type IIa
    — c. type IIb
    — d. type IV
    — e. type V

52. Pharmacologic therapy should be started in which of the following individuals?
    — a. 26-year-old healthy female with LDL cholesterol of 137 mg/dL
    — b. 54-year-old male with LDL choles-

terol of 127 mg/dL and history of two myocardial infarctions, who has been on diet therapy for several months
    — c. 46-year-old female with a total cholesterol of 276 mg/dL that was obtained at a local health fair
    — d. 42-year-old male with type 2 diabetes and triglyceride level of 4230 mg/dL who is unwilling to follow diet plan
    — e. 32-year-old asymptomatic male with LDL cholesterol of 227 mg/dL who has normal body weight

53. Which of the following are true of the endogenous lipid pathway?
    — a. Chylomicrons from the liver transfer triglyceride to IDL via lipoprotein lipase.
    — b. Triglycerides are stored in adipose tissue and oxidized for energy.
    — c. Cholesterol esters are transferred to cells via HDL.
    — d. VLDL is delipidated to IDL by means of lecithin-cholesterol acyltransferase (LCAT).
    — e. HDL is involved in the conversion of VLDL to IDL.

54. Which of the following are true of the reverse cholesterol pathway?
    — a. Cholesterol ester is added to spherical HDL by lecithin-cholesterol acyltransferase (LCAT), resulting in nascent HDL.
    — b. Cholesterol is transferred to apo-B-rich lipoproteins by cholesterol ester transfer protein (CETP).
    — c. Its proper function helps prevent atherosclerosis.
    — d. Cholesterol is disposed as bile acids in the intestine and recycled.
    — e. HDL_3 is a larger, more "mature" HDL than HDL_2.

IV. MATCHING

Match each item with the appropriate answer. Each may be used only once.

55. ___ A. Simvastatin
    ___ B. Gemfibrozil
    ___ C. Nicotinic acid
    ___ D. Probucol
    ___ E. Cholestyramine
    a. may cause hyperglycemia, flushing, and hyperuricemia
    b. lowers HDL
    c. may interfere with absorption of other drugs
    d. prolongs action of warfarin
    e. may cause myositis; most potent at lowering LDL

56. ___ A. Tendon xanthomas
    ___ B. Eruptive xanthomas
    ___ C. Orange tonsils
    ___ D. Palmar xanthomas
    a. triglyceride level of 5000 mg/dL
    b. type III dyslipidemia
    c. LDL cholesterol of 330 mg/dL
    d. very low HDL levels

57. ___ A. Low-density lipoprotein (LDL)
    ___ B. Very-low-density lipoprotein (VLDL)
    ___ C. High-density lipoprotein (HDL)
    ___ D. Chylomicrons
    ___ E. Intermediate-density lipoprotein (IDL)
    a. transports dietary triglyceride to peripheral cells
    b. transports cholesterol from the liver to peripheral cells
    c. transports triglycerides made in the liver to peripheral cells
    d. transports cholesterol from peripheral cells to the liver for disposal
    e. its delipidation forms LDL

58. ___ A. Apo B-100
    ___ B. Apo C-II
    ___ C. Apo A-I
    ___ D. Apo-E
    a. ligand (binding site) for lipoproteins (except LDL) to their receptors
    b. cofactor for activation of lecithin-cholesterol acyltransferase (LCAT)
    c. ligand (binding site) for LDL; atherogenic
    d. cofactor for activation of lipoprotein lipase

59. ___ A. Corneal arcus
    ___ B. Xanthelasma
    ___ C. Acanthosis nigricans
    ___ D. Eruptive xanthoma
    ___ E. Tendon xanthoma
    a. pustular lesion on buttocks, arms, and legs; seen in severe hypertriglyceridemia
    b. whitish band around cornea near limbus; may indicate hypercholesterolemia if seen in young adult
    c. tendinous thickening in extensor tendons
    d. yellowish plaque near eyelids; nonspecific for dyslipidemia
    e. grayish-brown, raised hyperpigmentation on back of neck and skin folds; often an indicator of insulin resistance

60. ___ A. Lecithin-cholesterol acyltransferase (LCAT)
    ___ B. Lipoprotein lipase
    ___ C. Cholesterol ester transfer protein (CETP)
    ___ D. Hepatic-triglyceride lipase (HTGL)
    a. transfer of cholesterol from mature HDL to VLDL, LDL, and chylomicron remnants
    b. esterification of cholesterol in immature HDL to form larger, mature HDL_2 particles
    c. triglyceride removal from IDL and LDL
    d. triglyceride removal from VLDL and chylomicrons

ANSWERS

1. List three: provide long-term fuel (triglyceride); are structural component of cell membranes; are necessary for steroid and sterol hormone synthesis (cholesterol); solubilize nonpolar compounds (bile acids)

2. chylomicrons, very low-density lipoprotein (VLDL), low-density lipoprotein (LDL), high-density lipoprotein (HDL)

3. chylomicrons, triglyceride; triglyceride, intestine

4. VLDL, triglyceride; triglyceride

5. LDL, cholesterol

6. HDL; cholesterol

7. apolipoproteins; ligands, cofactors, structural integrity

8. A-I, lecithin-cholesterol acyltransferase (LCAT); C-I; C-II, lipoprotein lipase

9. B-100; LDL; atherogenic

10. lipoprotein(a); atherogenic

11. exogenous; endogenous

12. chylomicrons; chylomicron remnants; lipoprotein lipase; triglycerides

13. VLDL; triglyceride, cholesterol ester; lipoprotein lipase, triglyceride, IDL; LDL, hepatic-triglyceride lipase (HTGL)

14. 3-hydroxy-3-methylglutaryl-CoA (HMG-CoA), mevalonate, HMG-CoA reductase

15. HDL; nascent HDL, HDL_3; lecithin-cholesterol acyltransferase (LCAT), HDL_2; cholesterol ester transfer protein (CETP), liver, intestine

16. primary, secondary; Fredrickson

17. chylomicrons, I; triglyceride; familial lipoprotein lipase deficiency

18. chylomicrons, VLDL, V; familial apo C-II deficiency; triglyceride

19. IIa, familial hypercholesterolemia; LDL

20. IIb, familial combined hyperlipidemia; VLDL, LDL, triglyceride, cholesterol

21. IV; VLDL; triglyceride

22. secondary; diabetes mellitus

23. familial hypercholesterolemia; atherosclerosis; familial defective apo-B

24. IIb, familial combined hyperlipidemia; triglyceride (VLDL), LDL

25. III, familial dysbetalipoproteinemia; palmar xanthomas

26. familial hypertriglyceridemia, IV; diabetes mellitus

27. V; triglyceride; pancreatitis

28. tendon xanthomas; eruptive xanthomas; lipemia retinalis; palmar xanthomas; type III hyperlipidemia (dysbetalipoproteinemia); tuberous xanthomas

29. familial hypobetalipoproteinemia; decreased; abetalipoproteinemia

30. Tangier disease; familial hypoalphalipoproteinemia; familial hyperalphalipoproteinemia

31. dietary therapy

32. HMG-CoA reductase inhibitors; LDL, VLDL (triglycerides); hepatitis, myositis

33. fibric acid derivatives; clofibrate; gemfibrozil; fenofibrate

34. bile acid sequestrants (resins), enterohepatic circulation, cholesterol; gastrointestinal (constipation, bloating)

35. nicotinic acid (niacin); LDL, triglyceride; flushing, prostaglandins; glucose tolerance

36. omega-3 fatty acids, hypertriglyceridemia; hyperglycemia; bleeding disorders

37. (e). Familial combined hyperlipidemia (type IIb) is the most common and occurs in 1 in 300 individuals. Heterozygous familial hypercholesterolemia (type IIa) occurs in 1 in 500 persons; the homozygous form is more rare (1 in 1,000,000).

38. (c). By the Friedewald equation, LDL = Total C − HDL-C − TG/5 = 245 − 45 − 250/5 = 200-50 = 150 mg/dL.

39. (b). Chylomicrons consist of approximately 90% triglyceride.

40. (e).

41. (*a*). Cholesterol is a necessary building block of many substances.

42. (*a*). This is a classic history for familial hypercholesterolemia.

43. (*b*). High HDL levels are cardioprotective.

44. (*a*). She has acute pancreatitis precipitated by severe hypertriglyceridemia.

45. (*c*). Hypertriglyceridemia often results in decreased HDL levels.

46. (*c*). Bile acid sequestrants may actually exacerbate hypertriglyceridemia.

47. (*b*). The extremely low HDL level suggests hypoalphalipoproteinemia.

48. (*e*). This is the classic presentation of LCAT deficiency. Fish-eye disease may present with corneal opacities but not renal insufficiency and anemia.

49. (*d*). Probucol lowers HDL and may theoretically increase the risk of CAD. Although it has antioxidant properties, no clinical study has demonstrated improved CAD outcomes.

50. True (*a, b, c, e*); False (*d*). Hepatotoxicity may potentially occur with all antihyperlipidemic agents except bile acid sequestrants, which are not absorbed.

51. True (*a, e*); False (*b, c, d*). A cream layer denotes chylomicronemia, present in types I and V hyperlipidemia.

52. True (*b, d, e*); False (*a, c*). (*a*) The woman's LDL cholesterol is within target range for her age and physical condition. (*b*) The man, despite having a lower LDL cholesterol, has a different goal (< 100 mg/dL) because of his cardiac disease. Many feel that LDL should be reduced to < 100 mg/dL in diabetics as well, as we may presume that many already have cardiovascular disease. (*c*) This woman needs a lipid profile to further define the disorder. The high total cholesterol could be from elevation of LDL, VLDL, or HDL cholesterol. (*d*) This man should be on therapy to lower triglycerides. (*e*) This patient probably has familial hypercholesterolemia; his LDL exceeds the range for his age.

53. True (*b, e*); False (*a, c, d*). VLDL, not chylomicrons (*a*), transfers triglyceride to IDL in the endogenous pathway. LDL transfers cholesterol esters to cells, not HDL (*c*). Triglyceride is removed from VLDL by lipoprotein lipase, not LCAT (*d*). The delipidation of VLDL (*e*) does involve transfer of lipid, phospholipid, and apoprotein to HDL.

54. True (*b, c, d*); False (*a, e*). Nascent HDL is converted to spherical HDL by cholesterol esterification (*a*). HDL_2 is larger and more mature than HDL_3 (*e*).

55. A (*e*); B (*d*); C (*a*); D (*b*); E (*c*).

56. A (*c*); B (*a*); C (*d*); D (*b*).

57. A (*b*); B (*c*); C (*d*); D (*a*); E (*e*).

58. A (*c*); B (*d*); C (*b*); D (*a*).

59. A (*b*); B (*d*); C (*e*); D (*a*); E (*c*).

60. A (*b*); B (*d*); C (*a*); D (*c*).

CHAPTER 9

POLYENDOCRINE DISORDERS AND PARANEOPLASTIC SYNDROMES

Q: What are the polyendocrine disorders?

A: Polyendocrine disorders involve more than one endocrine system. They may be divided into the immunoendocrine or immunodeficiency syndromes and the multiple endocrine neoplasia (MEN) syndromes. With few exceptions, the former are disorders of endocrine *deficiency*, while the latter are syndromes of endocrine *excess*.

Q: What are the immunoendocrine syndromes?

A: **Immunoendocrine syndromes** are autoimmune disorders that affect multiple endocrine organs. The first was described in 1926 by Schmidt, who reported autopsy findings in two patients with "a two-gland illness" (adrenal insufficiency and hypothyroidism). This syndrome, which may also be associated with other disorders, is commonly called Schmidt's syndrome or polyglandular autoimmune syndrome type II (PGA II). A less common syndrome is polyglandular autoimmune syndrome type I.

It is important to recognize these syndromes, as the patient may be at risk for developing further endocrine disorders. These disorders are also genetically transmitted, so genetic counseling and surveillance of family members is important.

Q: What is polyglandular autoimmune syndrome type II (PGA II)?

A: **Polyglandular autoimmune syndrome type II** (PGA II), sometimes called Schmidt's syndrome, is the occurrence of two or more of the following autoimmune disorders in the same individual:

Addison's disease

Autoimmune hypothyroidism (Hashimoto's thyroiditis or autoimmune atrophic thyroiditis)

Graves' disease

Type 1 diabetes mellitus

Myasthenia gravis

Primary gonadal failure

Other associated features (but by themselves not diagnostic of PGA II) include:

Vitiligo (Fig. 9-1)

Alopecia

Parkinson's disease

Pernicious anemia

Celiac disease

Graves' disease is unique in that it is an autoimmune disorder of hormonal *excess;* the others are *deficiency* syndromes.

The disorders must be autoimmune; that is, adrenal failure due to histoplasmosis, hypothyroidism due to thyroidectomy, and type 2 diabetes do not apply.

Inheritance is autosomal dominant with incomplete penetrance, so not all family members who are carriers will manifest a disease. In addition, affected family members may have different diseases; for example, a father may have type 1 diabetes, his daughter have Addison's disease, and her sister have Graves' disease. Susceptibility is related to certain HLA types on the 6th chromosome; these include HLA-DR3 and DR4 (type 1 diabetes), HLA-DR3 (Addison's disease and autoimmune atrophic thyroiditis); HLA-B8 and DR3 (Graves' disease), and HLA-DR3 and DR5 (Hashimoto's thyroiditis). Like all autoimmune diseases, incidence is higher in females. The disorder usually becomes evident during adolescence or adult life.

The individual diseases are identical to those that occur individually, but one disease may commonly exacerbate another. Thus, adrenal insufficiency aggravates hypoglycemic responsiveness in type 1 diabetics, or hyperthyroidism aggravates adrenal insufficiency. The diseases typically present at different times in life.

Q: What is polyglandular autoimmune syndrome type I?

A: **Polyglandular autoimmune syndrome type I** (PGA I) is much less common than PGA II and manifests as Addison's disease associated with mucocutaneous candidiasis and hypoparathyroidism. It is also called hypoparathyroidism-Addison's disease-mucocutaneous candidiasis (HAM) or autoimmune polyendocrinopathy-candidiasis-ectodermal dystrophy (APECD) syndrome. Other endocrine abnormalities are rarely seen (much less commonly than in PGA II), including hypothyroidism, Graves' disease, gonadal failure, and diabetes mellitus. Other associated disorders may include chronic active hepatitis, alopecia, pernicious anemia, and keratoconjunctivitis.

Only siblings are characteristically affected, as opposed to type II in which multiple generations are affected. Type I is inherited in autosomal recessive fashion. Unlike most other autoimmune endocrine disorders, there is no HLA association.

Q: What is the treatment of the PGA disorders?

A: Current treatment is directed at therapy of the individual disorders. Eventually, immunomodulation and gene therapy may be able to alter the development of these diseases.

Q: What are the multiple endocrine neoplasia (MEN) syndromes?

A: The **multiple endocrine neoplasia syndromes,** or MEN, were described early in the 20th century and are syndromes associated with multiple endocrine tumors, benign and malignant, producing a wide variety of endocrine manifestations, typically of hormonal excess. Hormone deficiency may occur as the result of destructive effects of a

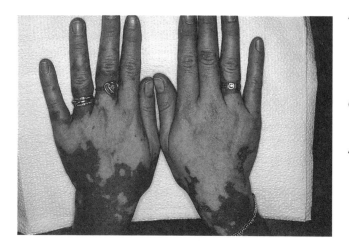

Figure 9-1. Vitiligo in woman with Graves' disease.

large tumor (e.g., a pituitary macroadenoma). They are divided into two broad categories: MEN I and MEN IIa/IIb.

MEN I and II share certain characteristics in that the cells typically produce one or more specific polypeptides or amines. The cells are typically amine precursor uptake and decarboxylation (APUD) cells. The APUD cells are derived from neuroectoderm and have certain neuron-like properties. Not all tumors are comprised of APUD cells (e.g., lipomas in MEN I). There is a pathological progression from hyperplasia to adenoma and, rarely, to carcinoma.

Q: How are the MEN syndromes inherited?

A: The MEN syndromes are usually autosomal dominant. MEN IIb is frequently sporadic.

Q: What is MEN I?

A: **MEN I,** also called **Wermer's syndrome,** is characterized by the "three Ps": pituitary, pancreatic islet, and parathyroid tumors. Two or more tumors in the same individual are diagnostic for MEN.

Hyperparathyroidism is the most common manifestation, occurring in over 95% of those affected. Hypercalcemia may appear as early as age 17 (isolated hyperparathyroidism is unusual in a person so young). By age 40, almost all individuals carrying the gene have hypercalcemia. It differs from the more common hyperparathyroidism usually seen in the normal population, as those with MEN typically have diffuse hyperplasia, whereas those with isolated hyperparathyroidism typically have a solitary adenoma (80%). Patients with MEN typically do not respond as well to surgery.

Pancreatic islet cell tumors are the second most common manifestation, occurring in up to 80% of patients. The tumors are typically multicentric, and thus surgical cure is difficult. Pharmacologic treatment of the hormone excess is often required.

The most common pancreatic tumor is a **gastrinoma,** leading to the Zollinger-Ellison syndrome and gastric acid hypersecretion. This results in solitary or multiple peptic ulcers and diarrhea, and is a major source of morbidity and mortality in MEN I. Patients usually have a greatly elevated gastrin level. Gastrinoma can be confirmed by the calcium or secretin infusion test; there is a great rise in gastrin with gastrinoma, but minimal elevation with other hypergastrinemic states. Treatment includes histamine-2 (H_2) antagonists (e.g., cimetidine, ranitidine) or proton pump inhibitors (omeprazole); gastrectomy may be required. As the pancreatic peptide somatostatin inhibits gastrin secretion, the long-acting somatostatin analog octreotide may be useful.

Insulinoma is the second most common islet cell tumor. This results in severe fasting hypoglycemia with inappropriately elevated serum insulin and C-peptide concentrations. Seizures and death may occur if the condition is untreated. As these tumors are usually multicentric, total pancreatectomy may be required. The antihypertensive agent diazoxide has potent antagonism and is the medical treatment of choice. Streptozotocin is toxic to islet cells and may be used in severe cases. Octreotide does not work as well as in gastrinoma.

Other tumors include **glucagonoma,** which may produce hyperglycemia and a characteristic rash (necrolytic migratory erythema). Pancreatic polypeptide secreting tumors and vasoactive intestinal peptide (VIP) tumors may occur, producing watery diarrhea.

Pituitary adenomas are the third most common manifestation and occur in over 50% of patients with MEN I. These include prolactinoma, growth hormone, and ACTH-secreting tumors, with the associated clinical manifestations. Tumors may also be nonfunctional and cause compressive symptoms if they are large enough.

Carcinoid tumors also may occur, but these are the least common tumor type. These tumors produce large amounts of serotonin and cause severe flushing and diarrhea. Lipomas (subcutaneous and visceral) are also associated, but do not produce hormones.

Q: What is MEN IIa?

A: **MEN IIa,** or **Sipple's syndrome,** is the association of medullary thyroid carcinoma with pheochromocytoma and, less commonly, hyperparathyroidism.

Medullary thyroid carcinoma is a multicentric neoplasm of parafollicular or C-cells. Therefore, it is usually associated with elevated calcitonin levels or exaggerated response of calcitonin to an infusion of calcium or pentagastrin stimulation testing. Severe calcitonin excess may cause vasoactive symptoms (e.g., flushing). It is much more aggressive than the epithelial thyroid cancers (papillary or follicular) and does not accumulate radioiodine. Treatment is total thyroidectomy. Medullary carcinoma may also occur as a familial syndrome not associated with MEN.

Pheochromocytoma presents with the typical manifestations of hypertension, tachycardia, headaches, hyperhidrosis, and cardiac arrhythmias. Clinical history and elevation of serum or urine catecholamines and metabolites typically establish the diagnosis. MRI or CT may localize the tumor. ^{131}I-metaiodobenzylguanidine (MIBG) is a catecholamine analogue selectively concentrated in adrenal chromaffin tissue and may be used to identify tumors. [111]I-labeled octreotide is also useful in identifying tumors not visible on MRI or CT. Whereas sporadic pheochromocytomas usually are unilateral, those in MEN II are more often bilateral.

Hyperparathyroidism may also be seen, although much less commonly than in MEN I (10% to 20% of MEN IIa patients as opposed to over 90% in MEN I patients).

Q: What is MEN type IIb?

A: **MEN type IIb** is the combination of medullary thyroid carcinoma, pheochromocytoma, multiple mucosal neuromas, and a characteristic marfanoid habitus (long, thin body habitus with arachnodactyly). Hyperparathyroidism is much rarer in this disorder than in type IIa.

Q: Are there any other MEN syndromes?

A: **"Overlap type" MEN** syndromes have been seen, with features of two or more MEN syndromes. This would include the familial occurrence of two or more endocrine tumors:

Pheochromocytoma

Islet cell tumors

Medullary thyroid carcinoma

Neurofibromatosis and pheochromocytoma

Von-Hippel-Lindau disease and pheochromocytoma

Q: How are patients screened for MEN syndromes?

A: Biochemical testing (e.g., for gastrinoma, insulinoma, and hyperparathyroidism) and imaging studies (i.e., MRI to screen for pituitary tumors) may be done in patients with a known family history. These studies may be repeated every 5 years in asymptomatic persons. DNA markers are being developed to screen for MEN I, but biochemical screening today represents the best method of detection. Mutations in the *ret* proto-oncogene on chromosome 10 can be detected in individuals with MEN IIa and IIb, as well as those with familial medullary thyroid carcinoma.

Q: What are paraneoplastic syndromes?

A: **Paraneoplastic syndromes** are also called **ectopic** or **"out of place" endocrine syndromes,** as the hormones are produced by tumors that are not of endocrine origin. For example, hypercalcitoninemia caused by medullary thyroid carcinoma is not a paraneoplastic syndrome because the tumor normally makes this substance. These disorders were first recognized in 1941 by Fuller Albright who noticed the association of hypercalcemia with certain malignancies. Verification that it is indeed an ectopic syndrome is supported if the manifestation subsides after specific treatment of the tumor, and if hormone levels from the tumor are higher than that of the parent gland. Messenger RNA coding for the particular hormone is found in the ectopic tissue. By definition, the syndrome returns if the tumor recurs.

Q: What types of hormones are made by these tumors?

A: Tumors in ectopic endocrine disorders typically produce peptides (of APUD or neuroendocrine origin). Some also make prostaglandins and sterol hormones (calcitriol). Table 9-1 lists the syndromes and their manifestations.

Q: What are the most common ectopic syndromes?

A: Hypercalcemia, the most common ectopic syndrome, is usually caused by secretion of parathyroid hormone-related peptide (PTH-rP); this syn-

TABLE 9-1.   Paraneoplastic Syndromes

SYNDROME	HORMONE	TUMOR
Humoral hypercalcemia of malignancy (HHM)	PTH-related peptide	Squamous cell carcinoma Renal cell carcinoma
Local osteolytic hypercalcemia (LOH)	Osteoclast-activating factors, (tumor necrosis factor, interleukins, PTH-rP)	Breast carcinoma Multiple myeloma
Vitamin D-dependent hypercalcemia	$1,25(OH)_2D_3$	Lymphoma
SIADH	ADH (vasopressin)	Small cell lung carcinoma
Cushing's syndrome	ACTH	Small cell lung carcinoma Bronchial carcinoids Islet cell tumors Pheochromocytoma Medullary thyroid carcinoma
Hypoglycemia	? IGF-2	Large mesenchymal sarcomas (fibrosarcomas, rhabdomyosarcomas) Hepatomas Carcinoids
Acromegaly, gigantism	GHRH GH (rare)	Neuroendocrine tumors of pancreas, lung, gut
Osteomalacia	? humoral factor	Mesenchymal tumors (usually benign tumors of the extremities)
Hyper-reninism	Renin	Wilms tumor (nephroblastoma) Renal hemangiopericytoma Renal cell carcinoma Pancreatic adenocarcinoma Ovarian carcinoma Small cell lung carcinoma
Sexual precocity; gynecomastia	Human chorionic gonadotropin (hCG)	Trophoblastic and germ cell tumors

drome is termed **humoral hypercalcemia of malignancy** (HHM). This accounts for approximately 80% of patients with paraneoplastic hypercalcemia. Native parathyroid hormone (PTH) hypersecretion by tumors has been reported in very rare instances.

Another type of paraneoplastic hypercalcemia is called **local osteolytic hypercalcemia** (LOH), which accounts for most of the remaining 20% with paraneoplastic hypercalcemia. LOH is caused by **osteoclast activating factors** (OAFs); these compounds include tumor necrosis factor α, bone-resorbing cytokines (interleukins 1 and 6), transforming growth factor α, and, interestingly, PTH-rP itself. Hypercalcemia is common in those with breast carcinoma and extensive bony metastases, and PTH-rP appears to be the OAF. Patients with multiple myeloma also may present in this fashion—a cytokine appears to be responsible. Very rarely, some hematologic malignancies (lymphomas) may produce calcitriol, resulting in a vitamin D-dependent hypercalcemia.

The syndrome of inappropriate antidiuretic hormone (SIADH) is the next most common paraneoplastic syndrome, followed by Cushing's syndrome due to ectopic ACTH secretion. Other syndromes are much rarer.

Q: What tumors cause paraneoplastic hypoglycemia?

A: Non-islet cell tumors that are known to produce hypoglycemia include large, bulky mesenchymal sarcomas (fibrosarcomas, rhabdomyosarcomas, and mesotheliomas), hepatocellular carcinomas, and carcinoids. These tumors do not appear to produce insulin, but some other humoral factor; an insulin-like growth factor (perhaps IGF-2) has been postulated.

Q: How is humoral hypercalcemia of malignancy (HHM) distinguished from hyperparathyroidism?

A: In most cases of HHM, the tumor makes PTH-rP (which has PTH-like actions), so PTH levels will be suppressed because of normal feedback on the parathyroids. PTH-rP levels are elevated. HHM is very aggressive, whereas hyperparathyroidism typically presents with mild hypercalcemia that progresses slowly over several years.

Q: How does Cushing's syndrome due to ectopic ACTH secretion differ from other causes?

A: With Cushing's syndrome due to ectopic ACTH secretion, the tumor (usually small cell lung carcinoma) is typically quite aggressive; thus, the effects of cortisol on muscle, fat, and skin (truncal obesity, moon facies, striae) often do not have time to develop, despite levels of cortisol that are much higher than in other forms of Cushing's syndrome. Therefore patients may not have the typical somatic features of classic Cushing's syndrome. The typical presenting signs are hypokalemia (from the mineralocorticoid effects of cortisol) and weight loss. Patients are often hyperpigmented as a result of the very high ACTH levels.

Bronchial carcinoids are less aggressive, and these patients often follow a more indolent course that can be difficult to distinguish from Cushing's disease. Tumors that secrete corticotropin-releasing

hormone (CRH) are another, extremely rare cause of ectopic ACTH syndrome. These may be distinguished from the other causes by the elevated CRH levels.

Q: How is ectopic Cushing's syndrome distinguished from the other causes?

A: Cortisol and ACTH levels are usually much higher in ectopic ACTH syndrome than in Cushing's disease, as ACTH-producing pituitary tumors are inhibited somewhat by the high adrenal corticosteroid levels. Patients with ectopic ACTH syndrome typically do not suppress with the high-dose dexamethasone suppression test, whereas those with Cushing's disease do. These tests are not infallible, however, and some overlap may occur. Adrenocortical carcinomas may present aggressively, but ACTH levels are suppressed. Benign adrenal tumors and iatrogenic steroid excess also result in low ACTH levels.

In cases where the two cannot be separated by clinical criteria and dexamethasone suppression testing, petrosal sinus sampling is recommended. In Cushing's disease, a "step-up" in ACTH should occur in the petrosal sinuses as compared to peripheral blood.

Q: What is the treatment of the ectopic humoral syndromes?

A: The treatment of ectopic humoral syndromes is directed at the primary tumor. If tumor shrinkage occurs, hormone secretion also diminishes and the syndrome improves. Specific antagonist therapy may be required in conjunction with antitumor therapy.

SIADH usually is treated with fluid restriction and treatment of the underlying disease. In refractory cases, demeclocycline, which produces ADH resistance (and thus a state of nephrogenic diabetes insipidus), may be used.

Hypercalcemia of malignancy due to PTH-rP is best treated with inhibitors of bone resorption (pamidronate, etidronate). Salmon calcitonin is a weak antagonist and is of use in mild cases. More potent but toxic antiresorptive agents include gallium nitrate and the antitumor antibiotic plicamycin (mithramycin). These patients are usually dehydrated and normal saline administration promotes calciuresis. Radiation therapy may benefit those with local osteolytic hypercalcemia (LOH). Those with hypercalcemia due to immunologic factors (myeloma) or $1,25(OH)_2D_3$ (lymphoma) respond to glucocorticoids.

Ectopic ACTH syndrome may be treated with the antifungal agent ketoconazole, which, in large doses, inhibits adrenal steroid synthesis. Other agents such as aminoglutethimide and metyrapone may be useful. The aldosterone antagonist spironolactone aids in correcting the hypokalemia. If these measures are unsuccessful, bilateral adrenalectomy may be required. These patients typically have a poor prognosis.

BIBLIOGRAPHY

Becker KL, Silva OL. Paraneoplastic endocrine syndromes. In: Becker KL, ed. Principles and practice of endocrinology and metabolism. 2nd ed. Philadelphia: Lippincott, 1995:1842–1851.

Deftos LJ, Nolan JJ. Syndromes involving multiple endocrine glands. In: Greenspan FS, Strewler GJ, eds. Basic and clinical endocrinology. 5th ed. Stamford, CT: Appleton & Lange, 1997:753–767.

Eisenbarth GS, Verge F. Immunoendocrinopathy syndromes. In: Wilson JD, Foster DW, Kronenberg HM, Larsen PR, eds. Williams' textbook of endocrinology. 9th ed. Philadelphia: W.B. Saunders, 1998: 1651–1661.

Strewler GJ. Humoral manifestations of malignancy. In: Wilson JD, Foster DW, Kronenberg HM, Larsen PR, eds. Williams' textbook of endocrinology. 9th ed. Philadelphia: W.B. Saunders, 1998:1693–1706.

REVIEW QUESTIONS

I. SHORT ANSWER

1. Disorders involving more than one endocrine system include the _____ syndromes, which are usually disorders of endocrine deficiency, and the _____ syndromes, which are those of endocrine excess.

2. The first polyglandular endocrine disorder was described by _____ in patients with adrenal insufficiency and hypothyroidism. This syndrome is called _____ or _____. It is typically inherited in _____ fashion with _____ penetrance. These disorders are typically linked to certain _____.

3. List five disorders associated with polyglandular autoimmune syndrome type II.

4. A unique disorder often seen in PGA II that is a disorder of endocrine *excess* rather than *deficiency* is _____.

5. A polyendocrine deficiency disorder much less common than PGA II that occurs primarily in children is _____. The three disorders associated with this syndrome include _____, _____, and _____. Unlike PGA II, there is no _____ association.

6. Syndromes involving multiple endocrine tumors and hormonal excess are called the _____ syndromes. They are inherited in _____ fashion.

7. MEN I typically involves tumors of the _____, _____, and _____. The most common manifestation is _____. The second most common tumors include those of the _____; _____ is specifically the most common tumor of this type.

8. The second most common pancreatic tumor associated with MEN I is _____; these patients present with _____. Levels of _____, _____, and _____ are elevated.

9. MEN IIa is typically associated with _____ and _____. A third, less common disorder, is _____. MEN IIb is also associated with multiple _____ and a typical _____.

10. An endocrine syndrome resulting from a hormone made from a tumor not of endocrine origin is called a _____. The first such syndrome reported manifested as _____. Hormones made by these tumors are chiefly of _____ origin.

11. The most common paraneoplastic syndrome is _____, and 80% of cases are caused by secretion of _____, which is biologically related to _____ and has similar actions. The remaining 20% of cases are usually due to _____, a result of secretion of osteoclast-activating factors. Rarely, certain hematologic malignancies such as lymphomas may cause hypercalcemia by producing _____.

12. The second most common paraneoplastic syndrome is _____, typically caused by

_____. The third most common is _____, which is usually caused by _____.

13. Cushing's syndrome due to ectopic ACTH secretion may often be distinguished from Cushing's disease with the _____ dexamethasone suppression test. Those with _____ classically suppress with this test, whereas those with _____ do not. The definitive test is _____, in which ACTH levels are sampled from the pituitary and peripheral blood.

II. MULTIPLE CHOICE

Select the one best answer.

14. A 57-year-old cigarette smoking male presents with a 2-month history of weight loss, anorexia, hyperpigmentation, and severe hypokalemia requiring multiple hospitalizations. Examination reveals a blood pressure of 220/130 with diffuse hyperpigmentation, anorexic appearance, and absence of truncal obesity or striae. Serum potassium is 2.0 mEq/L (normal: 3.5–5.2). ACTH level is 6788 pg/mL (normal: 9–52), and 24-hour urine cortisol excretion is 23,435 μg (normal: < 50). A 7-cm lung tumor is seen on chest x-ray. MRI of the pituitary demonstrates a 5-mm pituitary tumor. All of the following except which one would be appropriate management at this time?
    a. biopsy of the lung mass
    b. spironolactone
    c. ketoconazole
    d. transsphenoidal pituitary tumor resection
    e. CT of the abdomen

15. Which presentation would not be consistent with any of the multiple endocrine neoplasia (MEN) syndromes?
    a. 45-year-old man with hypertension, striae, muscle weakness, urinary free cortisol of 400 μg/day (normal: 20–80)
    b. 23-year-old woman with serum calcium of 12.2 mg/dL (normal: 8.0–10.6), serum

parathyroid hormone of 210 pg/mL (normal: 10–65)
    c. 34-year-old man with hyperhidrosis, 3-size shoe increase, progressive enlargement of hands, hypertension, glucose intolerance, bitemporal hemianopsia
    d. 39-year-old man with large goiter, TSH 0.02 μU/mL (normal: 0.32–5.00), T_3 900 ng/dL (normal: 80–190), 67% 24-hour radioiodine uptake (normal: 20% to 35%)
    e. 41-year-old man with BP 240/120, headaches, palpitations, 24-hour urine norepinephrine 976 μg/24 hour (normal: 11–86)

16. A 24-year-old thin male complains of fatigue, anorexia, and excessive thirst. Blood pressure is 100/80 supine and 70/45 standing. There is melanin pigment in the palmar creases and the buccal mucosa. There is a small diffuse goiter and deep tendon reflexes are slowed.

    Serum Na^+: 121 mEq/L (normal: 135–145)

    Serum K^+: 6.2 mEq/L (normal: 3.5–5.0)

    Blood glucose (fasting): 301 mg/dL (normal: 70–110)

    Serum ACTH: 1800 pg/mL (normal: 10–50)

    Serum TSH: 80 μU/mL (normal: 0.35–5.00)

    The most likely diagnosis is:
    a. hypothyroidism
    b. Addison's disease
    c. Multiple endocrine neoplasia I
    d. Polyglandular endocrine deficiency II (Schmidt's syndrome)
    e. panhypopituitarism

17. A 56-year-old male with history of squamous cell lung carcinoma is found to be mildly hypercalcemic with serum total calcium of 11.8 mg/dL (normal: 8.4–10.2) and hypophosphatemic at 2.3 mg/dL (normal: 2.5–4.5). Serum intact PTH is elevated at 112 pg/mL (normal: 15–65); serum PTH-related protein is undetectable. Serum creatinine is normal. This man's hypercalcemia is due to:
    a. squamous cell lung carcinoma
    b. primary hyperparathyroidism

c. tertiary hyperparathyroidism
d. vitamin D toxicity
e. local metastases to bone

18. Which one statement is *not* part of the criteria for establishment of a paraneoplastic syndrome?
    a. The clinical manifestation subsides after treatment of the tumor.
    b. The specific tumor is known to be of a type that can cause the syndrome.
    c. Hormone levels are higher from the tumor than from the parent gland.
    d. mRNA coding for the hormone is found in the tumor.
    e. The syndrome returns after relapse of the tumor.

19. A 28-year-old woman with history of Graves' disease presents with secondary amenorrhea. Progestational challenge is negative. FSH and LH levels are both several times normal. This woman has:
    a. polycystic ovary syndrome
    b. polyglandular autoimmune syndrome type I
    c. polyglandular autoimmune syndrome type II
    d. hypothalamic amenorrhea
    e. multiple endocrine neoplasia I

20. The most common paraneoplastic syndrome is:
    a. humoral hypercalcemia of malignancy
    b. local osteolytic hypercalcemia
    c. ectopic ACTH syndrome
    d. SIADH
    e. ectopic gonadotropin secretion

III. TRUE OR FALSE

21. Which of the following statement(s) regarding PGA II (Schmidt's syndrome) is true?
    ___ a. They are inherited in autosomal recessive fashion.
    ___ b. Hypoparathyroidism is a common presentation.

___ c. A patient may present with exophthalmos and hyperthyroidism.
___ d. Two different diseases often present at different times in the same patient.
___ e. Children, if affected, always have the same diseases as the parent.

22. Clinical disorders that may be seen with MEN I include the following:
    ___ a. hypocalcemia
    ___ b. Cushing's disease
    ___ c. pheochromocytoma
    ___ d. acromegaly
    ___ e. hyperglycemia

23. A 29-year-old African-American woman was recently diagnosed with hypothyroidism and placed on L-thyroxine, 100 µg daily. After several days she began experiencing nausea, vomiting, and dizziness. Exam demonstrates a thin woman with blood pressure of 90/60 and diffuse goiter. Which of the following should you do now?
    ___ a. Examine the gingiva and buccal mucosa.
    ___ b. Measure the serum ACTH level.
    ___ c. Increase the L-thyroxine to 150 µg daily.
    ___ d. Measure the serum cortisol level before and after cosyntropin.
    ___ e. Measure the serum potassium level.

24. Which of the following patients qualify for a diagnosis of an immunoendocrine syndrome?
    ___ a. A 21-year-old male with type 1 diabetes, hyperpigmentation, and peak cortisol of 3 µg/dL after synthetic ACTH.
    ___ b. A 48-year-old woman with type 2 diabetes, low T_4, and elevated TSH level.
    ___ c. A 56-year-old man with elevated calcium and intact parathyroid hormone levels, low TSH level, elevated T_3 level, and exophthalmos.

___ d. A 6-year-old boy with low calcium and PTH levels, high ACTH level, hyperpigmentation, and mucocutaneous candidiasis.

___ e. A 60-year-old male with coarse facial features, large hands and feet, elevated growth hormone level, and a large pituitary tumor.

25. Which of the following patient(s) meets the criteria for a paraneoplastic syndrome?

___ a. A 24-year-old man with ecchymoses, striae, hypertension, and diabetes. His urine free cortisol is seven times normal and serum ACTH is three times normal. MRI demonstrates a 5-mm pituitary tumor and petrosal sinus ACTH is greater than peripheral ACTH.

___ b. A 56-year-old man with metastatic squamous cell lung cancer. He has severe hypercalcemia, with low intact PTH and elevated PTH-related peptide levels. Calcium levels improve after irradiation of the lung tumor.

___ c. A 63-year-old woman with metastatic medullary thyroid carcinoma. She has severe diarrhea due to hypercalcitoninemia (10,000 times normal).

___ d. A 73-year-old man with small cell lung cancer and severe hyponatremia. He is euvolemic, and hypothyroidism and adrenal insufficiency have been excluded. Serum vasopressin level is inappropriately elevated for the low serum osmolarity.

___ e. A 34-year-old woman with recurrent hypoglycemia, seizures, and elevated serum insulin and C-peptide levels. CT scan of the abdomen demonstrates a small pancreatic tumor. Drug screen is negative for oral hypoglycemic agents.

ANSWERS

1. immunodeficiency or polyglandular autoimmune deficiency; multiple endocrine neoplasia

2. Schmidt; polyglandular autoimmune deficiency II, Schmidt's syndrome; autosomal dominant, incomplete; HLA haplotypes

3. List five: Addison's disease; autoimmune hypothyroidism (Hashimoto's thyroiditis or autoimmune atrophic thyroiditis); Graves' disease; type 1 diabetes mellitus; myasthenia gravis; primary gonadal failure

4. Graves' disease

5. PGA I; hypoparathyroidism, Addison's disease, mucocutaneous candidiasis; HLA

6. multiple endocrine neoplasia (MEN); autosomal dominant

7. parathyroids, pituitary, pancreas; hyperparathyroidism; pancreas; gastrinoma

8. insulinoma; hypoglycemia; insulin, proinsulin, C-peptide

9. pheochromocytoma, medullary thyroid carcinoma; hyperparathyroidism; multiple mucosal neuromas, marfanoid habitus

10. paraneoplastic syndrome; hypercalcemia; neuroendocrine (APUD)

11. hypercalcemia, PTH-related protein, parathyroid hormone; local osteolytic hypercalcemia; vitamin D metabolites (calcitriol)

12. SIADH, small cell lung carcinoma; ectopic ACTH syndrome, small cell lung carcinoma

13. high-dose; Cushing's disease, ectopic ACTH syndrome; petrosal sinus sampling

14. (*d*). This man's clinical history of rapidly progressive hypokalemia and hypercortisolism is most consistent with the ectopic ACTH syndrome, likely due to lung carcinoma. These levels of cortisol and ACTH are not typical of Cushing's disease. The pituitary tumor is probably an incidental finding and of no consequence. If there is any question, petrosal sinus sampling could be done. The aldosterone antagonist spironolactone (*b*) and inhibitor of steroid synthesis ketoconazole (*c*) will ameliorate the symptoms of steroid excess.

15. (*d*). Graves' disease is an autoimmune disorder, not one of endocrine neoplasia. All the other disorders could be explained by endocrine tumors associated with MEN: (*a*) Cushing's disease, MEN I; (*b*) hyperparathyroidism, MEN I or IIa; (*c*) acromegaly, MEN I; (*e*) pheochromocytoma, MEN IIa or IIb.

16. (*d*). This man has Addison's disease, type 1 diabetes, and primary hypothyroidism, establishing a diagnosis of PGA II. Panhypopituitarism (*e*) is excluded by the high ACTH and TSH levels.

17. (*b*). Primary hyperparathyroidism is common (1 in 1000) and may occur coincidentally in patients with cancer. True PTH-secreting tumors have been described but are extraordinarily rare; most malignancies produce hypercalcemia via increased PTH-related peptide (PTH-rP). Tertiary hyperparathyroidism (*c*) is seen in patients with long-standing renal insufficiency and autonomous PTH production; this man's creatinine is normal. Vitamin D toxicity (*d*) and local osteolytic hypercalcemia (*e*) result in a low PTH level.

18. (*b*). The mere presence of a tumor known to cause the syndrome does not mean that it is the cause, as the tumor may be hormonally inactive.

19. (*c*). She has premature ovarian failure, as gonadotropin levels are high. This along with Graves' disease establishes a diagnosis of PGA II. Patients with polycystic ovary syndrome (PCOS) (*a*) are anovulatory and should respond to progestational challenge. PGA I is usually seen in children and presents with hypoparathyroidism, Addison's disease, and mucocutaneous candidiasis. Women with hypothalamic amenorrhea (*d*) have low gonadotropin levels. MEN I (*e*) is not associated with these disorders.

20. (*a*).

21. True (*c, d*); False (*a, b, e*). Graves' disease (*c*) is common, and diseases often present at different times (*d*). They are inherited as autosomal

dominant, not recessive (*a*). Penetrance is incomplete, so affected family members often have other endocrine diseases. Hypoparathyroidism (*b*) is seen in PGA I.

22. True (*b, d, e*); False (*a, c*). Hypocalcemia (*a*) is not seen in the MEN syndromes; patients with medullary thyroid carcinoma (MEN IIa, IIb) may have hypercalcitoninemia, but this does not cause hypocalcemia. It may cause flushing and diarrhea because of the vasoactive properties of calcitonin. Hypercalcemia (due to hyperparathyroidism) is the most common laboratory manifestation of MEN I. Cushing's disease (*b*) and acromegaly (*d*) are due to pituitary tumors. Hyperglycemia (*e*) may develop in those with GH excess (acromegaly) or a glucagonoma. Pheochromocytoma (*c*) is a component of MEN IIa and IIb.

23. True (*a, b, d, e*); False (*c*). Patients who decompensate after starting thyroid hormone should be strongly suspected of having coexistent Addison's disease and PGA syndrome II. Thyroid hormone will increase the metabolism of the already marginal levels of glucocorticoids and may precipitate an adrenal crisis. Skin pigmentation is not helpful in dark-skinned persons, but the gingiva and buccal mucosa (*a*) should not normally show hyperpigmentation; they are often hyperpigmented in Addison's disease.

ACTH level (*b*) should be elevated, and K^+ (*e*) is often elevated. The diagnostic test is the cosyntropin stimulation test (*d*). Increasing thyroxine (*c*) would only make the problem worse.

24. True (*a, d*); False (*b, c, e*). The patient in (*a*) has type 1 diabetes and Addison's disease which confirms a diagnosis of polyglandular autoimmune (PGA) syndrome II (Schmidt's syndrome). The patient in (*d*) has hypoparathyroidism, Addison's disease, and mucocutaneous candidiasis, establishing a diagnosis of PGA I. Type 2 diabetes (*b*) is not an autoimmune disorder. Hyperparathyroidism (*c*) and acromegaly (*e*) are due to endocrine neoplasia and not endocrine deficiency. Graves' disease alone (*c*) does not qualify for PGA II.

25. True (*b, d*); False (*a, c, e*). This patient (*a*) has classic Cushing's disease, not paraneoplastic Cushing's (ectopic ACTH secretion). The patient in (*b*) has classic humoral hypercalcemia of malignancy. Medullary thyroid cancer (*c*) is a carcinoma of parafollicular or C cells, which normally make calcitonin; thus, it is not a paraneoplastic syndrome. The patient in (*d*) has SIADH due to small cell lung cancer. The woman in (*c*) has an insulinoma, which is not a paraneoplastic syndrome, as insulin is normally made in the islet cells.

INDEX

Note: Page numbers with an *f* indicate figures; those with a *t* indicate tables